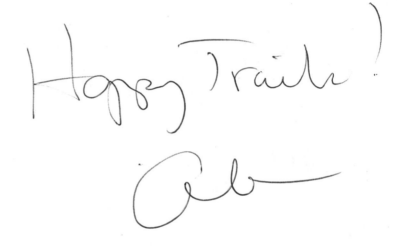

Happy Trails!

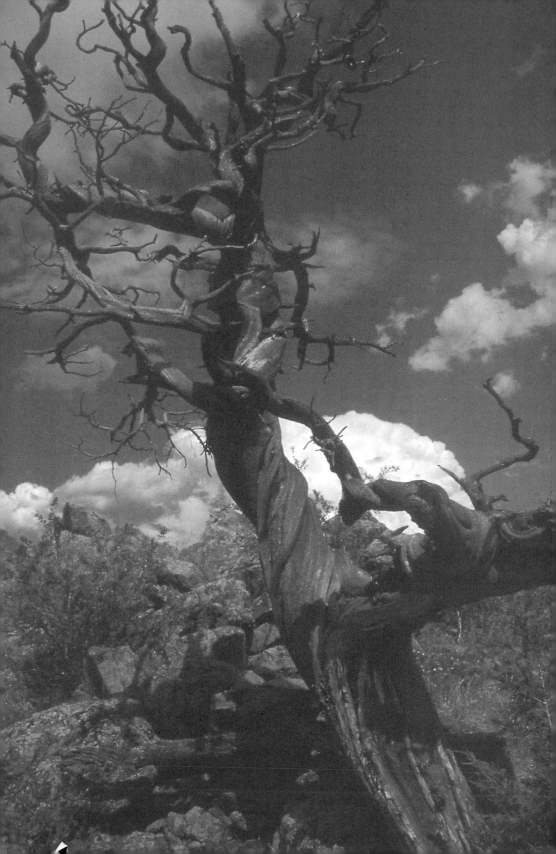

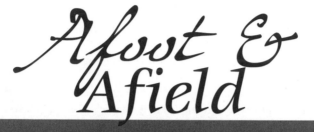

Afoot & Afield

Denver/Boulder
& Colorado's Front Range
A comprehensive hiking guide

Alan Apt

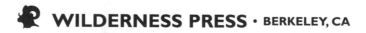

🐏 **WILDERNESS PRESS** · BERKELEY, CA

Lone pine on Chasm Lake Trail (Chapter 8: Trip 2)

Afoot & Afield Denver/Boulder & Colorado's Front Range: A Comprehensive Hiking Guide

1st EDITION February 2008

Front cover photo copyright © 2008 by Alan Apt
Photo on frontispiece copyright © 2008 by John Bartholow
Interior photos, except where noted, by Alan Apt

Maps: Ben Pease, Pease Press
Cover design: Andreas Schueller and Larry B. Van Dyke
Book design and layout: Andreas Schueller, Larry B. Van Dyke, and Lisa Pletka
Book editor: Laura Shauger

ISBN 978-0-89997-406-4
UPC 7-19609-97406-2

Manufactured in Canada

Published by: **Wilderness Press**
1200 5th Street
Berkeley, CA 94710
(800) 443-7227; FAX (510) 558-1696
info@wildernesspress.com
www.wildernesspress.com
Visit our website for a complete listing of our books and for ordering information.

Cover photo: A-Basin Ski area from Sniktau Mountain (Chapter 12: Trip 7),
Loveland Pass

To my children
and their children's children

Acknowledgments

I'd like to thank the many terrific people who accompanied me on these hikes over the years or offered advice: my family, Amy Johnston, Kate Apt, Laura Apt, Ryan Apt, and Jeremiah and Lylah Johnston, and my friends: Gina Apt, Alan Bernhard, Bill Black, Debra Beasly, David Bye, Dan Bowers, Larry and Margie Caswell, Joel Claypool, Nancy DuTeau, Jeff and Catherine Eighmy, Lars and Becky Eisen, Lenny and Susan Epstein, Phil and Joanie Friedman, John Gascoyne, John and Ann Hunt, Alan (ex-hiking partner) and Linda Stark, Rodney Ley, Ward Luthi, Jim and Shereen Miller, Robin Nielsen, Brendt, Nick, and Paul Orndorff, Joe Piesman, Mike Roggy, Sharon Roggy, Dian Sparling, Jay Stagnone, Jim Welch, and Jerry White. I especially want to thank Nancy Martin, who accompanied me on countless occasions over the last three years.

I also thank John Gascoyne for the excellent job he did producing draft maps for the book.

John Bartholow and Joe Grim provided a wide variety of excellent photos for the book, and I thank them for their valuable contributions. Thanks also to Jeff Eighmy and Alan Stark for photos.

Thanks to Jennifer Ackerfield, at the Colorado State University Herbarium, for her excellent reference on mountain climate zones.

I appreciate the enthusiasm, support, patience, and knowledgeable advice of the staff at Wilderness Press: Roslyn Bullas, Laura Keresty, and Laura Shauger. On the publishing front, this book certainly wouldn't have happened without the help of Alan Stark, and his virtual literary agency.

Thanks to the many friendly and helpful employees and volunteers of Colorado State Parks, Rocky Mountain National Park, the U.S. Forest Service, City of Fort Collins, Boulder County, El Paso County, and Larimer County, including Larry Frederick, Diana Barney, Maribeth Higgins, Becky Kelly, Jeff Maugans, Vicki McClure, Dick Putney, and Kristi Wumkres, just to mention a few.

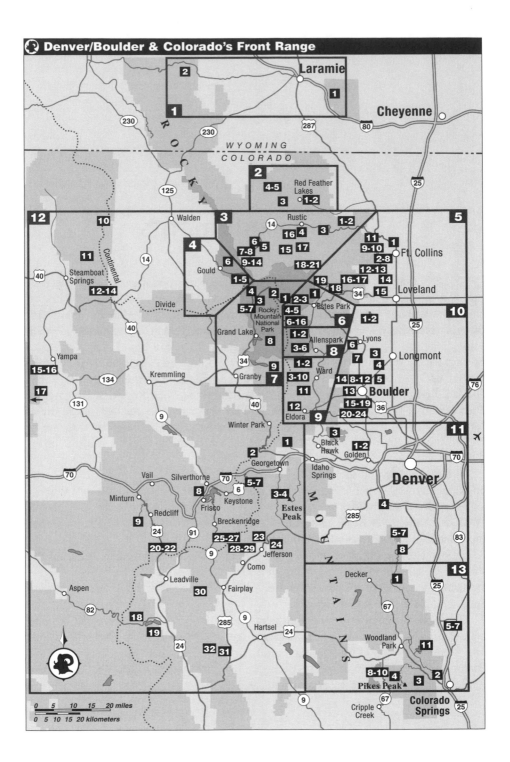

Denver/Boulder & Colorado's Front Range

Contents

PREFACE xii

INTRODUCING THE DENVER/BOULDER AREA 1

COMFORT, SAFETY, & ETIQUETTE 3

USING THIS BOOK 13

CHAPTER 1 WYOMING: MEDICINE BOW NATIONAL FOREST 17
  Trip 1 Aspen, Middle Aspen, & Pole Creek Trails 19
  Trip 2 Libby Creek Trail 21

CHAPTER 2 RED FEATHER LAKES AREA 23
  Trip 1 Mount Margaret Trail 24
  Trip 2 Dowdy Lake Trail 26
  Trip 3 North Lone Pine Trail to Mount Baldy Overlook 27
  Trip 4 Trappers' Loop to Trappers'/Renegade Trails 29
  Trip 5 Trappers' Pass to Buckskin Trail 31

CHAPTER 3 POUDRE CANYON & CAMERON PASS AREAS 32
  Trip 1 Grey Rock 34
  Trip 2 Hewlett Gulch 36
  Trip 3 Mount McConnel 37
  Trip 4 Lower Dadd Gulch 39
  Trip 5 The Big South Trail 41
  Trip 6 Green Ridge Trail 42
  Trip 7 Sawmill Creek Trail to Clark Peak 45
  Trip 8 Blue Lake Trail to Clark Peak 47
  Trip 9 Trap Park Trail to Iron Mountain 48
  Trip 10 Zimmerman Lake Trail 50
  Trip 11 Meadows Trail 53
  Trip 12 Montgomery Pass 56
  Trip 13 Diamond Peaks 57
  Trip 14 Cameron Connection 59
  Trip 15 Brown's Lake 60
  Trip 16 Mineral Springs Gulch to Prospect Mountain 62
  Trip 17 Fish Creek & Little Beaver Creek Trails 62
  Trip 18 Signal Mountain Trail 65
  Trip 19 Stormy Peaks Trail 67
  Trip 20 Emmaline Lake Trail 69
  Trip 21 Mummy Pass Trail 71

CHAPTER 4 COLORADO STATE FOREST..73

Trip 1 Michigan Ditch Trail to Thunder Pass Trail 74
Trip 2 Lake Agnes Trail 77
Trip 3 Seven Utes Trail 78
Trip 4 Mahler Mountain Trail 79
Trip 5 Ranger Lakes Trail 81
Trip 6 Grass Creek Yurt Trail 82

CHAPTER 5 FORT COLLINS AREA 84

Trip 1 Poudre River Trail 86
Trip 2 Spring Creek Trail 90
Trip 3 Cathy Fromme Prairie Natural Area 91
Trip 4 Foothills Trail: Pineridge Natural Area 93
Trip 5 Foothills Trail: Maxwell Natural Area 96
Trip 6 Foothills Trail: Centennial Drive 97
Trip 7 Foothills Trail: Reservoir Ridge Natural Area 99
Trip 8 Reservoir Road/Centennial Drive 100
Trip 9 Arthur's Rock Trail 101
Trip 10 East & West Valley Trails 106
Trip 11 Eagle's Nest Natural Area 107
Trip 12 Horsetooth Rock Trail 109
Trip 13 Horsetooth Falls & Connecting to Lory State Park 112
Trip 14 Coyote Ridge Trail 113
Trip 15 Devil's Backbone, Blue Sky, & Coyote Ridge Trails 116
Trip 16 Bobcat Ridge Natural Area: Valley Loop Trail 118
Trip 17 Bobcat Ridge Natural Area: Ginny Trail 119
Trip 18 Crosier Mountain Trail 121
Trip 19 North Fork Trail 123

CHAPTER 6 ROCKY MOUNTAIN NATIONAL PARK: EAST........................ 126

Trip 1 McGregor Ranch 129
Trip 2 Horseshoe Park 132
Trip 3 Deer Mountain 133
Trip 4 Cub Lake 135
Trip 5 Fern Lake 136
Trip 6 Mill Creek Basin 137
Trip 7 Glacier Basin & Sprague Lake 140
Trip 8 Around Bear Lake 143
Trip 9 Nymph, Dream, & Emerald Lakes 144
Trip 10 Flattop Mountain & Hallet Peak 145
Trip 11 Odessa Lake 149
Trip 12 Bierstadt Lake 151
Trip 13 Alberta Falls 152

Trip 14 The Loch 154
Trip 15 Jewell & Black Lakes 155
Trip 16 North Longs Peak Trail 159

CHAPTER 7 ROCKY MOUNTAIN NATIONAL PARK: WEST 161

Trip 1 Ute Trail 162
Trip 2 Toll Memorial Trail 164
Trip 3 Mount Ida 165
Trip 4 Colorado River Trail to Little Yellowstone Canyon 167
Trip 5 Baker Gulch to Mount Nimbus & Mount Stratus 169
Trip 6 Holzwarth Trout Lodge 171
Trip 7 Coyote Valley Trail 172
Trip 8 East Inlet & Thunder Lake Trails 173
Trip 9 Monarch Lake to Brainard Lake 175

CHAPTER 8 ROCKY MOUNTAIN NATIONAL PARK: SOUTH 178

Trip 1 Estes Cone 179
Trip 2 Chasm Lake 181
Trip 3 Copeland Falls 183
Trip 4 Allenspark & Finch Lake Trails to Wild Basin 183
Trip 5 Calypso Cascades, Ouzel Falls, & Ouzel Lake 186
Trip 6 St. Vrain Mountain 188

CHAPTER 9 BOULDER AREA: INDIAN PEAKS 189

Trip 1 Middle St. Vrain 190
Trip 2 Coney Flats Trail & Beaver Reservoir 192
Trip 3 Red Rock Picnic Area to Beaver Reservoir 194
Trip 4 Red Rock Picnic Area to Rainbow Lakes 196
Trip 5 Red Rock Lake 197
Trip 6 Mitchell Lake & Blue Lake Trail 199
Trip 7 Long Lake Trail 201
Trip 8 Lake Isabelle 201
Trip 9 Pawnee Pass & Peak 202
Trip 10 Niwot Mountain & Ridge 204
Trip 11 Rainbow Lakes & Arapaho Glacier Overlook Trails 205
Trip 12 Woodland Lake Trail 208

CHAPTER 10 BOULDER AREA: PLAINS & FOOTHILLS 211

Trip 1 Little Thompson Overlook Trail 212
Trip 2 Eagle Wind Trail 213
Trip 3 Pella Crossing 215
Trip 4 Lagerman Reservoir 217
Trip 5 Walden & Sawhill Ponds 218

Trip 6 Hall Ranch   219

Trip 7 Heil Valley Ranch   222

Trip 8 Cobalt, Sage, & Eagle Loop   225

Trip 9 Left Hand Reservoir: North Rim Loop   227

Trip 10 Foothills Trail: Hogback Ridge Loop   228

Trip 11 Foothills Trail: Wonderland Lake Loop   229

Trip 12 Anne U. White Trail   230

Trip 13 Red Rocks Trail & Mount Sanitas   230

Trip 14 Switzerland Trail   233

Trip 15 Mesa Trail: Northern Segment   234

Trip 16 Mesa Trail: Southern Segment   237

Trip 17 Doudy Draw Trail   237

Trip 18 Royal Arch Trail   239

Trip 19 South Boulder Creek Trail   240

Trip 20 Streamside Trail   241

Trip 21 Fowler Trail   242

Trip 22 Rattlesnake Gulch Trail   243

Trip 23 Eldorado Canyon Trail   245

Trip 24 Walker Ranch   247

CHAPTER 11   DENVER AREA: PLAINS & FOOTHILLS 250

Trip 1 White Ranch: Belcher Hill Trail   251

Trip 2 White Ranch: West Access Trails   253

Trip 3 Coyote, Mule Deer, & Elk Trails Loop   254

Trip 4 South Valley Park: Coyote Song Trail   257

Trip 5 Fountain Valley Trail   258

Trip 6 Carpenter Peak   260

Trip 7 Willow Creek & South Rim Trails   262

Trip 8 Ringtail Trail   263

CHAPTER 12   DENVER AREA: MOUNTAINS 264

Trip 1 St. Mary's Glacier & James Peak   266

Trip 2 Jones Pass   268

Trip 3 Silver Dollar Lake Trail   269

Trip 4 Mount Bierstadt   270

Trip 5 Baker Mountain   271

Trip 6 Grizzly Peak   273

Trip 7 Sniktau Mountain   274

Trip 8 Lily Pad Lake   275

Trip 9 Lake Constantine   276

Trip 10 Wyoming Trail (#1101)   279

Trip 11 Hinman Creek Trail (#1177)   281

Trip 12 West Summit Loop 1A   283

Trip 13 West Summit Loop 1B 285

Trip 14 North Walton Peak 286

Trip 15 Spronk's Creek Trail 287

Trip 16 Chapman Bench Trail 289

Trip 17 Mandall Lakes Trail (#1121) 291

Trip 18 Twin Lakes Reservoir & Colorado Trail 293

Trip 19 Black Cloud Trail to Mount Elbert 293

Trip 20 Vance's Hut Trail 297

Trip 21 Taylor Hill Trail 298

Trip 22 Mitchell Creek Loop 299

Trip 23 Colorado Trail: West Branch 300

Trip 24 Colorado Trail: East Branch 302

Trip 25 Boreas Pass Road 304

Trip 26 Gold Dust Trail: Southern Segment 304

Trip 27 Gold Dust Trail: Northern Segment 306

Trip 28 French Pass Trail 307

Trip 29 Bald Mountain 309

Trip 30 Limber Grove Trail 310

Trip 31 Salt Creek Trail (#618) 311

Trip 32 McQuaid Trail (#631) 313

CHAPTER 13 COLORADO SPRINGS AREA..315

Trip 1 Devil's Head Lookout 316

Trip 2 Garden of the Gods 317

Trip 3 Pikes Peak 320

Trip 4 The Crags 323

Trip 5 What in a Name Trail 325

Trip 6 West Loop 326

Trip 7 North Loop 327

Trip 8 Peak View, Elk Meadow, & Livery Loop 328

Trip 9 Homestead Trail 330

Trip 10 Revenuer's Ridge 330

Trip 11 Rainbow Gulch Trail to Rampart Reservoir 331

Appendix 1: BEST HIKES BY THEME..333

Appendix 2: RECOMMENDED READING 335

Appendix 3: AGENCIES & INFORMATION SOURCES..................336

Appendix 4: CONSERVATION & HIKING GROUPS 338

INDEX 340

ABOUT THE AUTHOR...348

Preface

"Our life is marked by many uncompleted journeys. Everywhere we go there is a place we could have gone. If we were true walkers, and had the courage to follow these unknown canyons into the interior terrain, we might possibly walk right into Eden."
—James Work, author, naturalist, and Colorado State University professor emeritus of literature

This book takes anyone who lives near or visits Denver, Boulder, Fort Collins, Colorado Springs, and other Front Range cities on an unparalleled tour into the majestic foothills, rivers, and plains of the Colorado Rocky Mountains. It offers a comprehensive and unique collection of trails that includes easy dayhike commutes, as well as far-flung mountaineering adventures, for weekends or vacations. The array of natural wonders will engage you for years to come. If you're willing to explore on foot, bike, or boat, just a small distance from the nearby parking lot, trailhead, or river bank, you can become immersed in the captivating trails and enchanted forests of the Rocky Mountain State.

When you venture into the higher reaches of these mountains—higher than trees can grow—you enter a magical place where space and time are suspended; you can almost reach out and touch the clouds scudding by. The natural heritage and beauty of Colorado is comparable to any on the planet. Fortunately much of the state is freely accessible public lands, secured for all to enjoy in city and county open spaces, state and national parks, and national forests and monuments. This invaluable bounty will only stay in public ownership if we let our representatives at all levels regularly know how much we treasure and enjoy this stewardship and do not want our children's legacy sold off for development of any kind.

Wherever you live in the Front Range, you are always close to a trailhead that offers an escape from the challenges of yard work or crowded highways. In this book I share the discoveries I've made over the past 30 years. There are millions of acres of public lands to explore that have been set aside with generous taxpayers' dollars by cities, counties, and the state of Colorado. Add to this the legacy of public lands set aside by the federal government, for all to use, and we enjoy millions of acres of priceless places to roam and hopefully pass on to future generations. This book spans from the Wyoming border on the northern border of Colorado to as far south as Pike's Peak and Fairplay in South Park. I have included hikes for kids of all ages and levels of ambition. There are abundant choices for everyone, from families with small children, to experienced hikers, to mountaineers, and hikers looking for a relaxing trip. Anyone who wants to revel in the nearby wonderlands of the Colorado Rocky mountain environment will find something to explore in this book. You don't have to limit your possibilities to hiking—run, bike, kayak, swim, or crawl on your belly, but get out there and enjoy the hills and vales of paradise. This is heaven, and you don't have to wait.

Introducing the Denver/Boulder Area

The recreational options in Colorado are virtually limitless because of the varied terrain, and spectacular geology. Ancient uplift created the lofty peaks of the Front Range, including countless mountains over 12,000 feet and Colorado's 54 14ers. Glaciers carved the magnificent high mountain valleys and cirques from uplifted highlands and mountains. Rivers carved canyons that tumble down from the rolling 12,000-foot highlands. The rugged backdrop of the Colorado Rockies Front Range starts at the Colorado-Wyoming border and spills south of Colorado Springs. The present mountain range of the Rockies was born nearly 55 million years ago, with the final uplift happening as recently as 10 million to 20 million years ago. Rocky Mountain National Park contains some rocks that are almost 1 billion years old; 1,750 million to be more precise. There is evidence of volcanoes, ancient seabeds, and more than one ice age; the last of which ended only 10,000 years ago. The dinosaurs were but a minor event in the geologic drama.

The high mountains contrast sharply with the unexpected gently rolling high plains, where Colorado's Front Range cities are located, that seem to stretch forever to the Colorado borders with Nebraska and Kansas. Most visitors are very surprised to find the cities residing on the flats. The unexpected gift of the Rockies is their superb foothills zone, where the transition from plains to mountains occurs. In most other states, the foothills would be considered a major mountain range. They could rival the Appalachian Mountains, which are much lower in elevation though broader. That is to say, the foothills aren't really hills; they are a set of delightful "mountains"

Bear Lake

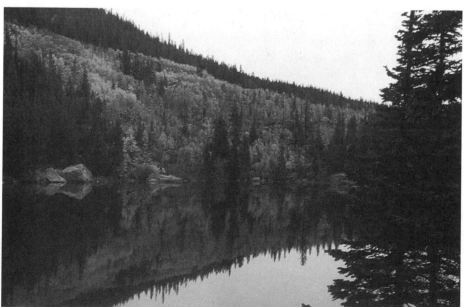

John Bartholow

1

unto themselves, as well as gracious and impressive gateways to the true monarchs of the state. The foothills also offer a refreshing landscape—soaring cliffs, scenic canyons, enchanting flora and fauna, and sculpted rock formations of their own; making it easy to stay closer to home and yet escape the urban. The foothills are also easier to enjoy because of their lower elevations.

The foothills zone is familiar to anyone living along the Front Range of Colorado, and some of the lofty "hills" climb up to 9000 feet. This zone is generally dominated by shrubs such as mountain mahogany, skunk brush, and wild plum, although species composition is highly diverse and ponderosa and lodegepole pine forests are common. In the north to central portions of the state, these species dominate. Farther south, fragrant juniper becomes more common. This vegetation type is commonly called pinyon-juniper woodland. Great expanses of this vegetation type are found throughout southern Colorado. High in the foothills region, forest vegetation becomes more important and that is where ponderosa and lodgepole pine, and even a spruce and nonnative Russian olive appear.

The subalpine zone is what many people envision as Colorado vegetation. This zone starts at about 9000 feet in elevation and covers a vast region in the center of the state. Although it is generally considered a single zone, plant species vary widely. The magical quaking aspen stands occur near the lower boundary of the subalpine. They are typically thought of as being transitional and not long lived, giving rise to spruce-fir forest after about 75 to 100 years. Higher in eleva-

tion, lodgepole pine replaces aspen as the primary tree species. The most common type of vegetation is the spruce-fir forest. This forest type is present at all altitudes in the subalpine zone and can grow under most conditions. Although not as common as other vegetation types, subalpine wetlands provide important biodiversity as well as habitat for elk and moose. Also interesting are the broad, flat, high-elevation "parks" like North and South Park between the mountain ranges. These beautiful parks are framed by towering mountain ranges, and frequently have short grass prairie type of vegetation, contrasting with the spruce-fir forest.

The alpine zone in Colorado begins at about 11,400 feet. Around 11,000-plus feet is what is known as the treeline, the point at which large trees cannot grow. Characterized by long, cold winters and a short growing season, it is challenging for flora, fauna, and humankind. The plants that have adapted to these harsh conditions frequently take on novel growth forms. The contorted growth of the stunted krumholtz species is a striking example of one such adaptation. A krumholtz, or krummholz, formation (from German *krumm* meaning "twisted" and *holz* meaning "wood") is a feature of subarctic and subalpine treeline landscapes with low-growing, twisted, dwarf pine trees. Tundra vegetation is frequently dominated by islands of dwarf krumholtz trees, expansive stands of shrubs, and a field layer of grasses, shrubs, and cushion plants.

Hike the trails in this book to experience the varied geology, geography, and stunning beauty of this landscape.

Comfort, Safety, & Etiquette

Most of the adventures in this book do not require special equipment. All you need is a good pair of walking shoes, a willing pair of legs, and a small sense of daring and adventure. The weather in Colorado is, however, always interesting, because it can and does change rapidly and unpredictably. Early fall or late spring blizzards are especially sneaky; as are thunderstorms, or weather fronts that can sneak up on you at any time of the day. I have experienced 40- to 50-degree temperature swings, with sun and heat being replaced by wind and freezing hail in a matter of minutes, compliments of a thunderhead mushrooming into the stratosphere, fueled by water from as far away as the Gulf of Mexico and the fires of the sun. It is always wise to be prepared for the unexpected if you are going to wander far. When the weather is in doubt, head back to your car or cabin! Lightning, freezing downpours, and whiteouts have been deadly for many recreationists.

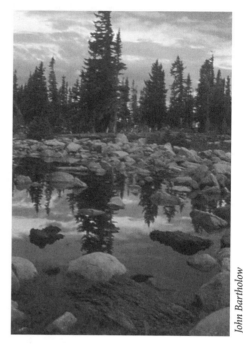

John Bartholow

Snowy Lake

Surviving in Style: Clothing & Equipment

High fashion standards have not made an impact in the world of hiking, unless you're in the vicinity of Vail or Aspen, where you will likely encounter uniformed tourists who feel the right clothing labels or styles are essential. Wear what you find comfortable, but be prepared for any kind of weather. If you are dressed appropriately, dramatic temperature drops, unseasonable snow, and high winds can be entertaining. Bundle up and amble down the trail cozy and smug in spite of Mother Nature's tricks; don't go high and far in only a T-shirt and shorts because hypothermia can be deadly. The first symptom of hypothermia is uncontrollable shivering followed by a loss of coordination and slurred speech (see page 10 for more information). People have died from it in air temperatures in the 40s and 50s—getting caught in a downpour or falling into a lake or stream and then being unable to get warm and dry or even simply dressing inadequately and experiencing dropping temperatures, strong wind, snow, or rain. Taking along extra clothing is very important.

When you pack, imagine hot, sunny, morning weather followed by an afternoon of cold, driving wind and three inches of hail. Dress in layers, and avoid cotton altogether if you can, opting for moisture-wicking clothing—nylon or synthetic fabrics. Although wool doesn't wick, it'll keep you warmer than cotton would. Carrying a daypack, or at least a fanny pack, is essential. You'll be chilly when you start if it is early, but as you walk you'll warm up nicely. You'll need the pack for peeling off your layers so you don't overheat. If you allow yourself to overheat and sweat, you will be chilled to the bone when you stop, especially if it is fall or spring. When you stop for lunch, you'll cool off quickly and want to put some layers back on. Cotton is not recommended because when it gets wet or damp it does not dry out easily nor does it insulate you against the cold.

On your average day, polypro, or synthetic composite, long-sleeved and short-sleeved shirts are recommended. Then a backup of wool sweaters or fleece with a water- and windproof jacket will work. I suggest an outer layer that is breathable and waterproof. Start off dressed so that you feel a little chilly and keep a warmer layer in your pack for when you stop for lunch, or a snack break. You'll warm up quickly. If jeans are your only option, be sure to pack a waterproof poncho or pants to put over them in case it rains or snows. I prefer pants with zip-off legs for maximum flexibility.

Headgear is especially important; you will lose most of your body heat through your head if it isn't covered with a good wool or polypro hat. A hat or cap that shields you from the strong, high-altitude sun is essential. Sunglasses are a must to avoid damaging sun and radiation. Goggles will also be important for an enjoyable experience in hail, snow, or high wind. Mittens are generally warmer than gloves, but whichever you bring should be waterproof if possible. If you don't have waterproof mittens or gloves, bring an extra pair in case they get soaked. An extra pair of dry socks is a good idea, too.

Boots

A good pair of well-designed walking or running shoes or waterproof boots will make your trip much more enjoyable. Lightweight, low-cut summer hiking boots or running shoes that are somewhat waterproof can work very well if you're planning a very short trek close to your car. Surviving a thunderous downpour in comfort will require more. I highly recommended that you use high-top, waterproof boots and polypro (synthetic composite) or composite wool socks if you're going very high or very far. Getting caught in a cold rain and hailstorm with soaking wet feet far from civilization can be very bone chilling. A pair of short gaiters is also a very good idea to keep the rocks, stickers, mud, and early- or late-season snow out of your boots and away from your Achilles tendons that are supposed to carry you a very long, pain-free, happy-go-lucky way.

Every pound on your feet, however, is equivalent to two on your back, so footgear weight is a consideration. Light- to mid-weight boot options are almost unlimited; many are lightweight like running shoes with their technology and cushioning and the additional protection of high-tech fibers, including waterproof fabric like Gore-Tex. Leather boots, though old technology and somewhat heavier, can be as waterproof as or even more so than synthetic boots, with a good coating of snow sealant or other waterproofing treatments. It is wise to waterproof all boots according to the manufacturers' recommendations before going on an all-day or multi-day trip since you'll likely be rained on. The disadvantage of some lightweight boots and shoes is that they offer less support for heavy backpacks and protection from the elements. Try to imagine how your footgear will feel after an all-day hike when you are bounding downhill on a rocky trail with weary feet and legs.

I've Got Blisters on Me Feet!

Blisters can ruin the day for you and your friends and family, cutting short a nice excursion. Regardless of the boots or shoes you decide to wear, break them in for a couple of weeks, at a minimum, before you wear them on a long dayhike or a backpacking trip. The leather or fabric adjusts and conforms to your toes, heels, and ankles as you wear them the first few times. Wearing them at home or on short jaunts around town will also tell you if they fit comfortably—something you cannot determine in a store.

Cover potential "hot spots" on your heels, toes, or ankles with moleskin, duct tape, or band-aids, especially if you are wearing new boots. It is always a good idea to apply moleskin or duct tape to your heels before you begin hiking to prevent blistering. When you feel a hot spot, don't wait until it becomes a blister to cover it up. Stop immediately and avoid injury that could ruin your trek.

Do not use cotton socks to avoid getting cold feet if your socks get soaked. Polypro and wool are much better insulators. Polypro socks also wick sweat to some degree. The primary advantage of cotton is it can keep your feet cooler, but thin synthetic socks can do that as well.

When you hike, get into a nice rhythm not unlike cross-country skiing or skating. Establishing a steady rhythm is much more enjoyable and easier on the body than lots of sprints and stops and starts.

If, after all of the above you still get a blister, it is medically advisable to break it. Then clean and disinfect it and cover it with duct tape, a band-aid, or moleskin until it heals.

The Advantages of Trekking Poles

Many avid hikers do not use trekking poles, but I find them very useful, particularly when I go off-trail or on a steep slope. When traversing downhill, I especially like the extra stability and power of using cross-country ski poles or a pair of the modern, shock-absorbent trekking poles. Some people see poles as an unnecessary appendage. The choice is yours. If you have cross-country ski poles, they work fine for hiking as long as they aren't too long. They are really only necessary when you are planning to climb or descend very steep slopes. Even then, you can survive without them though you may be much more likely to do a face-plant.

I enjoy using poles when descending because they take thousands of pounds of pressure off of your knees. That is a major asset of poles for hiking, particularly if you have had knee, hip, or ankle problems or if you are carrying a heavy backpack. Using poles also gets more of your body involved and provides an upper body workout that can burn more fat if that's a secondary goal.

Don't use poles that are too long though or you will stress your elbows. Your arms should be bent at 90 degrees when you use the poles. If someone in your party thinks your use of poles is humorous, have them walk in front of you and motivate them with a few carefully-placed, supportive prods.

Food & Water

Take plenty of food and drink. Also take water, at least 2 liters if you plan a multi-hour walk; assume a rate of 1 liter or quart per hour on very hot days when exercising strenuously. Bring easy-to-access snacks such as energy bars, trail mix, etc. You'll burn lots of energy and calories hiking uphill; some people estimate that a hiker can burn up to 800 calories per hour. Eating something with a little fat in it will also help keep you warm. Because of the extreme conditions they experience, Arctic explorers often eat large quantities of butter, lard, or blubber, but you would probably prefer chocolate. Bring extra food in case of an emergency, and ask your companions to bring enough for themselves as well.

Much has been made of the new high-protein diets and foods for exercise. Though eating something that contains protein along with carbohydrates will work well, carbohydrates are still the key ingredients for energy. You don't have to overeat, however, since excess calories from either carbohydrates or protein will simply be stored as fat. Exercising aerobically for longer than 40 minutes will cause your body to use fat stores as energy. If you don't want to deplete your glycogen (the fuel your muscles use) supply and want to stay as fresh as possible, have a small snack about once an hour or add a sports drink mixture or fruit juice to your water. Also try to exercise at an aerobic pace (a pace at which you are not out of breath), so you won't accumulate lactic acid, which will give you sore muscles. Always include some extra high-calorie food for emergencies.

As mentioned, drink plenty of water but don't drink directly from mountain streams and lakes. Though crystal clear and inviting, they are not creature free. The coldness of mountain water does not purify it; a parasite called giardia actually thrives in cold water. If you want to drink from streams and lakes, then take along a water filter or purification system or water-purifying tablets. Without tablets or a filtering system, water must be boiled for 10 minutes to kill giardia. Drinking tainted water can cause all of the following symptoms: diarrhea, nausea, cramp-ing, fever, foul belching or gas, chills, and weight loss (contracting giardia is not a good diet strategy). These symptoms might not manifest themselves until a week or two after you drink the tainted water. To prevent them, take along lots of water from home or the right equipment and know how to use it.

Here Comes the Sun

The harmful effects of the sun are magnified at high altitudes so cover up and avoid direct sunlight between the hours of 10 AM and 2 PM. Even on a cloudy day, you can end up with a terrible sunburn. Use a sunscreen with a sun protection factor, or SPF, of at least 15, and be sure to reapply it frequently. Sunburns can set the stage for skin cancer at a later age, and this is coming from a former sun worshipper. Your friendly dermatologist will tell you that there is no such thing as a healthy tan. Excess sun also adversely affects the immune system.

Things that Bite

An assortment of wild beasts can be found in the Colorado woods; the least trustworthy is usually on two legs, but the most likely to affect you are insects. Most of the animals that live in the forest would prefer not to encounter you at close quarters, nor would they find you as appetizing as their normal gourmet fare. (They are wild animals, not tame, so keep your distance.) The exceptions are mosquitoes and ticks, who want very badly to dine on your blood. Mosquitoes can carry West Nile virus, a nasty bug that can cause flu-like symptoms, partial paralysis, or even death. Ticks can carry Rocky Mountain spotted fever, a multi-week experience that is not enjoyable. You can avoid ticks by using repellents, wearing long-sleeved shirts and pants, and checking your warm

John Bartholow

A moose in the Trap Lake area

and fuzzy body parts frequently during and after your hike.

Insect repellent works very well for mosquitoes, the higher the DEET content the better. A new alternative to repellents containing DEET is products containing picaridin, which doesn't dissolve plastic as DEET does and smells better. Lemon of eucalyptus is more fragrant than picaridin and DEET but is not quite as effective or as long lasting.

Some people feel that DEET has a negative impact on skin, but there is no scientific evidence to support this when products containing it are used within manufacturer's guidelines. It's prudent to select the lowest concentration effective for the amount of time spent outdoors and apply it just once a day—it isn't water soluble and lasts up to 8 hours. Don't use products that combine DEET with sunscreen because you will likely need to reapply them for effective sun protection. Apply DEET on clothing when possible and sparingly on exposed skin; do not use under clothing. Don't use it on the areas around the eyes and mouth, on cuts or wounds, or on the hands of young children. Wash treated skin with soap and water and treated clothing after returning indoors. Avoid spraying in enclosed areas, and don't use it near food.

Larger carnivorous residents of the forests such as mountain lions, bears, and bobcats will generally avoid people if given the choice. They would much rather have normal, tastier diets of squirrels and other rodents. Mountain lions rarely attack or approach people; but if one does approach you for a lunch or dinner date stand tall, yell convincingly that you are big and bad, and don't run. Keep your children and pets close by since the mountain lions see them as potential snacks.

Snakes, rattlesnakes in particular, have been given a bad reputation. You don't want to spend time with one, nor do they want to spend time with you. They will try to avoid you, and they are slow movers. Just try to encourage one to move off-trail; it doesn't happen quickly. Unless you are in literal striking distance, you are in no danger. Their sizzling rattle doesn't mean they want to chew on you; they are simply warning you to back off. If the snake is in vegetation, throw some small rocks or sticks at it and make some noise and they will slither away. If you are bitten, your life is only at risk if you have a severe allergic reaction. Stay calm, slowly walk to your car, and have someone drive you to a hospital. Dogs and small children are at more risk from snake bites, though unlikely to die; you should seek immediate medical care for them. Rattlesnakes are rare at higher elevations but common in foothills areas.

Safety Measures & Checklist

Do not hike alone; go with a companion and let others know where you will be going and when you will be coming back. Watch for trail markers and be very aware of your surroundings.

Extra clothing is essential not optional. Extra food and water is also necessary because cold temperatures and exercise will increase your caloric needs. Staying warm by dressing in layers of warm synthetic or wool clothing is the best way to prevent hypothermia. Wear sunblock and protect your eyes with ultraviolet-rated sunglasses. UV radiation is much more intense at higher elevations and snow reflects the rays making it even more intense. Avoid severe sunburns and snow blindness by being prepared. Use extreme caution whenever crossing streams—they are almost always stronger and deeper than they appear. Consult this clothing and equipment checklist before heading out on a trip:

❑ Wind- and waterproof outer coat or shell
❑ Extra fleece or wool clothing, polypro long underwear, and extra socks
❑ Warm hat, face mask, or baklava
❑ Warm, waterproof mittens or gloves
❑ Space blanket, tarp, or garbage bags big enough to crawl into
❑ Hand- and foot-warmer gel packets if you get cold easily
❑ UV-rated sunglasses, goggles, and a ski mask
❑ Prescription glasses or extra contacts
❑ Sunscreen (SPF 15 or more)
❑ Extra food and water and water purification tablets
❑ First aid kit
❑ Knife
❑ Waterproof matches, lighter, and a candle
❑ Map and compass and, optionally, a GPS unit
❑ Headlamp or flashlight with spare batteries
❑ Ice ax and ski or trekking poles
❑ Insect repellent
❑ Mirror for signaling or a whistle
❑ Cell phone (Sometimes there is coverage, but frequently there is not.)
❑ Camera (for evidence of the fun you had!)

Effects of Altitude

If you live in Colorado and are accustomed to exerting yourself in the high country, then you have nothing to fear. If you or your companions, however, rarely venture above 5000 feet, then recognize your potential limitations at higher elevations. Keep in mind that altitude's effects are unpredictable, especially for those who are visiting from sea level. If you have visitors who have just arrived from a lower elevation, give them at least two days to acclimate before venturing above 5000 feet. If you live at 5000 feet, you need less time to adjust to higher altitudes. Taking 250 milligrams of the prescription medication acetazolamide (Diamox) twice daily for two days before going to higher elevations and for the first two days you are at altitude will also help. Don't take it if you don't need it, and as always check the possible side effects before taking any medication.

Above 8000 feet, plan easy adventures until you determine how well everyone acclimates. Physical conditioning can ease the impact but doesn't prevent altitude sickness. It is risky to drink a lot of alcoholic beverages the evening before or during a high-country adventure. Alcohol's impact is enhanced at altitude; plus, the dehydration and oxygen deprivation alcohol consumption will cause is likely to give you a headache. Alcohol will slow your metabolism and make you feel colder on a chilly day, not warmer. Wait until you're back at camp or lower elevations to enjoy your favorite alcoholic beverages.

Drinking a lot of water before and during high-altitude exercise is a good preventive measure, though not foolproof. Your body needs as much as 8 quarts of water per day if the weather is hot and your exertion strenuous. You will need a minimum of 2 quarts or liters per person for an all-day excursion to avoid headaches. Take along some headache remedies, such as aspirin, and nausea medication (some people feel that Tums have ingredients that can prevent the effects of altitude) just in case. One benefit of aspirin, if your stomach tolerates it, is blood thinning, which can carry more oxygen to your brain and help you avoid an altitude headache. Whatever you choose, take it along with food to avoid stomach upset. Altitude and elevation gain definitely slow you down. Assume at least 1 hour per mile or 1000 feet of elevation gain if you aren't well conditioned.

The most common symptoms of altitude sickness, which can last a couple days, are severe headaches, nausea, loss of appetite, insomnia or poor sleep with strange dreams, lethargy, and a warm, flushed face. Resting, hiking at lower elevations, eating lightly, and drinking more liquids can help. Avoid taking barbiturates since they can aggravate the illness.

The most serious illness caused by altitude is high-altitude pulmonary edema (HAPE), which occurs when fluid collects in the lungs. Symptoms include difficulty breathing, a severe headache with incoherence, staggering, and a persistent hacking cough. If you or anyone in your party experiences these symptoms, they should be taken to a lower altitude immediately and see a physician as soon as possible. High-altitude cerebral edema (HACE), which occurs when your brain swells because fluid collects in it, is very serious; the symptoms include severe headache, delirium, and losing consciousness. This is a rare condition but does occur.

When traveling to higher altitudes, some people, most often women, experience swelling of the face, hands, and feet, with a weight gain of as much as 12 pounds. It is uncomfortable but harmless and will subside after returning to lower elevations. Although the cause is unknown, the condition can be treated with a low-salt diet and diuretics. Nose bleeds are more common at higher elevations because of the very dry air. Staying hydrated and avoiding getting a cold (good luck) are the best way to avoid them. The most effective way to stop a nose bleed is to gently pinch the nose shut for 5 minutes.

Weather & Road Conditions

High mountain weather can and does change rapidly and severely. Some of the most violent weather occurs after clear blue-sky mornings with no hint of rain or thunderstorms. Be prepared for the unexpected. Dramatic temperature swings are common year-round. In the early 20th century Colorado miners were known for commenting on the weather, "There are only two seasons in the mountains; winter and the 4th of July." Mountain weather can produce 90°F and snow or freezing hail in the same place on the same day. It's wise to plan to be on your way down by 11 AM or noon at the latest; most thunderstorms occur by midday, though they can happen earlier.

Colorado has one of the highest numbers of reported lightning strike deaths in the U.S., second only to Florida. The climate tends to produce highly volatile weather at high altitudes; we scrape much closer to the jet stream than most of the U.S. This doesn't mean you have to be afraid to venture up next to the clouds on our soaring summits; many people at lower elevations are struck while mowing the grass, playing golf, or playing softball. (No, drinking beer has nothing to do with attracting lightning.) It does mean that you should get below the treeline as quickly as you can when you hear the roll of thunder or see dark clouds forming near your route. Watch for high gathering cumulus clouds that tower high above, and the characteristic anvil shape that signals the dramatic uplift of moisture into the stratosphere, and its impending return journey from on high, to the ground you are walking on, accompanied by the thunderbolts of Zeus. As mentioned, it also means you should get an early start on your hike if you want to avoid thunderstorms so that you will have a leisurely stroll back to the trailhead. Assume a thunderstorm will occur on the trail by noon on most summer days, especially warm ones, and plan accordingly. The warmer the temperatures, the more likely there is enough energy for a thunderstorm. I generally like to turn around by 11:30 AM during thunderstorm season.

It is always a good idea to check road or trail conditions after major storms in the spring or fall, especially mountain passes, to make sure they are still open. To get road condition reports, call (877) 315-7623 for statewide information, (303) 275-5360 or (303) 371-1080 for Denver/Boulder weather and snow conditions, (303) 639-1111 for Denver roads conditions, and (719) 520-0020 for Colorado Springs roads. For winter avalanche and weather information, call the Colorado Avalanche Information Center in Fort Collins at (970) 482-0457 or in Denver at (303) 275-5360, Rocky Mountain National Park at (970) 586-1206. Call Roosevelt National Forest at (970) 498-2770 and Summit County at (970) 686-0600 for trail conditions.

Symptoms of Hypothermia

Hypothermia, which occurs when your body's core temperature drops below 98.6°F, is a serious and sometimes fatal condition that can severely impair the brain and muscles. If someone dresses inadequately or falls into a lake or stream, stop immediately and take steps to get them dry and warm. Preventing hypothermia is much wiser than waiting until the situation becomes life threatening. Some symptoms of this condition include: uncontrollable shivering, slurred or slow speech, fuzzy thinking, poor memory, incoherence, lack of coordination causing stumbling or vertigo, and extreme fatigue or sleepiness. If you observe any of these symptoms, take immediate action to warm the individual experiencing the difficulties. Stop and use your emergency supplies to make a fire and provide warm liquids, or wrap the individual in additional warm clothing and see if you can get them to move around enough to warm them up.

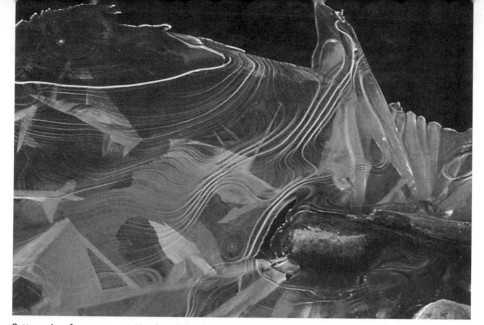

Patterns in a frozen stream, Hewlett Gulch (Chapter 3: Trip 2)   *John Bartholow*

Trail Etiquette

> *"This land is your land, this land is my land..."*
> —Woody Guthrie

Wilderness is the poetry of the physical world; untrammeled, pristine, and invaluable. There are few places on our small planet that have not been paved, plowed, built upon, sold off, or developed. Public wilderness is a limited and vanishing commodity; roads and all that they bring are not. Please let your elected officials know that you value wilderness for hiking, camping, fishing, hunting, and other low-impact pursuits and want it to be around and freely available for future generations of family and friends.

Public land is not owned by the government. It is land that we, the public, own that the government protects and keeps for us. This ownership comes with the opportunity for "re-creation" of the body and soul and the responsibility of care and maintenance. Many of the areas described in this book are wilderness areas and require extra precautions and work to prevent the deterioration of the wilderness experience. We should all try to apply the Leave No Trace philosophy to the use of all public lands so that we can all enjoy them without the negative impacts that heavy use can exact. The National Outdoor Leadership School (also known as NOLS) developed these basic principles:

- Avoid building a fire; bring a lightweight stove and extra clothing for cooking and warmth. Enjoy a candle instead of a fire. Where fires are permitted, use them only for emergencies and don't scar large rocks, overhangs, or trees. Use only down or dead wood and do not snap branches off of live trees. Minimize campfire impacts.

- Pack out whatever you pack in. Don't burn trash, pack it out. If you see unburned trash, pack it out.

- Dismantle structures and cover latrine pits.

- Get as far off the trail as possible when you have to urinate. Use toilet paper or wipes sparingly, and pack them out or bury them at least 9–12 inches deep. Dispose of human waste at least 200 feet from the trail or water sources. Use bare ground for burial or pack out human waste. Use backcountry toilets whenever they are available.

- Know the risks and regulations of the area you are visiting. Visit the backcountry in small groups. Try to avoid popular areas in times of high use.

- Be considerate of others. Be respectful of wildlife—don't approach it too closely, and control your pets.

- Wear clothing and use equipment that is natural hued unless it is hunting season, though bright colors would make it easier to find you if lost.

- Repackage food into reusable containers that won't leak.

- Do not remove trees, plants, rocks, or historical artifacts; they belong to everyone.

- Stay at least 200 feet from wildlife forage or watering areas. Camp at least 200 feet from the trail, water sources, and muddy areas. Save the water, trail, and vegetation from damage.

- Stay on trails unless you are hunting or fishing or have a unique destination that requires it. Shortcuts cause erosion and resource damage.

Friends of the Forest

You can help maintain our forests and have a great time by volunteering with the U.S. Forest Service or the National Park Service, as well as city and county open lands agencies. Check at your local Forest Service office or Rocky Mountain National Park for opportunities. The Fort Collins/Roosevelt/Arapaho U.S. Forest Service office sponsors a summer group called the Poudre Wilderness Rangers and a winter group called the Nordic Rangers. There are also the Diamond Peaks Mountain Bike and Ski Patrols. A variety of nonprofit organizations offer hiking and other outdoor activities, as well as volunteer opportunities, such as the Rocky Mountain Nature Association, Colorado Mountain Club, Sierra Club, and more. For contact information and their locations, see the appendix of organizations. Please consider contributing to or joining organizations that make a difference in preserving and enhancing outdoor recreation and environment.

Using This Book

This book includes everything from mountain climbs to easy strolls and wheelchair-accessible trails. Frequently, long, demanding hikes include a short segment at the beginning that can be easy and enjoyable for the less ambitious. So don't immediately rule out a hike if it includes climbing a mountain; the first mile or so could be quite easy and scenic.

A safe estimate for travel time is 1 hour per mile, or slower, when going uphill at higher altitudes, unless you are exceptionally fit and acclimated. Add time for every 1000 feet to be gained. If you are very fit and acclimated, your pace could be 20 to 30 minutes per mile. If the trail is fairly level and you live at 5000 feet or above and exercise regularly, then you can safely estimate 30 minutes per mile. Of course, the more you stop, the longer it will take you to hike the trail; fitness and experience levels and trail and weather conditions all have a significant impact on the amount of time it takes a particular person to negotiate a particular trail. Conditions vary, and your hiking time could double or even triple if you become caught in a severe storm that includes heavy rain, hail, or lightning. If novices are along, it is wise to have reasonable ambitions and monitor for potential blisters or fading energy levels. Use your watch to judge time out and back. Be conservative—you don't want to end up far from your car or cabin in the dark.

Conditions can vary dramatically and unpredictably. Trails that are normally relatively easy to negotiate can become very challenging in major rainstorms or late spring or early fall snow squalls, but conditions can vary greatly at any time of the year. Spring conditions can make a short jaunt exhausting because of wet, snowy, or slippery trails. One of my recent late fall hiking trips had some of the most variable conditions I have seen—all on the same trail. The south-facing slopes were bare, while the north-facing slopes were frozen and slick. And the part of the loop I faced last required the most work to avoid landing on my posterior. Needless to say it made for an interesting day that required twice the expenditure of energy I had expected.

Your First Adventure

Be conservative your first time out and emphasize enjoyment, not goals. Don't be like my friend "the Bear," who always lives on the edge and pushes himself or his friends beyond reasonable limits. He usually ignores weather forecasts, gets a late start, and insists on going off-trail and straight uphill at a rapid pace. In fact, I've even seen him go charging off into the wilderness late in the day only to become engulfed by thunderstorms well above treeline. Don't be a "Bear." Pick a short, easy round trip that will be an enjoyable half-day jaunt. That will give you a chance to see how your body will react on any given day. Have a good time and don't expect too much of anyone, including yourself.

Great for Kids

Within some trail descriptions, you'll notice "Great for Kids" boxes; these designate trails or trail segments that are appropriate for more relaxed family outings and children of all ages. They are often part of a longer, more challenging hike, but I have highlighted the portion works best for a laid-back stroll so that families may find a suitable hike. These trail sections include opportunities for scenery, picnics, and a bit of exercise without major effort.

Capsulized Summaries

Each trip entry includes a capsule summary, highlights, directions to the starting point, and the full description of the trail itself. The capsule summary at the beginning includes distance, a difficulty rating, elevation information, trail uses, governing agency, recommended maps, the location of nearby facilities, and any special notes.

DISTANCE

All distances listed have been cross-checked with multiple source maps, many of which are contradictory; so the mileage is a very close estimate. The mileages given are round-trip.

DIFFICULTY

All trips include a difficulty rating. Many trips have a range because you can always opt for traveling only a portion of the trail and thereby turn a moderate or challenging trail into an easy one. Many of the trails offer multiple options because even a short out-and-back trip offers a nice outdoor experience with pleasing scenery. Your primary goal is to do what is enjoyable to you at the optimal pace for you and your companions.

The difficulty ratings in this book are generally on par with those given by the U.S. Forest Service. It is

assumed that people using this book are reasonably fit and physically active or have been medically cleared for physical activity at altitudes above 5000 feet. If you have been leading a sedentary lifestyle and decide to start hiking, check in with a health care professional to make sure you're ready for strenuous activity.

Easy

Most of these trails are appropriate for beginners who have never hiked. The number of steep sections and the overall elevation gains are limited. To truly enjoy one of these treks, you should be physically active and exercising at least 2 times per week for at least 20 minutes per session. The ratings assume that you have determined that you are able to handle the elevated heart rate and lack of oxygen

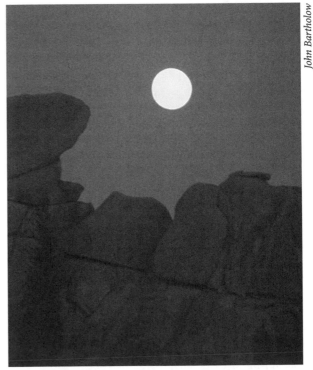

Vedauwoo, Wyoming, near Laramie

John Bartholow

at higher elevations. It also assumes you won't attempt the entire route but will cover what you can while still having fun and will turn around before you are exhausted. Decide how long you want to be out before you go. Then time your outbound trip and estimate how long it will take to return to the trailhead to avoid exceeding your comfort range. The physically active young are generally, but not always, going to have a slight advantage over an equally active "mature" adult.

Moderate

These trails include several steep sections and require a longer, more sustained effort. You will enjoy trails rated as moderate if you have a somewhat higher level of fitness. This doesn't mean you have to be a serious athlete. It just means you are physically active and exercise 20–40 minutes at least 3 times per week. You can, of course, choose to challenge yourself if you aren't currently at the "enjoyable" fitness level.

Challenging

Trails rated as challenging assume a high level of fitness to successfully enjoy them, and the experience to survive under the possibility of rapidly changing weather conditions. These trails will have many steep sections, which require sustained climbing. You should be challenging yourself with almost daily exercise if you want to enjoy this kind of all-day, strenuous trek to the mountaintops. You should also have good route-finding skills and bring and know how to use a topographic map and compass and even perhaps a GPS unit.

ELEVATION

This is the elevation gain to reach the high point or summit on a particular trip. It does not include possible elevation gains to get back to the trailhead. A rolling trail will require uphill climbs on the return, which are not included in this figure. In cases where it is relevant, the starting elevation is listed as well so that you know what general elevation range a particular hike covers.

TRAIL USE

While all of the trails are suitable for hiking, some are also good for backpacking, camping, fishing, horseback riding, motorized recreation, mountain biking, paddling, road biking, rock climbing, running, all of which I generally note. I point out which trails are accessible for wheelchair users and whether a trip is great for families hiking with kids or has an option that is appropriate for such groups, which is covered in a sidebar in the actual trip description.

Dogs are allowed in all national forests and Bureau of Land Management areas and most state, county, and city parks and open spaces. Within the summary information for the individual trails, I mention whether they are allowed. They usually have to be leashed to protect them from the wildlife and the wildlife from them. They are not allowed on trails in national parks, like Rocky Mountain National Park. Although dogs are allowed on many trails, it is often easier to leave them at home. If you do bring them, carry plastic bags to clean up after them if they leave waste on the trail. Be sure to control your pets at all times. Some dogs are too friendly or aggressive, and many people are intimidated by dogs, especially when they're barking or growling.

AGENCY

The name of the governing local, state, or national agency that you can contact for information is included; their contact information is listed in the appendices.

MAPS

Maps in the National Geographic Trails Illustrated series covering Colorado are generally the recommended maps in this section. If you are mountaineering, you should purchase the appropriate U.S. Geological Survey topographical map for the area you will be visiting.

FACILITIES

Any nearby facilities, such as restrooms or restaurants, are pointed out here, whether they're at a trailhead or perhaps a nearby visitors' center.

NOTES

This section covers regulations for areas where dogs are prohibited or restricted or other special information that you'll want to know before you go to the trailhead.

HIGHLIGHTS

This is a very brief overview of the trail and the main sights you will encounter.

DIRECTIONS

The driving directions provided are generally from the closest city or town. In some cases, driving times or distances from larger metropolitan areas are provided.

Map Legend

Featured Trail	▬▬▬▬▬▬
Cross-Country Route	•••••••••••••••
Other Trail	▬ ▬ ▬ ▬ ▬
Steep Terrain (dense contour lines)	
Gentle Terrain (sparse contour lines)	
Stream	*Creek*
Body of Water	
Boundary Line	▬ ▬ - - ▬ ▬
Limited Access Highway	═══════
Major Road	═══════
Road	───────
Unpaved Road	═══════
Railroad	┼┼┼┼┼┼┼

Trip Number	**1**
Featured Trailhead	**T**
Other Parking	**P**
Picnic Area	🛆
Campground	🛆
Ranger Station or Visitor Center	🏠
Restroom	👥
Point of Interest	■
Peak	▲
Pass	) (
Bridge	═
Interstate Highway	70
U.S. Highway	34
State Highway	14
County Road	34
Forest Road	395

North Arrow

Chapter 1
Wyoming: Medicine Bow National Forest

You might be wondering why a hiking book about hiking on the Front Range of Colorado includes Wyoming. The Wyoming state line is only 20 miles north of Fort Collins and only 90 miles north of Denver, and the Medicine Bow Mountains are no farther in time or distance from Fort Collins than the upper reaches of the Poudre Canyon, Rocky Mountain National Park, or the Indian Peaks. Laramie, Wyoming, is 65 miles north of Fort Collins, and the Happy Jack area is only another 5 miles east on Interstate 80. It takes about 1½ hours to drive from Fort Collins to the Medicine Bow National Forest.

The Medicine Bow National Forest was the beneficiary of President Theodore Roosevelt's exceptional vision of the need for wild places. Roosevelt set aside millions of acres of public land as Medicine Bow Forest Preserve in 1902, providing everyone with a multiuse legacy that could last for generations. As Roosevelt said, "Leave it as it is. The ages have been at work on it, and man can only mar it." While the origin of the Medicine Bow Mountains name is not known for certain, the legend that rings truest is that it evolved from the Native American practice of making bows from a mahogany forest in the area. The theory that the arrows were treated with medicine or poison doesn't fit with the typi-cal practices of the tribes, primarily the Shoshone, who peopled the high plains. Friendly tribes often gathered in the area to hold powwows to try to cure diseases, in an effort that was known as "making medicine" in 1800s slang. Making bows and making medicine were apparently combined by the immigrant settlers into

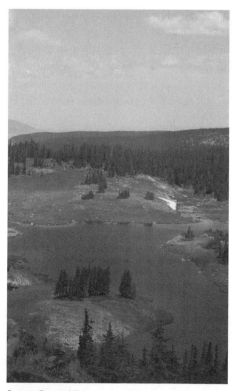

Snowy Range View

the name "Medicine Bow" for the area. The contemporary national forest covers 1,093,750 acres and is an inheritance people can enjoy in the nonconsumptive style of the Native Americans who treasured its unique beauty. Medicine Bow National Forest includes parts of three mountain ranges—the Medicine Bow, Laramie, and Sierra Madre—as well as four different wilderness areas.

Happy Jack

Though Happy Jack was created as a cross-country ski area, it is also used the rest of the year by hikers and mountain bikers, as well as snowshoers. It features the unique geography and geology of the Laramie foothills with craggy rock outcrops, grassy meadows, and thick stands of aspens and conifers that give it a sense of wilderness very near civilization. Happy Jack is so relatively small that it would be difficult to get lost in the area and not intersect a trail rather quickly, though you might end up on a much longer trek than you wanted if you didn't bring a map. Grab a map at the trailhead if one is available and have fun.

The trails roll over the foothills in every compass direction and provide interesting viewpoints and vistas at almost every turn. I describe only one of the many fun options, most of which are fairly short. If you have more than 2 hours, you can probably take in two trails or loop one twice since they are short and of easy to moderate intensity. You can design a trek of any length or intensity depending on who is with you. Most of the trails are loops and intersect each other except the Summit Trail, which is an independent out-and-back loop.

Snowy Range

This area is primarily known for the Snowy Range Downhill Ski Area but has lots of summer recreation opportunities, too. Snowy Range Pass features several nice U.S. Forest Service campgrounds that are popular with cross-country travelers and locals. Fortunately the Forest Service has done a nice job of separating the motorized and nonmotorized users. You will encounter all-terrain vehicles (ATVs) and off-highway vehicles (OHVs) as you enter some of the trails and the roads and parking areas. You can escape both the sight and sound of ATVs and OHVs on the nonmotorized trails.

Though I only describe my favorite trail, Libby Creek, there are several nice routes in the Snowy Range. You might also want to check out Round Mountain, which is a good route for beginners. You can combine this trail with the Libby Creek Campground Loops to create three different loops, the longest of which is a moderate 7 miles over rolling terrain that is more of an intermediate-level adventure. Barber Lake Trail is also worth exploring and is a moderate venture for mountain bikers.

Other Places to Explore: Vedauwoo

About 80 miles or 1½ hours north of Fort Collins and between Laramie and Cheyenne, Wyoming, are magical rock formations that look like they have been airlifted from Moab, Utah, and dropped for local amusement. One of the rare attractions that has retained its Native American name, Vedauwoo is very popular with rock climbers, campers, and hikers. A small area east of Happy Jack, it is certainly worth a visit if you want to enjoy a great natural rock sculpture garden but don't want to drive very far to do so.

TRIP 1 Aspen, Middle Aspen, & Pole Creek Trails

Distance	2.0 miles, Loop
Difficulty	Easy
Elevation Gain	253 feet (starting at 8340 feet)
Trail Use	Mountain biking, great for kids, leashed dogs OK
Agency	Medicine Bow National Forest
Map	*Medicine Bow National Forest*
Note	Dogs are not allowed on the Middle Aspen, Ridge Loop, Lower UW Loop, and Blackjack Trail Loops. There is a $2 day-use fee per person.

HIGHLIGHTS One of the main routes at Happy Jack, these trails travel through a variety of scenery while twisting, turning, and gently rolling up, down, and through the forest. You will enjoy vistas of foothills, pretty meadows, and rock gardens along the way. The trails are good for beginners and intermediate-level mountain bikers; they don't require any technical skills.

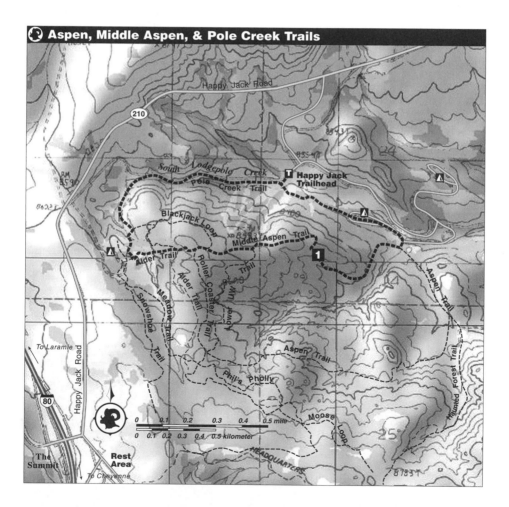

Aspen, Middle Aspen, & Pole Creek Trails

DIRECTIONS Drive to Laramie, Wyoming, north on U.S. Highway 287 to Interstate 80 and then east on I-80 to the Happy Jack exit (Highway 210), the first exit after you climb a very long hill east of Laramie. The extra elevation means that Pole Mountain receives much more early and late snow than Laramie. Drive over I-80 and notice an excellent visitors center on the right with some interesting natural history and map displays and restrooms that have ample space for a wardrobe change.

Turn left if you don't need the rest area, and you will see the Happy Jack area about 0.5 mile up on the right. Pay the $2 per person day-use fee at the east end of the parking lot, and pick up a good map of the many trail options. There are usually smaller maps of the area in one of the wooden boxes on the display.

The Aspen Trail is one of the well-marked main trails that you will see after you leave the parking lot. Go up a slight hill and then bear left until you come to a fence and a crossroads with the University of Wyoming Trail. Take the Aspen Trail about 0.5 mile to the intersection of the Middle Aspen Trail. I recommend the Middle Aspen option because it not heavily used and offers some nice open vistas. The trail features lots of twists and turns that allow you opportunities to wander into the woods if you are on foot. Some of the hills are steep enough for intermediate mountain biking, but most are easy. Eventually you will pass through a more open area and then head steadily downhill until you intersect the Pole Creek Trail. Turn right on it and enjoy the bottom of the arroyo before climbing back up the hill to the parking area.

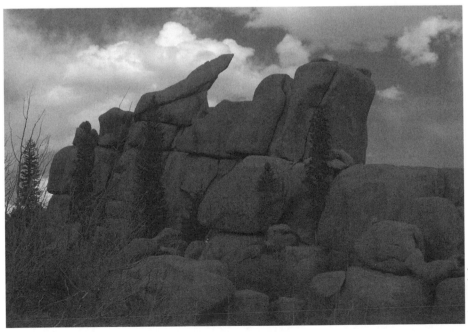

John Bartholow

Happy Jack

TRIP 2 Libby Creek Trail

Distance	Up to 6.0 miles, Loop
Difficulty	Easy
Trail Use	Mountain biking, motorized recreation, leashed dogs OK
Elevation Gain	400 feet (starting at 9800 feet)
Agency	Medicine Bow National Forest
Map	*Medicine Bow National Forest*

HIGHLIGHTS One of the most scenic in the area, this trail features great views of the mountains, petite Libby Canyon, and the expansive, picturesque, high, and lonesome Wyoming plains. It is well separated and buffered from off-highway vehicles (OHVs) after the first 0.25 mile.

DIRECTIONS Drive 27 miles southwest from Laramie, Wyoming, on the Snowy Range Highway (State Highway 130) to Centennial. Continue west on State Highway 130 to enter Snowy Range Recreation Area. Continue on 130, which becomes Snowy Range Road, to the Green Rock Picnic Ground.

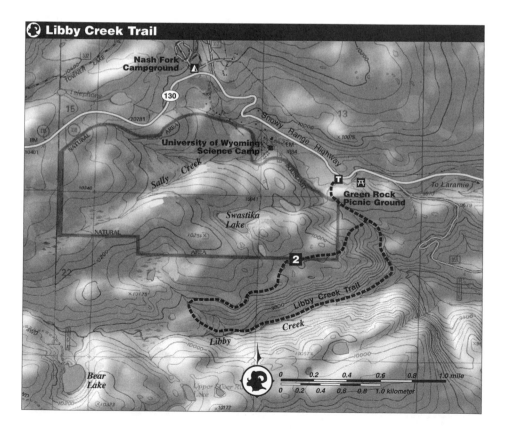

The entire trek is a moderate round-trip that features some short, steep climbs and descents of limited distance and duration at the beginning and end of the loop. If you just want to see the great view from the ridge on top of Libby Creek Canyon, you can do so by starting at the Green Rock Picnic Ground and going counterclockwise on the loop. You will gain about 200 feet in 0.5 mile to get to the viewpoint. To pick up the trail, walk to the right of the restrooms and then walk west (right) for about 50 yards on Barber Lake Trail, a four-wheel-drive road that is sometimes heavily used by OHVs. Then go left (southwest) along the edge of the trees. Follow the blue diamonds that mark the nonmotorized trail on the right. Very well marked as it enters the trees, the trail starts level and then goes downhill for about 0.25 mile. Follow the trail sign on the right as you descend the hill on the Barber Lake Trail.

After veering off to the right, you start the fairly steady climb that is broken up by some short, flat stretches. You are in the thickly wooded forest until you start to reach the top of the ridgeline. When the trees thin out, you are able to see the canyon rim on your left. When you have almost topped out completely, you see a faint trail going toward the rim for the view that you can follow, but almost any route works for a departure from the trail to see the rim.

After enjoying the views, return to the trailhead or rejoin the trail as it descends and climbs through varied tree cover. The trail reaches a small open bowl and then a side trail descends into the canyon. The main trail goes straight, rounds a bend to the left, and then descends less steeply and more gradually to the canyon floor than the side trail. From there it is a level jaunt through the canyon before the trail climbs back out to the Barber Lake Trail and then the starting point.

Chapter 2
Red Feather
Lakes Area

The Red Feather Lakes Area is bordered on the northwest by the beautiful Medicine Bow Mountains that grace this part of northern Colorado and southern Wyoming and the majestic Rawah Range that looms to the southwest. It offers unique vistas that ease the soul. Rolling foothills and low mountains are transformed into the limitless horizons of the high plains of southern Wyoming. The lakes are petite but comely, and festooned by the rocks left behind when the glaciers retreated at the end of the last ice age. The region is approximately 45 miles northwest of Fort Collins, close to the Wyoming-Colorado border, and the trails are not as heavily used as those in the Poudre Canyon. The lakes region features unique and striking terrain that combines the rolling characteristics of the foothills and hogbacks with the conifer forests of the high mountains. The vistas are crowned with interesting rock formations, and the picturesque valleys and canyons are as varied as they are beautiful. Popular for camping, fishing, and horseback riding, the area isn't overwhelmed with throngs of hikers and mountain bikers.

Beaver Meadows Resort

If you want a good place for beginners or families with easy-to-use, difficult-to-lose trails and the convenience of a low-key rustic lodge and restaurant, check out Beaver Meadows Resort. The day-use fee is only charged in the winter. The resort offers a variety of overnight accommodations. If you complete all of the hiking routes outlined on the resort map, you will have a satisfying day with a wide variety of views and trails that climb, roll, ascend, and descend through an aspen and pine forest and cross some beautiful sunny meadows.

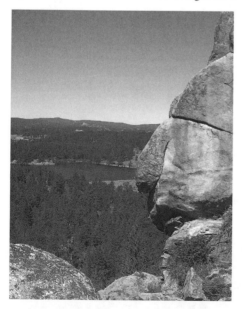

Profile Rock near the Mount Margaret Trail (Trip 1)

TRIP 1 Mount Margaret Trail

Distance	8.0 miles from the Red Feather Road Trailhead, 7.0 miles from the Dowdy Lake Trailhead, Semiloop
Difficulty	Easy
Elevation Gain/Loss	257 feet/130 feet to summit (starting at 7700 feet)
Trail Use	Mountain biking, horseback riding, leashed dogs OK
Agency	Canyon Lakes Ranger District, Roosevelt National Forest
Map	Trails Illustrated *Red Feather Lakes & Glendevey*
Note	Campground and restrooms at Dowdy Lake

HIGHLIGHTS The round-trip to the summit can be a pleasant half-day-plus adventure, but it is very worthwhile to hike or bike even a small section of this scenic trail. You don't have to bag the anticlimactic Mt. Margaret summit, which is lower than the trailhead, to enjoy a feeling of satisfaction. This popular summer hiking route has a relatively low altitude of 7700 feet and limited shade, so it can be very warm in midsummer. It is ideal for hiking in spring, early summer, or early fall, unless you get an early start and beat the heat. If you do arrive in early spring, be prepared for the marshy area at the beginning of the trail and a slightly wider stream crossing.

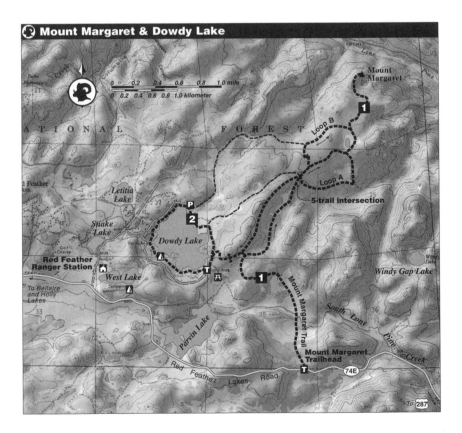

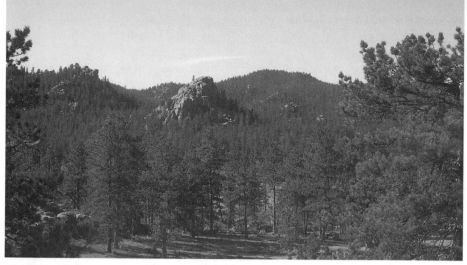
Mt. Margaret Trail

DIRECTIONS From Fort Collins drive north on U.S. Highway 287 toward Laramie. After 10 miles, you pass the turnoff for Poudre Canyon (State Highway 14); keep going north another 10 miles until you reach the junction with Red Feather Lakes Road (County Road 74E) known as The Forks near Livermore, which many maps show as Livermore. At the bottom of a long hill where Highway 287 veers to the right, turn left (west) onto paved CR 74E. It's another 23 miles to the Red Feather and Dowdy Lakes area on a road with lots of curves and climbs and a speed limit of generally 45 miles per hour. Allow at least 30 minutes from Livermore or 1 hour or more for a leisurely, low-stress drive from Fort Collins. The trailhead is approximately 20 miles from Livermore on the right (north) side of the road.

To reach an alternate route, take Red Feather Lakes Road to the trailhead 1 mile before the Dowdy Lakes area on the north (right) side of the road. It is easy to miss if there aren't any cars in the small parking lot, and there is a fence since the area is sometimes used for grazing.

The trail has some nice stands of aspens and a variety of evergreens but is mostly open. It features nice vistas of the foothills, rock outcroppings that are good for minor scrambles (or bouldering), peaceful mountain meadows guarded by stately conifers, and the smaller but very scenic canyons and valleys of North Larimer County.

The trail first goes gently uphill and then gently downhill into the Lone Pine Creek drainage. It crosses Lone Pine Creek in 0.5 miles, which can be part of a marshy area in the late spring or early summer. The trail passes a footbridge to the right (east) side of the trail as it continues through some fairly tall willows. Negotiating the narrow board bridge is easier with hiking poles. The marsh surrounding the stream area may get your feet wet early in the season if you don't have waterproof boots.

After crossing the creek, the trail passes the first of the dramatic rock formations and one of many pretty meadows often covered with wildflowers in the spring. The trail travels north for about 1 mile and then turns west and north again to reach the Dowdy Lake Connector Trail on the left (west). Continue to the right (northeast) as the trail levels and trees and rock formations become more common. In about 0.75 mile you come to the Loop A and Loop B trails. For variety, though it adds a bit of distance, take Loop B on the left on the way out and Loop A on the way back. In both cases, you rejoin the main trail after taking very pretty and somewhat different side jaunts. The extra mile this route adds is insignificant if you are mountain biking.

After the end of Loop B, you see a sign for Mt. Margaret. The trail broadens and the trees thin, passing more dramatic rock formations as the trail goes downhill, uphill, and then downhill—a gentle roller coaster to the base of the summit. If you make it all the way to Mt. Margaret, you are treated to views of canyons and valleys that surround the rocky summit. The actual summit rock requires a bit of technical climbing skill and a rope for complete safety but can be easily observed from and politely ignored for the broad and flat adjacent rock.

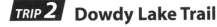 **Dowdy Lake Trail**

Distance	1.5 miles, Loop
Difficulty	Easy
Elevation Gain	Negligible (starting at 7700 feet)
Trail Use	Camping, paddling, fishing, great for kids, leashed dogs OK
Agency	Canyon Lakes Ranger District, Roosevelt National Forest
Map	Trails Illustrated *Red Feather Lakes & Glendevey*
Note	This fee area has a campground and restrooms.

HIGHLIGHTS A pleasant, easy, and scenic stroll heads around a most comely mountain lake punctuated by striking rock outcrops dating from the last ice age. I imagine the lake was a favorite watering hole for the Ute Indians who inhabited the area from about 4000 years ago until the 1860s when they were forced to leave. The nice campground is very popular, so reservations are necessary.

DIRECTIONS From Fort Collins drive north on U.S. Highway 287 toward Laramie. After 10 miles, you will pass the turnoff for Poudre Canyon (State Highway 14); keep going north another 10 miles until you reach the junction with Red Feather Lakes Road (County Road 74E) known as The Forks near Livermore, which many maps show as Livermore. At the bottom of a long hill where Highway 287 veers to the right, turn left (west) onto paved CR 74E. It's another 23 miles to the Red Feather & Dowdy Lakes area on a road with lots of curves and climbs and a speed limit of generally 45 miles per hour. Allow at least 30 minutes from Livermore or an hour or more for a leisurely, low-stress drive from Fort Collins. The trailhead is approximately 20 miles from Livermore on the right (north) side of the road. Then continue on the Red Feather Lakes Road (County Road 74E) to the Dowdy Lake turnoff. Turn right toward the campground and look for a place to park at an unused campsite.

Walk through the campground to the edge of the lake and circumnavigate in either direction. I prefer clockwise since you are less likely to encounter as many people. The trail crosses one or two stream crossings, but they are generally trickles. As the trail rounds the lake, the view is ever changing, with the some of the best views from the far side of the lake. You can get a peek at the Rawah Peaks from the far side if you want to circumnavigate.

You might also walk along a beautiful, less-visited trail across the road from the Dowdy Lake Trailhead that wanders through some gorgeous meadows while rolling over hill and dale before joining the Mt. Margaret Trail described above.

TRIP *3* North Lone Pine Trail to Mount Baldy Overlook

Distance	5.0 to 12.0 miles, Out-and-back
Difficulty	Moderate
Elevation Gain	400 feet (starting at 9300 feet)
Trail Use	Leashed dogs OK
Agency	Canyon Lakes Ranger District, Roosevelt National Forest
Map	Trails Illustrated *Red Feather Lakes & Glendevey*

HIGHLIGHTS This lightly used trail passes through 20-foot-tall fir trees and 2-foot-tall pines in a part of Roosevelt National Forest that has recovered from forest fires and logging. Its topography is similar to that of Beaver Meadows and Mt. Margaret, but it climbs higher and provides views of the high plains and canyons as they climb steeply into the stark terrain of southern Wyoming in the distance. The North Lone Pine Trailhead is well marked, but the trail is not and requires good route-finding skills to be navigated successfully.

DIRECTIONS From Fort Collins drive north on U.S. Highway 287 toward Laramie. After 10 miles, you pass the turnoff for Poudre Canyon (State Highway 14). Then go north another 10 miles until you reach the junction with Red Feather Lakes Road (County Road 74E) in Livermore. At the bottom of a long hill where Highway 287 veers to the right, turn left (west) onto paved CR 74E. Follow CR 74E another 24 miles (on a road with curves

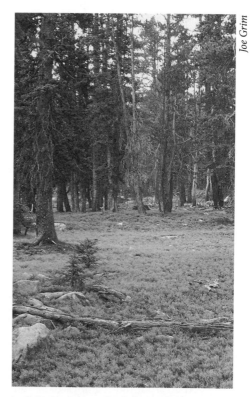

Joe Grim

Lodgepole pines on the Lone Pine Trail

North Lone Pine Trail to Mount Baldy Overlook

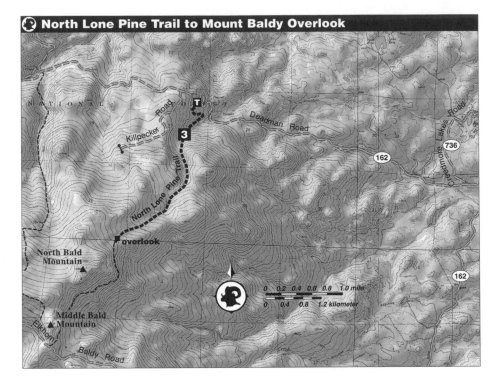

and climbs and a speed limit of 45 miles per hour), and pass the Creedmore Lakes Road (County Road 180) turnoff. The road becomes gravel Deadman Road (County Road 162). The trailhead and the picnic area are on the right (north) side of the road. It is an ideal place, weather and wind permitting, for photos or a lunch or snack break before beginning to hike the trail.

You are fairly high up on the mountain when you reach the trailhead. Very well marked and impossible to miss on the south (left) side of the road, the trailhead is fairly obvious from the trail marker and information board, but the trail is unmarked after that. Follow the trail by tracing the small tree tunnel it forms. It climbs steadily and roller coasters some as it meanders through the thick tree cover and goes from 9300 feet up to 10,400 feet. As you travel to the higher reaches of the trail, some breaks in the trees offer views.

After approximately 2 miles on the trail, you cross an old logging road. You cross the road again about 0.75 mile later. Assume it will take you at least two hours round-trip to reach and return from the Mt. Baldy overlook from the trailhead. The trail levels somewhat and has a view of one of the Baldy Mountains on the left, staying high on the ridge. Leave the trail when you reach a rock outcropping on the left, and climb the rock carefully for the best view of the Baldys. The trail continues and eventually dead-ends at the Elkhorn-Baldy four-wheel-drive road, but I suggest turning around at this point and finding your way back to the trailhead.

TRIP 4 Trappers' Loop to Trappers'/Renegade Trails

Distance	2.5 to 3.0 miles, Loop
Difficulty	Easy
Elevation Gain	400 feet (starting at 8400 feet)
Trail Use	Horseback riding, leashed dogs OK
Agency	Beaver Meadows Resort
Map	*Beaver Meadows Resort Trails*
Facilities	Restaurant and restrooms in lodge

HIGHLIGHTS You can take any loop of the resort's 5 miles of trails you like; however, this beautiful route offers gentle climbs and descents, good views, and a nice mix of forest, rock outcrops, and small meadows.

DIRECTIONS From Fort Collins drive north on U.S. Highway 287 toward Laramie. After 10 miles, you pass the turnoff for Poudre Canyon (State Highway 14). Then go north another 10 miles until you reach the junction with Red Feather Lakes Road (County Road 74E) in Livermore. The resort is about 26 miles from Livermore. Continue west on Red Feather Lakes Road (County Road 74E) past the local landmark, the Pot Belly Restaurant, until the road forks, where CR 74E ends. Go right on County Road 73C, a dirt road, and bear left (straight) at the next intersection for another 4.3 miles. When you see the sign for the resort on the left, take the private resort road another 0.8 mile to the parking lot. Allow about 1 ½ hours to drive from Fort Collins. All of the trails begin across the meadow south of the lodge and up the hill next to it.

One of the beautiful meadows at Beaver Meadows Resort

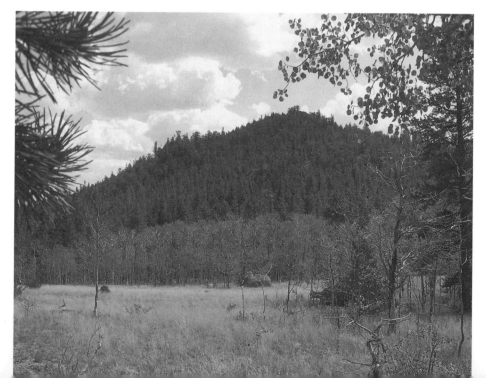

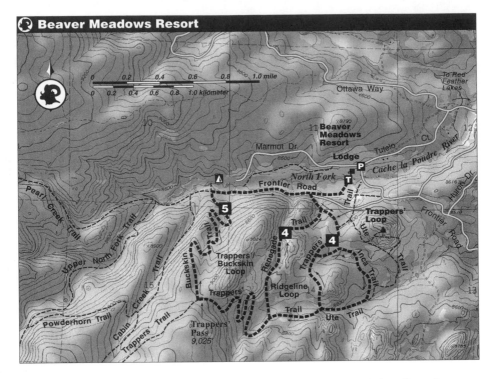

Beaver Meadows Resort

Walk uphill, and at the top turn right onto Frontier Road. Go left at a yellow sign and up another short hill to reach Trappers' Loop Trail. The trail goes gradually uphill through thick trees with a small rock formation on the right. Follow it to the left until you reach the top of the first hill with a very nice view of the mountain panorama across the valley. A small plane crash and fire that leveled the forest on the mountainside across the valley more than 20 years ago is virtually undetectable.

If you'd like a different route, try the Renegade Trail, which is the first option on the right (west). Otherwise, you'll be on the Trappers' Trail, winding through a mixed aspen and pine forest. Red flags mark the top of the ridgeline. To stay on the trail turn sharply right—a pretty meadow filled with aspen trees will be your reward. It is always fun to watch the aspen leaves "quaking" in the soft summer breezes or to appreciate their golden color in the fall. Follow the signs for the Trappers' Trail when you cross the meadow and then climb a bit of a switchback through nice variety of lodgepole pine, spruce, and aspen.

The intersection with the Inca Trail will come into view. It takes a little more than an hour to combine the Trappers' and Inca trails and wander downhill to a valley framed by several large rock outcroppings. This valley has a colorful mixture of mature aspen and fairly tall lodgepole pine trees and is a good place for a rest stop for a snack or lunch. You can then go left on the Inca Trail back to the base area or go right on Trappers' to extend your trek.

If you extend your trip on Trappers' Trail, go right (west) from the Inca/Ute trails and then up and down rolling terrain in and out of trees in a narrow meadow nicely framed by trees on both sides. Most of the trail on this backside of the area is open with good views. The meadow is long but not very wide.

After less than 0.5 mile, the trail reaches the well-signed junction for a return to base camp via the top of the Trappers' Trail. The latter goes uphill a little and then downhill back where you started at the Inca-Trappers' intersection. If you continue straight past the sign, you will eventually intersect the Renegade Trail. Take it right uphill. You crest the ridge after 0.5 mile and then can enjoy a good view of the base valley far below. The trail descends gradually into a soothing forest. When you reach the Trappers' Trail, go left to return to the lodge or try another loop if you have the time and energy.

TRIP 5 Trappers' Pass to Buckskin Trail

Distance	3.5 to 4.0 miles, Loop
Difficulty	Easy
Elevation Gain	800 feet (starting at 8400 feet)
Trail Use	Horseback riding, leashed dogs OK
Agency	Beaver Meadows Resort
Map	*Beaver Meadows Resort Trail*
Facilities	Restrooms in lodge

HIGHLIGHTS This additional adventure features more elevation gain than Trappers' Pass and Inca Trail route and a different panoramic view from one of the highest ridges in the resort.

DIRECTIONS From Fort Collins drive north on U.S. Highway 287 toward Laramie. After 10 miles, you pass the turnoff for Poudre Canyon (State Highway 14). Then go north another 10 miles until you reach the junction with Red Feather Lakes Road (County Road 74E) in Livermore. The resort is about 26 miles from Livermore. Drive west on Red Feather Lakes Road (County Road 74E) approximately 20 miles, past the local landmark, the Pot Belly Restaurant, until the road forks, where CR 74E ends. Go right on County Road 73C, a dirt road, and bear left (straight) at the next intersection for another 4.3 miles. When you see the sign for the resort on the left, take the private resort road another 0.8 mile to the parking lot. Allow about 1 ½ hours to drive from Fort Collins. All of the trails begin across the meadow south of the lodge and up the hill next to it.

Walk up the hill, and at the top of the hill turn right onto Frontier Road. Go down the opposite side of the hill. At the bottom of the hill, go left at a yellow sign up the hill onto the Trappers' Loop Trail.

If, like me, you occasionally can't resist the urge to get to the top of the highest point, continue uphill to the top of Trappers' Pass at around 9000 feet. It is a very reasonable switchback—not recommended for small children, but is certainly doable for ambitious families. After enjoying the view, walk along the short top of the ridgeline to the Buckskin Trail. It goes gradually downhill, losing 400 feet of elevation, meandering through the trees with occasional nice views of the base area and surrounding hills.

Red Feather Lakes

Chapter 3

Poudre Canyon
& Cameron Pass Areas

Colorado is graced with some of the most magnificent canyons in the world, and the Poudre Canyon is one of them. Long and spectacular, it offers some of the best hiking and biking trails. Some trails near the bottom of the canyon are very close to Fort Collins, and some are usable almost year-round. Its upper reaches will be wet from spring snowmelt in the late spring and early summer, but the trails are a treat after they dry out. In the winter the trails are nirvana for snowshoeing, backcountry skiing, and snowboarding.

Cameron Pass is over 10,000 feet, and most of the trails described start at elevations of 7000 to 9000 feet. At 9000 feet you are in a Rocky Mountain climate zone roughly equivalent to the climate found at sea level 100 miles north of the Canadian border. Being in this climate zone generally translates to cool summer breezes on even the hottest days but almost daily afternoon thunderstorms in July and August in the higher elevations. Fortunately, these trails are generally well protected by stately evergreens that offer abundant shade on hot summer days, and break the not-uncommon winds when temperatures cool in the fall. There are a lot of ideal, warm, sunny days with welcome cool breezes moving down from the mountaintops.

Cameron Pass is bordered on the south by Rocky Mountain National Park's (RMNP) well-named Never Summer Range, which is crowned by the jagged Noku Crags, and on the south by the seldom-seen and little-known Rawah Range, and its monarch, Clark Peak. West of the pass are the Colorado State Forest and the stark beauty of North Park.

To reach Poudre Canyon, take U.S. Highway 287 north from Fort Collins and exit west onto State Highway 14 at Ted's Place. The high mountain trails are at least 1¼ hours from Fort Collins on this National Scenic Byway through the canyon. The trip features the largely unfettered Poudre River, winding through towering rock canyon walls, alternating with some of the most striking mountain meadows anywhere. The lower canyon trails are 20 to 30 minutes from Fort Collins. Cameron Pass and Pingree Park are at least 1½ hours without motor home traffic.

Pingree Park Area

A branch summer campus of Colorado State University and research and conference center, Pingree Park is not open to the public for visits, except for scheduled conferences or meetings. It enjoys a spectacular setting that features the majestic mountain backdrops of the Cache la Poudre Wilderness, Comanche Peak Wilderness, and RMNP. The surrounding area is Roosevelt National Forest and is open to the public with no permits required. This

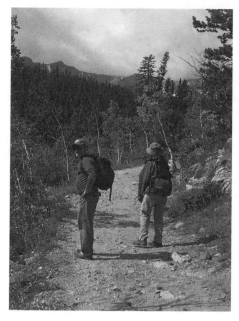
Hikers in Pingree Park

area also offers access to RMNP, which requires permits for camping. The Pingree Park area is approximately 27.5 miles from the entrance of the canyon at Ted's Place on U.S. Highway 287. The Pingree Park County Road (131) turnoff is on the left (south) side if you are driving west, and the road network accesses trails for the aforementioned wilderness areas, some of which start at 8000 feet and offer less-busy access to some unique summits and lakes on the north side of RMNP.

Long Draw Road

Though Long Draw Road can be rough and is heavily used by vehicles on weekends, it offers good access to several nonmotorized routes through some exquisite old-growth forests of stately fir and spruce trees. It begins 60 miles west of Fort Collins on State Highway 14 across from the parking lot for Blue Lake. The trip is an enjoyable 19-mile drive to Long Draw Reservoir as the road rolls, climbing short hills at times. Fairly flat,

it is a tree tunnel at times until it nears the edge of Long Draw Reservoir. Long Draw Campground has a very dramatic setting in the Never Summer Range on the northern edge of RMNP and is a very worthwhile destination. Long Draw Campground is located approximately 9 miles east of State Highway 14 on the Long Draw Road at an elevation of 10,030 feet. The campground's 25 sites enjoy the shade of many spruce and lodgepole pines. The campground offers excellent dayhike access to RMNP and Thunder Pass via the Michigan Ditch Road and can be used for a car shuttle thru-hike to Trail Ridge Road destinations, via backpack or long dayhike. For more information, see the descriptions for Little Yellowstone on page 167 since that is where you can end up.

Mountain biking is possible on the road if you don't mind lots of weekend vehicle traffic or can use it during the week when traffic is light. The traffic is a fraction of what you see on State Highway 14 (Poudre Canyon Road). This road also accesses several great hiking or biking options—the Meadows Trail, Trap Park or Peterson Lake, RMNP at Corral Creek, Comanche Peak, Thunder Pass, and Never Summer Range summits.

Other Areas of Interest: Gateway Park

Between the Grey Rock and Hewlett Gulch trails is the turnoff for this city recreation site—a wonderful place for a riverside picnic. It is at the confluence of the North Fork and Main Stem of the Poudre River. A fee area that costs $6 at the time of this writing, it includes some very scenic, very short (1.5 miles) walking trails and a picnic area and can be used as a launching point for paddlers.

TRIP 1 Grey Rock

Distance	7.0 miles, Semiloop
Difficulty	Moderate
Elevation Gain	2000 feet (starting at 5500 feet)
Trail Use	Rock climbing (off-trail), leashed dogs OK
Agency	Canyon Lakes Ranger District, Roosevelt National Forest
Map	Trails Illustrated *Cache La Poudre & Big Thompson*
Note	Restrooms next to the parking lot

HIGHLIGHTS Grey Rock is one of the most popular trails in Poudre Canyon because of its close proximity to Fort Collins and the spectacular scenery and varied terrain it offers. Starting at the river, you climb through a diverse mixed conifer forest and savor the ever-widening panorama of the canyon at your feet. Summiting buys you a stunning 360-degree view from the top.

DIRECTIONS Take U.S. Highway 287 north from Fort Collins and exit west onto State Highway 14 at Ted's Place. Drive approximately 8.5 miles west on Highway 14 from Ted's Place. The parking area is elevated from the roadway and easy to miss on the left (south) side of the highway.

The trail is actually on the north side of the highway. Walk down the steps, cross the road carefully, and take the footbridge across the sparkling Poudre River. The trail goes west and veers away from the river into a creek drainage that is usually dry. It starts to climb immediately and crosses the creek. The trail is fairly rocky and bumpy before it recrosses the creek, smoothes out, and climbs more steeply. After approximately 1 mile the trail comes to an intersection, where you can take either direction for a long, beautiful, mountainside loop. If it is a warm day and you want to end the hike in more shade, go straight (bear left) to take the more open west side loop first. If the heat and shade are not factors, then go right (east) and end up in the open on the

return. The loop to the west is a bit longer because it travels through pretty Grey Rock Meadow. If you aren't planning to hike all the way to the summit and want a moderate, less challenging hike, start on the west side and make the meadow your destination. If your goal is to summit and you want the shortest route, take the easterly route out-and-back.

East Route

The trail traverses toward the drainage and parallels it for more than 0.5 mile. It then tracks west, away from the drainage and on to some broad switchbacks, breaking out of the thick tree cover and affording some nice views across the canyon. After the switchbacks the trail goes northeast and then descends gradually to the level area that borders the meadow; this is the intersection with the meadow route. For a direct route to the summit, take the trail northeast (bear right), rather than taking the west loop down to the meadow.

Great for Kids

The meadow is a good turnaround point for families with small children. The rest of the trail to the top is steep and rocky and requires scrambling and route-finding.

Grey Rock Mountain & Hewlett Gulch

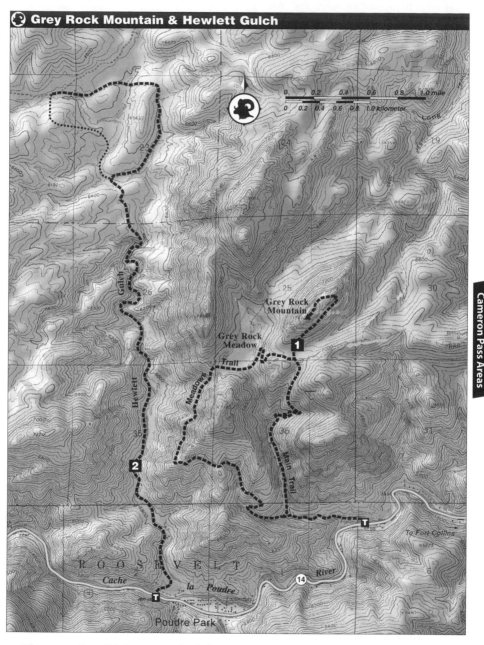

The summit trail is better marked than ever, but it is still deceptive and it can be easy to get off-trail and become lost. A small child was lost several years ago and never found. Keep your children and hiking partners in view at all times. The trail levels for a little while after the intersec- tion and then climbs through some steep sections. It traverses to the north for less than 0.5 mile and then takes sharp turns to the west and then south, as it switch- backs and requires some rock scrambling. There is more than one route through this section, but try to take the marked trail if possible. You eventually emerge on a rocky ridge with a view of a small pond that dries up during very hot and dry summers. The summit rock is visible to the southwest and requires another hour round-trip from this point unless you are fast and don't stop and enjoy the view.

West Route

The trail heads west and then northwest and follows an informal drainage as it steepens and emerges from the trees in about 0.5 mile. You enter sweeping switchbacks and reach a nice overlook for Hewlett Gulch. The switchbacks track north and east before leading you to a path that goes north, enters trees, narrows, and descends easterly toward the

meadow. When you reach the meadow, a great place for a picnic, you'll have a terrific view of the Grey Rock summit and the technical climbing routes to the top.

Whether you want to complete the loop or reach the summit, continue to the east as the trail climbs gently to the intersection of the east side trail. Turn right (south) to return to your starting point; go straight/left (north) to start the rocky summit climb. As described above, pick a route to the southwest around the water; then go west and find an easy scrambling route to the top. If you find the climb has become technical, you have strayed off course—no technical skills are needed for the final short scramble to the summit.

 Hewlett Gulch

$\overset{\text{see}}{\underset{\text{p. 35}}{\text{map on}}}$

Distance	6.0 miles, Semiloop
Difficulty	Easy
Elevation Gain	570 feet (starting at 5672 feet)
Trail Use	Mountain biking, horseback riding, leashed dogs OK
Agency	Canyon Lakes Ranger District, Roosevelt National Forest
Map	Trails Illustrated *Cache La Poudre & Big Thompson*

HIGHLIGHTS Just west of the Grey Rock Trail, this trail is a rewarding, easy canyon/arroyo hike or bike through pretty meadows and lofty ridges, in a rocky environment that climbs to some nice viewpoints. An optional loop climbs to the open high point and sweeping views. The steep and rocky section of the loop can be avoided by taking the out-and-back route on the east (right) side of the loop.

DIRECTIONS Take U.S. Highway 287 north from Fort Collins and exit west onto State Highway 14 at Ted's Place. Drive approximately 10.5 miles west on Highway 14 from Ted's Place. The parking area is elevated from the roadway and hard to miss across the river on the right (north) side of the highway.

The trail goes northerly from the parking lot, rolling and climbing gradually through the gulch. After less than 0.5 miles it descends and crosses the creek for the first of several crossings. Enjoy some tall cottonwoods, and after another 0.25 mile see the ridge tops and

cliffs soaring above. The stream is much deeper, but passable, during the spring, and dries up to a trickle as summer progresses. After approximately 1.5 miles, if you look carefully at the top of the ridge on the east, you can see one of the routes up to Grey Rock high above.

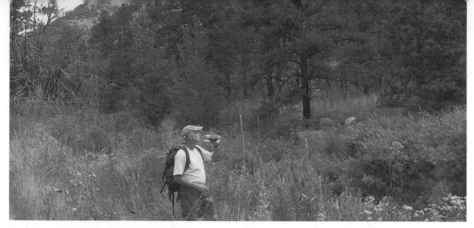
Hydrating on the Hewlett Gulch Trail

After wandering through the narrowing gulch, the trail opens up into a broad meadow area good for a picnic. Then it goes downhill to a trail intersection; bear right or plan to go straight uphill, very steeply on a very rocky, old four-wheel-drive road on the west side of the loop. Bear right for the east side of the loop and travel through a small arroyo with pretty rock formations with the generally dry streambed on the right. The trail winds and begins to climb in earnest over lots of rocks and through some trees. Then it goes much more steeply uphill, opens up considerably, and turns into a double-track trail. It tops out in a meadow area with a view of a rural subdivision to the north, an impressive rocky ridge to the east, and the jumbled canyon foothills to the south.

Turn around at any point along the way, especially if you have small children along or are not an expert mountain biker. In early spring this is a good trail for wildflowers and has lots of places for snack and water breaks. If you turn around after topping out, you can avoid the unpleasant plunge on the narrow rocky road though you will walk a bit farther on the return.

TRIP 3 Mount McConnel

Distance	4-plus miles, Loop
Difficulty	Easy to moderate, depending on distance you hike
Elevation Gain	1240 feet (starting at 6660)
Trail Use	Camping, leashed dogs OK
Agency	Canyon Lakes Ranger District, Roosevelt National Forest
Map	Trails Illustrated *Cache La Poudre & Big Thompson*
Note	Restrooms at trailhead

HIGHLIGHTS This is a short, relatively easy hike with spectacular views of the Poudre Canyon and distant peaks. Its location next to a campground and the river make a weekend river reverie tempting. The trail includes some steep sections.

DIRECTIONS Take U.S. Highway 287 north from Fort Collins and exit west onto State Highway 14 at Ted's Place. Take State Highway 14 approximately 5.5 miles west of Stove Prairie Road (County Road 27). Park where you see the sign for Mountain Home Campground on the left (south) side of the road.

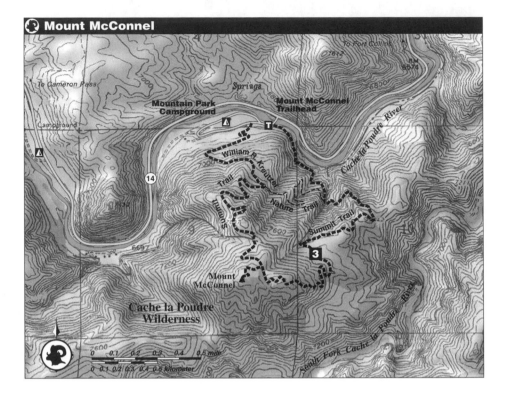

The trailhead is near the restrooms at the end of the parking lot loop road on the south side. The route described here includes the William R. Kreutzer Nature Trail, which can be used for shorter, easier excursions. The nature trail has many interpretive signs along the way. The steepest, sketchiest section of the main trail is the east side of the loop. If you don't have good soles on your boots or a good sense of balance, you might want to avoid it since parts of it are a slippery chute.

If you want to see all of the sites and avoid the steep sections, go out-and-back to the summit on the west side, return to the trailhead, and then take a short jaunt on the east side of the loop and turn around after you have seen the view and enjoyed a few informational nature trail signs. The west side loop is wide with frequent resting points and great views, one of which is a little more than 1 mile from the start. This is also a good turnaround point if you want to avoid steep climbing. The steep section is short and not that challenging and will take you just below the summit rocks. If you have a clear day, enjoy the distant Rawah Range peaks, as well as views of the canyon and river below. A side trail up to the summit is a very easy rock hop. The loop trail continues and plunges down the east side of the canyon slope, affording sweeping views of the canyon to the east. After you reach the summit, return to the trailhead the way you came, and enjoy a picnic lunch next to the whispering river.

TRIP 4 Lower Dadd Gulch

Distance	7.0 miles, Out-and-back
Difficulty	Easy to moderate, depending on distance you hike
Elevation Gain	1800 feet (starting at 7030 feet)
Trail Use	Mountain biking, horseback riding, leashed dogs OK
Agency	Canyon Lakes Ranger District, Roosevelt National Forest
Map	Trails Illustrated *Cache La Poudre & Big Thompson*
Note	Restrooms across the highway from the trailhead

HIGHLIGHTS This is a shady, delightful trail near Rustic that rolls and gently climbs its way through some uniquely beautiful foothills terrain, crossing several streams and weaving through ponderosa pines, tall cottonwood trees, lodgepole pines, and aspens. The top end of the trail opens up for some great views of the high foothills that would be a major mountain range in most other states. On the return, you will enjoy views of the rock outcrops that top the Poudre Canyon. The trail tops out on a ridge and Dadd Gulch Road comes up the other side from Crown Point Road. You can picnic next to the Poudre River after your hike is over and cool your heels.

DIRECTIONS Drive approximately 2 miles east of Rustic (1.5 miles west of the Indian Meadows Picnic Area) on State Highway 14. Parking areas are available on both sides of the road. The one on the right (north) side is next to a pretty mountain meadow and has restrooms.

The trailhead is on the left (south) side of State Highway 14. Pass through two livestock gates and travel gently uphill though nice shade. After the first stream crossing, the trail begins to climb more steeply and then opens up and widens with nice rocky views. After the third stream crossing, you will have hiked 0.5 mile. You'll likely hear birds singing and see violet columbine blooms if you visit in the spring or early summer as you cross the stream for the fourth and fifth times. Cross a small meadow under a tangle of power lines and see charred terrain from a fire that swept through the area high on the ridgeline above. In season, you'll likely see many butterflies at each of the eight stream crossings.

At approximately the 1.3-mile mark, bear right as the main trail separates from power lines, which follow a secondary trail, and you leave these signs of civilization behind. Enter an awesome

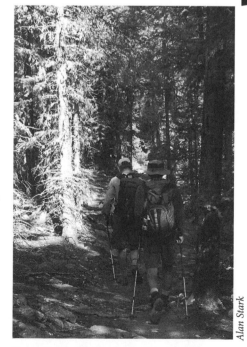

The author and a friend enjoy tree heaven.

Alan Stark

(margin tab) Poudre Canyon & Cameron Pass Areas

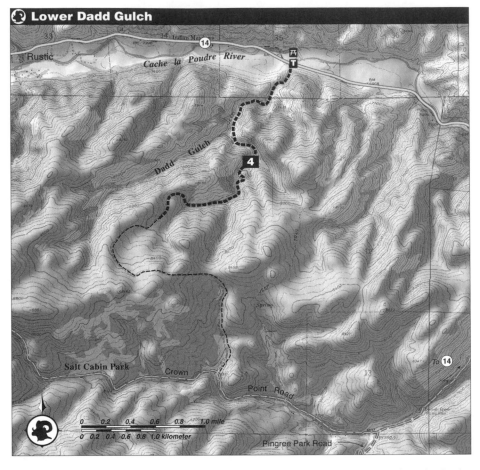

ponderosa pine forest and climb, noticing a small ridge on the right. If you want a nice view, detour off-trail and enjoy, but please avoid trampling, wildflowers; you'll see the distant mountain range to the west. The rest of the trail is a long traverse that ends at Dadd Gulch, which is open to motorized travel and accessible from Crown Point Road. (If you're looking for a challenging mountain bike route, try the round-trip from the trailhead to Crown Point Road.) Turn around, retrace your steps, and dip your toes in the Poudre River before you drive back down the canyon or visit Rustic for a snack.

TRIP 5 The Big South Trail

see
map on
p. 43

Distance	6.0 to 16.0 miles, Out-and-back
Difficulty	Easy to moderate
Elevation Gain	960 feet (starting at 8440 feet)
Trail Use	Camping, leashed dogs OK
Agency	Canyon Lakes Ranger District, Roosevelt National Forest
Map	Trails Illustrated *Poudre River & Cameron Pass*

HIGHLIGHTS The Big South is the sparkling south fork of the Cache la Poudre River that winds through a beautiful canyon as it rolls and tumbles and twists and turns its way down from its origin in Rocky Mountain National Park. The trailhead is where State Highway 14 and the river part company, so you can hike along the wild and scenic river in the Comanche Peak Wilderness in peace away from the highway. This is a rolling, gradually climbing trail offering the cascading river, a mixed conifer and aspen forest, and the experience of trekking up the ever-changing canyon until it vanishes into deep forest green. Sections of the trail are very rocky because it is skirts the edge of the compact arroyo, surrounded by richly stained colorful rock cliffs and rock falls. Three backcountry campsites a little more than 1 mile from the trailhead are nice for first-time backpacking experiences.

DIRECTIONS U.S. Highway 287 north from Fort Collins and exit west onto State Highway 14 at Ted's Place. Drive approximately 48 miles west and south on State Highway 14 from Ted's Place. The parking lot is on the left side of the road 1 mile past Poudre Falls.

Poudre Canyon & Cameron Pass Areas

The sparkling south fork of the Cache la Poudre River

Joe Grim

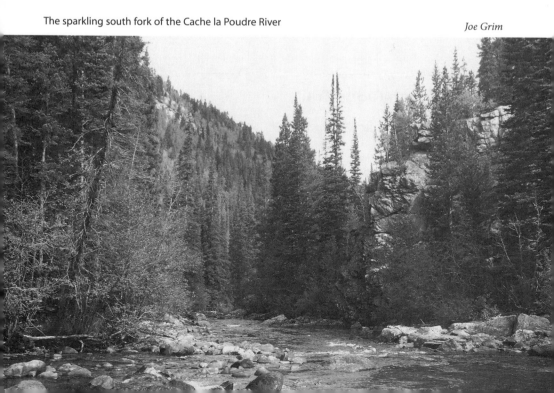

The trailhead is on the left or east side of the road just after the turnout for Poudre Falls. Poudre Falls can be very dramatic during the spring runoff or in early winter when portions of the waterfall freeze into unpredictable shapes and the sun glistens on the combination of ice and water. The Big South Trail offers a similar spring torrent and winter ice sculptures in its first 0.5 mile that often linger into early spring. The dazzling water is a treat in any season and is only a short stroll from the trailhead.

The beginning of the trail is very rocky because it skirts the edge of rockfalls and the narrowest section of the arroyo with small waterfalls and colorful rock outcrops. After 0.5 mile you enter the northeast corner of the Comanche Peak Wilderness; wilderness rules apply, which means biking is prohibited. The South Fork or Big South really isn't very big—more of a stream than a river but with a sweet melody. The trail stays on the east side of the river. It climbs slowly through the trees, over and around crumbling, picturesque rock walls, and quickly gains 100 feet. It then climbs a little more steeply over a narrow but short section of rocks that can be tricky early or late in the season if it's covered with snow or ice.

The trail drops down to the river for a nice flat stretch over the next mile that includes three backcountry campsites and then rolls back uphill through another rocky section. It breaks out of the trees for some great views of the soaring canyon foothills and then climbs another 100 feet to reach 8700 feet in elevation. It descends back to the river temporarily before traversing a large rockfall near 8800 feet in elevation.

At approximately 5 miles the canyon opens up and turns into a pleasing meadow that invites you to picnic. Relax and enjoy the view of the rock formations around you. In about another 2 miles you will see Flowers Road and a washed out footbridge. After this point choose when to turn around and retrace your steps. If you continue to the end of the marked route, the trail ends at the edge of the forest.

TRIP 6 Green Ridge Trail

Distance	200 yards to Lost Lake, 1.0 mile to Laramie Lake, 4.5 miles to North Twin Lakes, Out-and-back
Difficulty	Easy
Elevation Gain	497 feet (starting at 8993 feet)
Trail Use	Mountain biking, backpacking, fishing, motorized recreation, leashed dogs OK
Agency	Canyon Lakes Ranger District, Roosevelt National Forest
Map	Trails Illustrated *Poudre River & Cameron Pass*

HIGHLIGHTS This easy hike on a gradually climbing, rolling trail that accesses four lovely lakes—Lost, Laramie, and the Twin Lakes. Take in one, some, or all of them for a nice jaunt. The lakes are pretty, and there are nice views of the surrounding mountains from them. The trail is usually closed to vehicles until the Fourth of July; so use it early to avoid off-highway vehicles, but be prepared for some wet spots. Bring insect repellent for early season adventures.

The Big South & Green Ridge Trails

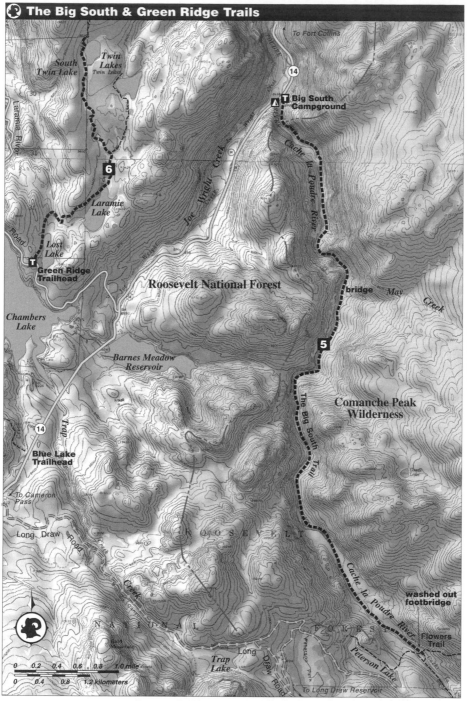

To Fort Collins

14

Big South Campground

South Twin Lake

Twin Lakes

Twin Lakes

Laramie River

6

Joe Wright Creek

Cache la Poudre River

Laramie Lake

Lost Lake

Green Ridge Trailhead

Road

Roosevelt National Forest

bridge *May*

Creek

5

Chambers Lake

Barnes Meadow Reservoir

Comanche Peak Wilderness

The Big South Trail

14

Trap

Blue Lake Trailhead

To Cameron Pass

Long Draw Road

ROOSEVELT

washed out footbridge

Creek

NATIONAL

Gan Mountain

FORES

Peterson Lake

Flowers Trail

Cache la Poudre River

Long Draw Road

Trap Lake

| 0 | 0.2 | 0.4 | 0.6 | 0.8 | 1.0 mile |
| 0 | 0.4 | 0.8 | 1.2 kilometers |

To Long Draw Reservoir

DIRECTIONS Take State Highway 14 approximately 50 miles west from Fort Collins. About 2.5 miles past the Big South Trailhead where the highway crosses the Poudre River, turn right (north) onto well-marked Laramie River Road. Closed in winter, this road goes by Chambers Lake Reservoir, is the access route for the Rawah Wilderness area and lakes, and continues all the way to Laramie, Wyoming, via Glendevey and Wood's Landing. Take Laramie River Road approximately 1.5 miles north to reach the trailhead on the right (east) side of the road at the Lost Lake parking lot. You are getting close when you crest the hill next to Chambers Lake. The trailhead is well marked, and the trail has alternating blue and orange U.S. Forest Service diamonds; the orange ones indicate that it can also be used for motorized recreation.

The Green Ridge Trail, which is sometimes used by off-highway vehicles, is found off of the Laramie River Road. The trail starts at Lost Lake and heads north through a thick lodgepole pine and fir forest along the lake's northwest shore for around 0.3 mile.

In 0.25 mile the trail forks with the primary four-wheel-drive road going

> **Great for Kids**
>
> If you're hiking with small children or are looking for a small adventure, explore the south and north shores of Lost Lake and call it a day. If you go just a bit farther, you can also see Laramie Lake.

straight (north) and the trail to the lakes going downhill to the right. Follow the orange and blue diamonds. Nice views of the Rawah Wilderness are your reward from the north access to Lost Lake where there is a small dam at around the 0.3-mile mark. Once you pass Lost Lake, the trail (former double-track four-wheel-drive road) meanders through thick trees as it tracks northeast. The trail rolls and climbs steadily and in another mile you can see part of Laramie Lake. Watch for a side trail down to the lake, which is virtually invisible from the trail. The side trail to the lake is unsigned.

From Laramie Lake it is another mile to South Twin Lake. The trail stays in the trees and heads north for 0.3 mile before taking the fainter side loop trail over to South Twin Lake. North Twin Lake is a bit farther and somewhat anticlimactic after visiting the larger lakes but offers its own brand of serenity. It is directly north from Laramie Lake, or you can take the loop to visit South Twin Lake and then return more directly.

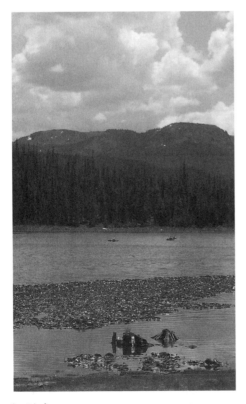

Lost Lake

TRIP 7 Sawmill Creek Trail to Clark Peak

Distance	3.0 to 10.0 miles, Out-and-back
Difficulty	Moderate to challenging, depending on distance and elevation gained
Elevation Gain	3500 feet (starting at 9480 feet)
Trail Use	Leashed dogs OK
Agency	Canyon Lakes Ranger District, Roosevelt National Forest
Map	Trails Illustrated *Poudre River & Cameron Pass*
Note	Restrooms at Meadows Trailhead

HIGHLIGHTS This relatively lightly used trail offers access to a high mountain panorama of the soaring peaks in the Rawah Range, including its monarch Clark Peak, with a short hike. Summiting Clark Peak is a challenging daytrip; it is more easily climbed from the west through the Colorado State Forest or from the end of the Blue Lake Trail (Trip 8), but this is one of the challenging routes for climbing it. Alternatively, the trail works for out-and-back trips of any length with enthralling views. The trail ends up in the Rawah Wilderness Area, with an endless network of former logging roads to explore and try to get lost on. At least one goes over the ridge to the Blue Lake Trail. The possibilities are endless for the addicted backcountry rambler with compass and topographic map or a GPS unit in hand who wants to go beyond the described route or off-trail.

DIRECTIONS Drive 60 miles on State Highway 14 west from Fort Collins to the Blue Lake parking area on the right or west side of the road, across from Long Draw Road. It is well marked but doesn't have any facilities. If you reach Zimmerman Lake before seeing Blue Lake, turn around because you missed it. Park in the lot for Blue Lake and walk 200 yards west on Highway 14; you will see the trailhead on the right (north) side of the road marked by a "road closed" gate. Do not park on the road or you might be ticketed or towed.

The trail, an old logging road, starts off in the trees for the first mile or so and gradually steepens. You can sometimes see a blue diamond marker up fairly high on the trees, directing you away from dead ends and incorrect old logging roads. (The markers may not be in place after a windy stretch of weather.) The trail turns sharply to the left (west) after the first 0.5 mile, which can be easy to miss since a faint logging road continues straight ahead as well. On this very sunny section of trail, you will warm up considerably. You can start to see nice views back to the southeast of the mountains and cliffs above Zimmerman Lake all the way to the dappled ridgeline of Comanche Peak and its surrounding

wilderness area. The trail then turns back to the Sawmill Creek drainage and travels primarily west-northwest.

After another mile of climbing, the trail levels somewhat and then goes slightly downhill to an intersection, which is a nice viewpoint for photos and a good place for a snack or lunch break. At this point the views of Clark Peak and its subpeak neighbors are nonstop and quite spectacular, but the wind can become a factor if it is a chilly early spring or fall day. If clouds are gathering on the summits, plan wisely for a retreat when you hear the first peal of thunder.

For the last 2 miles to the headwalls and steeper treks up toward Clark Peak, choose between the north or south routes

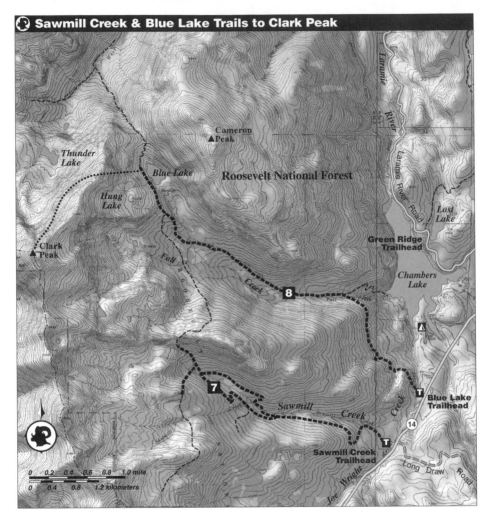

to reach the high mountain cirques. To journey beyond the end of these trails, you need good bushwhacking and route-finding skills; you will encounter multiple, sometimes confusing trails—a network of old logging roads that can suddenly disappear. If you keep traveling upslope to the southwest through the tall trees, you will eventually break through for a terrific sight. It is worth the extra effort to see the base of the Rawahs and the high bowls and peaks even if you don't plan to climb them. Either use a compass or carefully note the way back so you don't get lost. Aim for the drainage (downhill

to the east) if you get turned around, and you'll get back to the highway.

If you want to climb Clark Peak, you'll need more than one topographic map, a compass, and perhaps a GPS unit and the skills to use them. After the trails peter out, the terrain becomes extremely steep. Go north and west when in doubt and avoid climbing the dead-end ridges to the northeast as I did when I went with a friend. After going over a couple of ridges, you'll reach the cirque below the summit and follow the southwest ridge to the summit. Get a very early start to avoid thunderstorms, and plan on a very long, but rewarding day.

TRIP 8 Blue Lake Trail to Clark Peak

Distance	2.5 to 12.4 miles, Out-and-back
Difficulty	Easy to moderate/challenging, depending on distance hiked
Elevation Gain	1300 feet to Blue Lake, 3451 feet to Clark Peak (starting at 9500 feet)
Trail Use	Backpacking, leashed dogs OK
Agency	Canyon Lakes Ranger District, Roosevelt National Forest
Map	Trails Illustrated *Poudre River & Cameron Pass*

HIGHLIGHTS One of the most popular Cameron Pass area trails offers easy, short, round-trip excursions; a challenging all-day adventure; or a backpack trip to a pristine mountain lake surrounded by towering mountains. This trail offers almost everything—stately trees, pretty riparian areas, nice meadows, stream crossings, and a winding tree-covered path with striking views. It can be used for a relatively easy, 5-mile, out-and-back trip or moderate-to-difficult, 12.5-mile trip to the lake. Hiking all the way to the lake is an all-day adventure; don't attempt it if heavy weather is predicted unless you start early and are well prepared, or you may end up dodging lightning bolts. It is a popular overnight destination for backpackers but can also be a moderate to challenging and highly satisfying dayhike if you are fit. If you start at the crack of dawn, you can summit Clark Peak.

DIRECTIONS Drive 60 miles on State Highway 14 west from Fort Collins to the parking area on the right or west side of the road, across from Long Draw Road. It is well marked but doesn't have any facilities. If you reach the Zimmerman Lake trailhead before seeing Blue Lake, you missed it!

The trail starts at the edge of the parking lot and travels right (north) and then veers gradually to the northwest. It descends gradually for about 0.25 mile, quickly enveloping you in the beautiful forest, and then gradually climbs about 300 feet in the first mile after crossing the drainage. At a viewpoint a little more than 1 mile from the trailhead on the right side, you can see Chambers Lake and across the valley behind you.

The next 0.5 mile to the creek crossing is a gentle climb; you can see the Rawahs in the distance before you descend. After descending to a stream crossing, the trail climbs again, this time more steeply, reaching the wilderness boundary in short order in less than 0.5 mile. The trail rolls quite a bit for most of the trip to the lake, but after crossing Fall Creek and viewing a nice

---

Great for Kids

The first big viewpoint is a good turn-around point for small children. You might also consider continuing on the gentle climb to the creek crossing to enjoy a great view of the Rawah Mountains in the distance.

---

meadow area, it climbs steadily to almost 11,000 feet. The last 0.5 mile is an almost 200-foot descent to the lake that you will want to save energy for on the return trip. The sparkling lake is in a magnificent setting among some of the highest peaks of the Rawah Range, including its monarch, 12,951-foot Clark Peak and 12,127-foot Cameron Peak. The summits are obscured by the steep shoulders of the mountains that surround the lake.

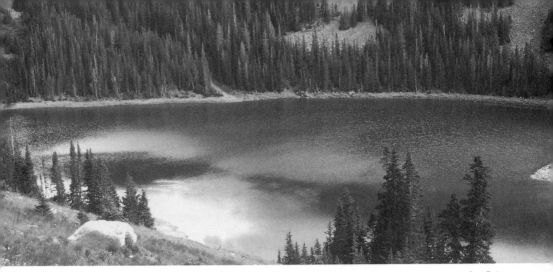

Blue Lake

Joe Grim

Clark Peak via Blue Lake

You can summit Clark Peak from Blue Lake if you are very ambitious and start at the trailhead at dawn. It's easier to ascend the east slope of Clark Peak than the west slope from the Sawmill Creek route, but the former is also difficult because of the longer distance to Blue Lake. It is a great backpack and nontechnical climbing opportunity if you have the time. If you don't, prepare yourself for a long, challenging trek; start at dawn and expect to have an 8- to 12-hour day, depending on your fitness level, pace, and route-finding skills. Once you reach the lake, continue north and mount the ridge, or steep hill, to the northwest. From there take a sharp left (south) and proceed southwest up very steep slopes to the summit and its commanding 360-degree view.

TRIP 9 Trap Park Trail to Iron Mountain

Distance	4.5 miles to end of Trap Park, 5.6 miles to Iron Mountain, Out-and-back
Difficulty	Moderate to challenging
Elevation Gain	1300 feet to Trap Park, 2743 to Iron Mountain (starting at 9522 feet)
Trail Use	Fishing, leashed dogs OK
Agency	Canyon Lakes Ranger District, Roosevelt National Forest
Map	Trails Illustrated *Poudre River & Cameron Pass*

HIGHLIGHTS This is a spectacular but little-known area off of Long Draw Road. The trail edges uphill through a beautiful riparian area following the Trap Creek drainage on a narrow trail. Peterson Lake is a possible side trail destination popular with fisherman. The park is a draw, or small canyon, and offers interesting, varied scenery and a rolling trail that climbs gently. After 1 mile, you reach the wide open, impressive "park" framed by a pretty mixed forest that opens into a series of high tundralike meadows, topping out with a great view of the mountains. You can hike all the way to the top of Iron Mountain

Trap Park Trail to Iron Mountain

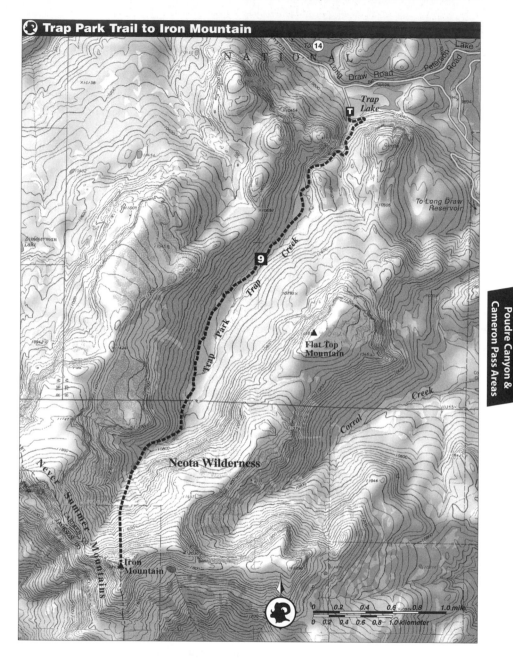

at the highest point. Be sure to wear bright colors in hunting season because the area is popular with hunters.

DIRECTIONS Take Highway 14 about 52 miles to Long Draw Road. The quickest access is to follow Long Draw Rd. Turn left and drive 2.7 miles until you see the turnoff to the Trap Park parking area on the right.

From the parking area, the trail goes west 0.25 mile to a fork where the Peterson Lake Trail goes left (south). Some informal game trails through the trees on the left meander to the lake. Please stay on the primary trails to avoid resource damage and help to preserve the semipristine environment. Like most of the canyon, this area is popular with hunters, especially during the elk and deer seasons, so be sure to wear bright colors. After approximately 200 yards, the Peterson Lake Trail is visible on the left and the Trap Park Trail switchbacks somewhat steeply up a rocky hillside that offers a nice photo opportunity and view of the lake. The trail then climbs more slightly above Trap Creek toward the open park area.

When you crest the top of the small arroyo that frames the creek, the park opens up with a magnificent view of the mountain ridgeline with Iron Mountain, on the north edge of the Never Summer Range, providing the dominant view to the southwest.

After a snack and water break, continue across the park to the 1.5-mile point, where a shortcut joins the main trail. From here, either descend to and follow a trail near the creek or stay high to climb the north-facing ridge for another mile to enjoy another natural spectacle. Climbing the slope southwest to the top of the ridge is a rewarding but challenging adventure, but don't proceed if thunderstorm clouds are looming. From the top of the pass, climb southeast to the top of Iron Mountain for spectacular views of the Rawahs and Michigan Reservoir. There is no trail on Iron Mountain, so route-finding skills are required.

Great for Kids

The top of this arroyo is a great place for a picnic and a turnaround spot for small children. You can see Iron Mountain and the beautiful park stretching out before you. There is a game trail across the drainage, which ends abruptly.

TRIP 10 Zimmerman Lake Trail

Distance	2.2 to 3.0 miles, Semiloop or Out-and-back
Difficulty	Easy
Elevation Gain	476 feet (starting at 10,019 feet)
Trail Use	Fishing, option for kids, leashed dogs OK
Agency	Canyon Lakes Ranger District, Roosevelt National Forest
Map	Trails Illustrated *Poudre River & Cameron Pass*
Facilities	Restrooms at trailhead

HIGHLIGHTS This is a short and steady climb to a small lake with great views of the surrounding remnants of the Never Summer Mountains. It is a very popular trail so expect company, but crowds thin out quickly when you reach the lake. The Rawah Wilderness and Never Summer Mountains that form the northwest border of Rocky Mountain National Park surround the lake. This can be the beginning of a mostly downhill car shuttle loop with the Meadows Trail. There is also a loop trail around the lake that features lots of trees and can be used to extend the short hike to the lake.

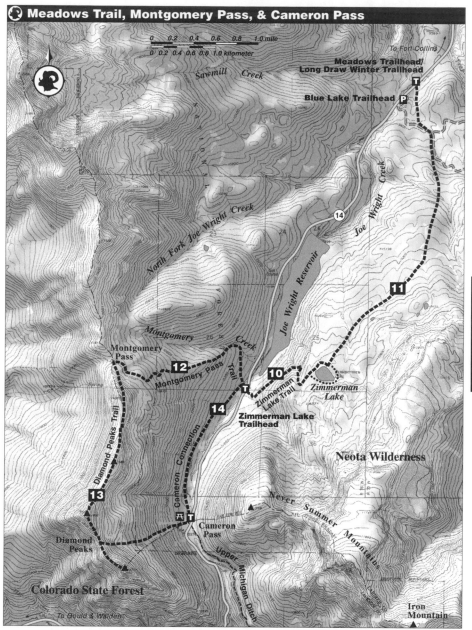

Meadows Trail, Montgomery Pass, & Cameron Pass

DIRECTIONS Take State Highway 14 west from Fort Collins for 58 miles, and park in the large parking lot, with restroom facilities, on the east (left) side of the road a few miles before reaching Cameron Pass, approximately 63 miles from Fort Collins. Highway 14 generally travels east-west when it first enters the Poudre Canyon and then dips dramatically to the southwest at Kinikinik. By the time you stop for the Zimmerman Lake Trailhead, the road is actually more north-south than east-west.

The parking lot is usually almost full, and the trail can initially be busy. You can achieve off-trail solitude once you reach the lake. The trail goes southeast (right) out of the parking lot and then immediately east (left) into tall pine trees. It climbs gently for about 200 yards and then gradually steepens and narrows into switchbacks. The trail climbs almost 400 feet over the next 0.75 mile before exiting the trees and leveling somewhat next to a very nice, tree-rimmed meadow. The trail widens on the right edge of the meadow. You will see an expansive view of the Rawahs to the east from the top of the meadow. At this point, you'll also need to decide whether you want a longer jaunt to the lake or not because you've reached the intersection for the loop trail.

If you do, bear right (straight) and take the tree-lined loop to the far side of Zimmerman Lake. Otherwise, bear left for the main trail that climbs and then levels as it goes north back into the trees. In another 0.25 mile you will reach the west edge of the lake. Either stay on the trail to reach the northeast edge of the lake or climb a short hill to the right to the lake's surface. You can extend your hike on paths around the north (left) or south (right) edges of the lake.

Bushwhacking to the top of the ridgeline of Iron Mountain to the south is fun

> ### Great for Kids
> The lake is a nice half-day activity for families with small children that can be extended with trails that lead north or east from the lake. Families with small children usually find making it to the lake enough fun and exercise for a day. Circumnavigating the lake, however, is an easy addition.

if you have good route-finding skills and like steep, challenging ascents. You can also survey the great scenery at the lake, have a snack, and reverse course if you've had enough. The trail continues north and then reaches a fork, where an easterly trail (right) heads to the north end of the lake and the northbound trail (straight or left) goes down to the Long Draw Reservoir Road via the Meadows Trail. You can circle the lake in either direction late in the season, but you'll encounter bogs early in the season. To access more loop trails, take the almost flat right fork. Once you reach the northeast corner of the lake, you can bushwhack your way from there into the hills and onto the ridgeline above the lake if you have good mountaineering and route-finding skills and use a map and compass and perhaps a GPS unit.

The Never Summer Range provides the backdrop for Zimmerman Lake.   *Joe Grim*

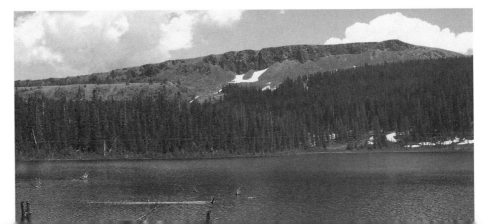

TRIP 11 Meadows Trail

see map on p. 51

Distance	10.0 miles, Out-and-back
Difficulty	Moderate
Elevation Gain/Loss	1296 feet from Meadows Trailhead (starting at 9200 feet), 1296 feet from Zimmerman Lake (starting at 10,490 feet)
Trail Use	Option for kids, dogs must be leashed in wilderness areas and under voice control on the rest of the trail
Agency	Canyon Lakes Ranger District, Roosevelt National Forest
Map	Trails Illustrated *Poudre River & Cameron Pass*
Facilities	Restrooms at Meadows and Zimmerman Lake Trailhead
Notes	Biking is prohibited because it's a wilderness area.

HIGHLIGHTS This trail winds through a superb old-growth forest of tall, stately fir and spruce trees. If you'd like a shorter trip, you can park a car shuttle at Zimmerman Lake Trailhead. If you start at Zimmerman Lake instead of at Meadows Trailhead, it is mostly downhill. It's a satisfying out-and-back from either end with nice viewpoints and picnic possibilities along the way. Visit in midsummer (after midsummer the wetlands have dried out). The trail enters the Neota Wilderness about halfway to Zimmerman Lake; from that point on you can follow the markers for the cross-country ski/snowshoe trail.

DIRECTIONS Take State Highway 14 approximately 60 miles west from Fort Collins to the parking area on the left side of the road, across from Long Draw Road. Poorly marked, it is just before you reach Long Draw Road and the Blue Lake parking lot on the right.

If you want a major all-day adventure and challenging workout, try the Meadows Trail up to Zimmerman Lake and back. For a calmer adventure, leave a car at Long Draw Reservoir Road or Meadows Trailhead and follow the Meadows Trail from the northwest side of the Zimmerman Lake loop. Look for red wooden arrows that mark the trail. From the Meadows Trailhead, go north to Long Draw Road, which will seem like it is east. A rolling trail with some moderate climbs and descents that is generally downhill from Zimmerman Lake, Meadows Trail requires at least a half-day commitment one-way or a full day for the round-trip, so you need an early start to make the trek without thunderstorms. The delightful trail winds through the stately spruce and fir trees of a dense forest and then opens up into several namesake meadows, and initially crests a ridgeline with great views

of the Rawahs as it winds through part of the Neota Wilderness.

When the wetlands have dried out for the year, you can park in the Meadows lot, southeast of the Blue Lake lot. The walk from the parking area adds about 0.5 mile to the hike but is a very pretty, winding section of trail with a small brook that eventually retreats into its banks, after inundating the trail during spring runoff.

When the wetlands are not dried out, it's easier to park on Long Draw Road about 0.25 mile from the Meadows Trailhead and hike from there. The trail is located on the right (northwest) side of the road on an uphill. You will see a white No OHVs sign on the right side of the road where the trail, actually a wide, former logging road, begins. After 100 yards it splits; take the right fork. The trail climbs gradually and then more

---

Great for Kids

The nice viewpoint after the wilderness boundary is a good family turnaround point since you won't see any great views again for some time, until you reach the first of the meadows; a very short 0.5 mile ahead, beyond the fork in the trail. Though the trail itself is a great place for communion with the magnificent old-growth trees, when you reenter the thick tree cover the trail levels and rolls gently to some nice picnic spots, before it gets steeper.

---

steeply uphill to the northwest through a tree tunnel. When it levels temporarily, a break in the trees allows you a great view of the Rawahs to the north and west. The trail bears left (south) past a meadow and then continues to climb, turning right (north) next to a large rock and then steepening. The trail continues to climb for the next 0.5 mile, and then levels again, goes downhill, reaches the wilderness boundary, and then switchbacks more steeply to the top of a small ridge where you get another nice view. It stays fairly level for the next 0.25 mile before starting to climb again.

When you reach another fork, look carefully for the brown marker with a black arrow, telling you to turn sharply right (north) to stay on the trail. It reenters thick trees and after about 100 yards winds through the trees, reaches a small meadow—a chief characteristic of this

trail and very suitable for a picnic—and then climbs again in earnest. It is still approximately 3.5 miles to Zimmerman Lake.

You climb through several switchbacks; it is very easy to lose the trail in this section unless you watch carefully for the light brown wood signs with black arrows that appear every 200 yards or less. After the sets of switchbacks, you reach an oblong hump where the trail turns sharply left and goes around a small hill. Be careful to avoid the false trail straight ahead. You will shortly see another arrow pointing the way. The trail then winds downhill to the first meadow where it exits the trees and travels along the left (south) edge of the meadow. The trail reenters the thick tree cover at the other end of the meadow; watch carefully for the break in the trees where it reenters and starts to climb again. Though it is easy to lose the trail, if you watch carefully you will see that it is one of the best signed trails in the area.

The trail wanders through more turns, passes a small meadow, and climbs again. It descends to the second meadow and exits the trees again, following the left edge of the forest until it reenters and starts to climb again about 100 yards at the end of the second submeadow. Do not continue straight up the middle of the top of the meadow. As you enter the trees, the trail continues its serpentine swivel through and then down to the third meadow.

The Zimmerman Lake loop is also excellent for snowshoeing and skiing.
Joe Grim

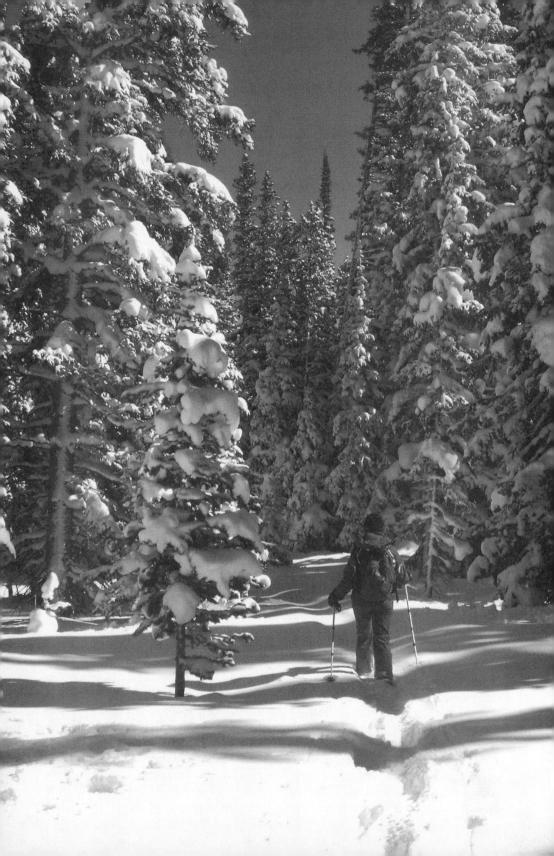

TRIP **12** Montgomery Pass

see map on p. 51

Distance	3.5 miles, Out-and-back
Difficulty	Moderate-plus
Elevation Gain	1000 feet (starting at 10,000 feet)
Trail Use	Leashed dogs OK
Agency	Canyon Lakes Ranger District, Roosevelt National Forest
Map	Trails Illustrated *Poudre River & Cameron Pass*
Facilities	Restrooms at Zimmerman Lake parking lot

HIGHLIGHTS The magnificent view from the top of the pass includes North Park, Clark Peak, the distant Zirkel Range, and the approach to Diamond Peaks, as well as the northern reaches of Rocky Mountain National Park. It is worth the steep, but short 1000-foot climb to the pass. You can descend the pass into the Colorado State Forest if you arrange a car shuttle or want a challenging out-and-back adventure, or once you have surmounted the pass, you can walk west into the ski bowls and enjoy a great view of the Nokhu Crags, Ute and Mahler Peaks, and Thunder Pass. Feel free to take a spectacular roller-coaster hike to the top of the Diamond Peaks if you have the time and energy in the summer; you don't have to worry about the avalanches that can make the peaks treacherous in the winter. The pass can also be climbed from the west side through Colorado State Forest; check for details at the Moose Visitors Center. Unfortunately, the west side access also allows off-road, motorized vehicles that share the good hiking and biking route to the top.

DIRECTIONS Take State Highway 14 west from Fort Collins for 58 miles to the Zimmerman Lake-Montgomery Pass Trailhead parking lot. Across from the Zimmerman Lake Trailhead, the trail is well marked but not easily visible from the road; it can be spotted in the trees down the road to the right from the Zimmerman Lake parking lot.

This intermediate trail gains 1000 feet of elevation in the almost 2 miles it takes to reach the pass. You'll have to wait until early July to enjoy it, unless you like sloshing through icy water and mud, which isn't a good idea anyway because it causes severe trail erosion.

The trail starts out climbing west gradually and then gets steeper quickly through thick tree cover, paralleling the Montgomery Creek drainage. It tracks to the left or slightly northwest after 0.25 mile. After another 0.25 mile you can momentarily relax before it gets steeper again in 100 yards. It essentially rolls steeply uphill—expect 200 feet of climbing per 0.25 mile with easy and difficult stretches. Because of its elevation change,

the trail isn't for the poorly conditioned. After approximately 1 mile you will come to a fork. The left takes you straight up to the bowls popular with skiers and snowboarders in winter, while the right takes you temporarily downhill and then gradually to the actual pass. The views from the bowls are just as good as or better than the pass and not to be missed.

Following the trail to the pass, you encounter broad switchbacks around 10,700 feet and see a meadow off to the left (south). The next 200 feet to the top of the pass takes you out of the trees and affords spectacular views in all directions—Zimmerman Lake and Joe Wright Reservoirs to the east and north; the Rawah range and its monarch, Clark

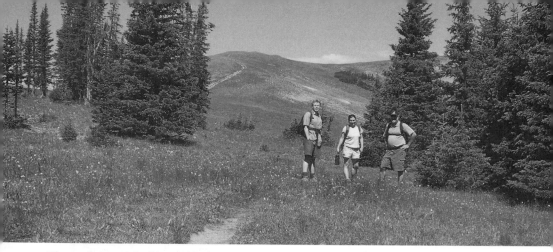

Hikers trek toward the Diamond Peaks.

Peak to the northwest; and the cliffs and Nokhu Crags in the Never Summer Range of Routt National Forest to the southwest. It is usually fairly breezy on top year-round, so be prepared for a distinct temperature drop. Sunglasses or even goggles and a hat, cap, or hooded jacket are often necessary to hang onto your hair, and afternoon thunderstorms are always an issue during the summer climbing season. The worst you can face is an uncommon horizontal hurricane-force hailstorm.

From the top of the pass, you can climb to the top of the ridgeline to the left (southwest) and the Diamond Peaks or continue down the other side on a very steep four-wheel-drive road toward the Michigan Reservoir in the Colorado State Forest. Otherwise, have a snack and drink and enjoy your return trip down the trail.

TRIP 13 Diamond Peaks

see map on p. 51

Distance	4.0 miles, Out-and-back and point-to-point options
Difficulty	Moderate-plus
Elevation Gain	1505 feet (starting at 10,276 feet)
Trail Use	Leashed dogs OK
Agency	Canyon Lakes Ranger District, Roosevelt National Forest
Map	Trails Illustrated *Poudre River & Cameron Pass*
Facilities	Restrooms at the parking lots for Zimmerman Lake and Montgomery Pass, as well as Cameron Pass

HIGHLIGHTS The Diamonds are prominent peaks on Cameron Pass with summits offering panoramic views of everything from North Park to the Never Summer Range. They can be climbed in a long, scenic traverse from Montgomery Pass or a more direct ascent from Cameron Pass. Summer and fall are much safer times to savor their summits since avalanches frequently scour their summits in the winter.

DIRECTIONS Take State Highway 14 west from Fort Collins for 63 miles to the Zimmerman Lake parking lot. The Montgomery Pass Trailhead is across from the east end of the Zimmerman parking lot. Well marked but not easily visible from the road, it can be spotted in the trees down the road to the left from the Zimmerman Lake parking lot. Alternatively, drive to the summit of Cameron Pass and park in the lot on the north side of the road.

From Montgomery Pass

Follow the directions to Montgomery Pass in Trip 12. From the summit of Montgomery Pass turn west and traverse on the right (northwest) side of the ridge. Stay below the top of the ridge to the right since it undulates and you would have to do more up and down climbing if you hiked across the top. The traverse on the north (right) side of the ridge is somewhat vertical tundra and there is no trail to speak of. After rounding the ridge, aim for a saddle between the high point of the traversed ridge and the bottom of the peaks. An alternate, but slower route with a faint trail is to go around the south (left) side of the ridge to the winter ski bowls and traverse much lower into the informal trail that then climbs up to the saddle. This route also rolls and descends as it approaches the peaks, making for more altitude to regain.

Once you reach the saddle just pick a route to the top of the first peak and create your own switchbacks to the top. Avoid hiking single file, preserving the tundra, and enjoy the wildflowers and nonstop views. You can return the way you came or go down and back to Montgomery Pass via the Cameron Pass and Cameron Connection trails.

Cameron Pass Route

You can do a car shuttle by going up Montgomery Pass and down to Cameron or vice versa, or just go round-trip from Cameron Pass. This is a shorter and more direct route than the Montgomery Pass route. More direct also means much steeper as in, short, sweet, and steep.

The trail begins at the back of the Cameron Pass parking lot. Bear left through the trees and generally follow the drainage. The trail is faint, and good bushwhacking skills are required. Once you are on top of the wettest part of the drainage, start climbing somewhat to the left (west). You will have to navigate through some marshy tundra if it is early in the season. Later in the summer it dries out. You will know if you are on track because veering too far to either the right or left takes you into the creek or onto terrain that is too steep. Once you are 1 mile from the trailhead and well above the drainage, it is easier to track toward the saddle that is more off to the right (northwest)—the direct route to the left (west-southwest) is very steep with a clump of trees. You don't have to veer very far northwest to hit the closest part of the saddle, and then you climb the peaks.

View from the top of North Diamond Peak

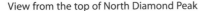

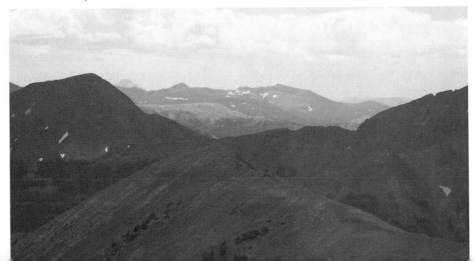

TRIP 14 Cameron Connection

see map on p. 51

Distance	3.0 miles, Out-and-back
Difficulty	Easy
Elevation Gain	200 feet (starting at 10,000 feet)
Trail Use	Leashed dogs OK
Agency	Canyon Lakes Ranger District, Roosevelt National Forest
Map	Trails Illustrated *Poudre River & Cameron Pass*
Facilities	Restrooms at Zimmerman Lake Trailhead and the top of Cameron Pass

HIGHLIGHTS This is a short, surprisingly scenic trail through an old-growth forest of spruce and fir. It shares its trailhead with the Montgomery Pass Trail and is often overlooked. It offers excellent shelter from prevailing winds and, though it parallels the highway, is far enough away to be completely buffered from its sound or sight. This trail is available only in the late summer and early fall because it crosses many streams and wetlands that don't dry out until the end of the summer hiking season.

DIRECTIONS Drive 58 miles on State Highway 14 from Fort Collins to reach the Zimmerman Lake parking lot on the left (east/south) side of the road. You can park here or 1 mile farther down the highway on the right (west/north) side of the road in the Cameron Pass parking lot.

This short scenic trail shares one of its trailheads with the Montgomery Pass Trail. From there it journeys southwest to the summit of Cameron Pass, paralleling Highway 14, but far enough from the highway to eliminate auto noise. It also features beautiful spruce and fir trees and three nice meadows with views near the pass. It is sheltered by trees most of the way to protect trail users on windy days. It climbs slowly and rolls gently making it a good trail for beginners. Turn left (west/south) at the Montgomery Pass Trailhead.

If you start at the Cameron Pass parking lot, the trail goes downhill at first and then uphill on your return at the end. Blue diamonds mark the trailhead and most of the trail, if they haven't been removed by weather, on the east (north) side of the Cameron Pass Parking area.

Cameron Pass

Just driving over Cameron Pass is a treat because you get to enjoy several

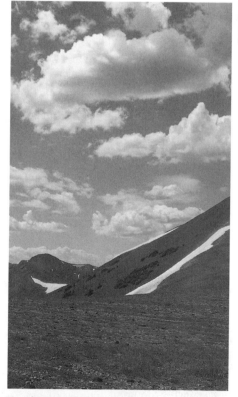

View from the Diamond Peaks

peaks on the northern border of Rocky Mountain National Park. First you are greeted by the rugged splendor of the Nokhu Crags, with their rooster top rocks. You see Mount Richtofen peering over the Crags shoulder, and daring you to try its scree slopes on another day. Then you see the tail end of the Never Summer Range, Seven Utes, Mahler Mountain, and the Diamond Peaks. The summit of State Highway 14 at 10,200 feet is one of the most popular destinations for hikers and bikers. You might also encounter some overlap with off-highway vehicles approaching from the Lake Agnes or Colorado State Forest area when you take the Michigan Ditch Trail. From the parking lot you can also bushwhack northwest up the Diamond Peaks after the snow is gone when there is no avalanche danger.

TRIP 15 Brown's Lake

Distance	8 miles, Out-and-back
Difficulty	Moderate
Elevation Gain	1500 feet (starting at 10,500 feet)
Trail Use	Leashed dogs OK
Agency	Canyon Lakes Ranger District, Roosevelt National Forest
Map	Trails Illustrated *Poudre River & Cameron Pass*

HIGHLIGHTS This beautiful rolling route has dramatic views of the Rawahs and Never Summer Mountains before it reaches two pristine mountain lakes surrounded by the rocky cliffs of a glacier-carved cirque.

DIRECTIONS Take U.S. Highway 287 north to State Highway 14. Then drive 26 miles west from Ted's Place to the Pingree Park Road. Drive 4 miles south; turn right (west) for Crown Point Road. Drive 12 miles to the Brown's Lake Trailhead; the parking area is on the right (north) side of the road and the trailhead on the left (south).

The Brown's Lake Trail goes gradually uphill from the trailhead and weaves through the trees. After around 0.25 mile it steepens considerably. After 200 feet of elevation gain, it gets much rockier and climbs approximately 500 feet more over 1 mile to almost the height of 11,462 foot Crown Point that is next to the trail. You will have great panoramic views from this point onward. Hike up to the left (east) toward the small rocky summit and find a nice spot to enjoy the view and declare victory.

Continuing toward Timberline Lake, the trail veers downhill to the right (west),

Great for Kids

If you have small children, the rocky summit near Crown Point is a good turnaround point after you enjoy a picnic spot. That gives you a 360-degree spectacular view, without the rest of the roller-coaster hike to the lake. The downside is that you don't see the lake.

crosses a valley, and then climbs another long hill ahead, regaining the 150 feet it lost and a bit more to reach the top of the next ridge at 11,400 feet. From there the trail descends again and doubles back on

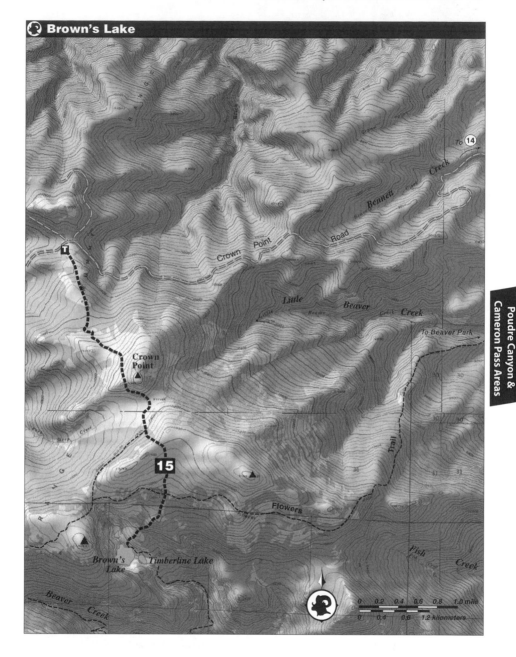

Brown's Lake

itself as it switchbacks through the trees. If you look carefully, you will glimpse the cliffs above the lakes. The long switchbacks take you down 200 feet to a high point overlooking the two small adjoining large lakes that make up this body of water captured in the cirque. From this point, continue your descent another 600 feet to the lakeshore at 10,600 feet. Timberline Lake is the smaller of the two adjoining lakes; Brown's Lake is the larger one.

TRIP 16 Mineral Springs Gulch to Prospect Mountain

Distance	4.0 miles, Out-and-back
Difficulty	Easy
Elevation Gain	500 feet (starting at 9300 feet)
Trail Use	Great for kids, leashed dogs OK
Agency	Canyon Lakes Ranger District, Roosevelt National Forest
Map	Trails Illustrated *Poudre River & Cameron Pass*

HIGHLIGHTS This pretty woodland meadow has beautiful aspen and pine trees and nice views of Poudre Canyon and the distant Rawah and Medicine Bow Mountains from the top of Prospect Mountain. A low-key adventure, it is a short, easy jaunt and could include a picnic on the summit.

DIRECTIONS Take U.S. Highway 287 north to State Highway 14. Then drive 26 miles west from Ted's Place to Pingree Park Road. Drive 4 miles south; turn right (west) for Crown Point Road. Approximately 4.5 miles from Pingree Park Road on the right (north) side of the road, the access road is after the two turnoffs for Salt Cabin Park.

Take the closed road uphill and ignore the first side road with a locked gate that you come to at around 0.25 mile. Stay to the left and eventually crest the hill after a little less than 1 mile. The trail meanders downhill through the trees. At the bottom of the hill, you reach the foot of a pretty meadow with the top of Prospect Mountain and the ridgeline visible to the right (north). Go left (west) and look for a faint road or trail on the right that heads to the top of the mountain at around 1.5 miles. The trail is in thick trees at the outset but breaks out into nice southern exposure on the 0.5-mile gradual uphill trek to the top. As you near the top, you see great views of the plains to the east and the top of Poudre Canyon to the north. The top affords nice views of the Rawah and Mummy Ranges to the west.

TRIP 17 Fish Creek & Little Beaver Creek Trails

Distance	4.0 to 10.0 miles, Out-and-back and semiloop options
Difficulty	Easy to moderate
Elevation Gain	600 feet (starting at 8012 feet)
Trail Use	Horseback riding, leashed dogs OK
Agency	Canyon Lakes Ranger District, Roosevelt National Forest
Map	Trails Illustrated *Poudre River & Cameron Pass*
Note	Biking is prohibited because this trail is in a wilderness area.

HIGHLIGHTS These lightly used trails are graced by the beauty of the Comanche Peak Wilderness towering magically above with the often snow-capped peak it's named for highlighting the view. This trail requires some route-finding because it is not well marked. It rolls up and over a large hill and then descends into the glade on the other side with

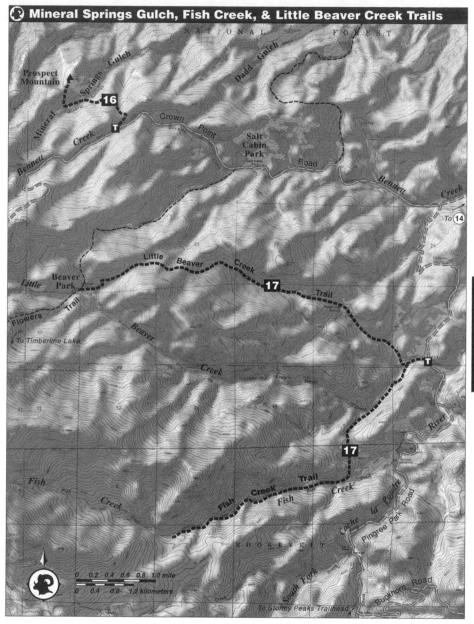

Mineral Springs Gulch, Fish Creek, & Little Beaver Creek Trails

nice peekaboo views along the way. You can choose from two very different options if you want to hike to the end of one of the trails.

DIRECTIONS Take U.S. Highway 287 north to State Highway 14. Then drive 26 miles west from Ted's Place to the Pingree Park Road. Take Pingree Park Road 8 miles from its intersection with State Highway 14 to the trailhead. Pass Crown Point Road and the Jack Gulch Campground. The well-marked trailhead is on the right (west) well beyond the campground. Cross the cattle guard and park near the largest trailhead sign, making sure you don't block the cattle guard gate. To get to the trailhead, walk back through the cattle

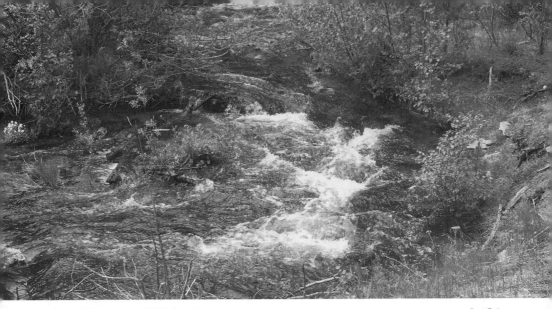

The frolicking water of Fish Creek   *Joe Grim*

guard and look for a mileage marker sign to the right of the fence that indicates that the Comanche Peak Wilderness is 1 mile and the Beaver Creek intersection is 2 miles. The trail goes up the hill to the left at a sharp angle.

This double trailhead starts off as Fish Creek Trail and then intersects Beaver Creek Trail. Both trails go into the Comanche Peak Wilderness Area. According to the trailhead U.S. Forest Service sign they intersect and part company after 2 miles. According to the map, however, they intersect and part company only 1.5 miles or so from the trailhead, which seems more accurate.

Choose between two options: the Little Beaver Creek Trail to Beaver Park where it intersects with Flowers Road or the Fish Creek Trail that ends at the Beaver Creek Trailhead on Beaver Road near Hourglass Reservoir. The trail is faint. If you keep in mind that it goes west and then northwest and that you should end up on top of the ridge to your right, it doesn't matter if you lose the trail. You will see a great view of Fall Mountain (12,258 feet), Comanche Peak (12,702 feet), and other mountains in the Mummy Range after 0.5 mile or less. Keep the drainage and peaks on your left

and make your way slowly to the top of the ridge watching for tree blazes (where bark has been removed). The ridgeline levels out around 8400 feet for a much more gradual climb. Then you enter the wilderness and turn right (north) and eventually go back to the west.

Stay on top of the ridge and you are en route; enjoy the thick lodgepole pine and spruce forest. You come to a power pole and telephone line for Pingree Park at around 8600 feet—not typical wilderness landmarks. As the trail swings back

---

Great for Kids

Since you have easily exceeded 1 mile when you reach 8600 feet and see the views of the Comanche Peak and the Mummies, you might want a break. Also, this is the last sunny viewpoint for awhile; the trail goes downhill about 0.25 mile to the intersection with the Little Beaver Creek Trail.

around to the west, you can see Coman-che Peak and the Mummies.

If you want a nice, short excursion, turn around there and retrace your route. Except for climbing back up the last hill, it's downhill to the trailhead. If you choose to go farther, the Fish Creek branch offers better views over the next mile or two. The Little Beaver Creek Trail stays in the trees for the most part and offers views of the heavily forested valley, while Fish Creek continues to have good views of the Comanche Peak summits.

TRIP 18 Signal Mountain Trail

Distance	Up to 10.0 miles, Out-and-back
Difficulty	Moderate-plus
Elevation Gain	2700 feet (starting at 8560 feet)
Trail Use	Fishing, backpacking, leashed dogs OK
Agency	Canyon Lakes Ranger District, Roosevelt National Forest
Map	Trails Illustrated *Poudre River & Cameron Pass*

HIGHLIGHTS This little used trail offers protection from winds and heat and a tour of a magical river arroyo. It starts off gently following the enchanting streambed for 2 miles. Signal Mountain is a steep climb from there as you accomplish most of the gain in the last 3 miles and climb above treeline and on to the tundra to enjoy the spectacular view. It offers a trip through a beautiful riparian area that features a mixed old-growth forest of aspen, pine, fir, and spruce and striking rock outcrops. It makes a nice any length out-and-back trip; climbing Signal Mountain, however, would be a serious all-day adventure.

Another access to Signal Mountain, via the Bulwark Ridge, is at the North Fork/Dun-raven Trailhead parking lot. It is 4 steep miles one-way to the summit on a ridge of Signal Mountain, with nice views of the Dunraven Creek valley below.

DIRECTIONS Take U.S. Highway 287 north to State Highway 14. Then drive 26 miles west from Ted's Place to Pingree Park Road. This trailhead is a bit closer to Highway 14 making for a somewhat shorter drive. There are actually two access points to this trail and mountain. One in Pingree Park and the south end of the trail near Glen Haven. For this one take Highway 14 to Pingree Park Road. The trail is on the left (east) side of the road approximately 10 miles from the entrance and 2 miles from the Pingree Park Campus. It is approximately 0.5 mile beyond the turnoff for Pennock Pass. Park alongside the road.

The trail runs along Pennock Creek. The trail drops down to the stream and then winds through the thick forest and is fairly level with nice views across the stream. At approximately 1 mile into the trek you cross Pennock Creek on a footbridge that goes across the creek. The trail begins to climb steadily and gains another 200 feet to reach 9000 feet in the next mile or so as it parallels the stream. Bear right when the trail meets an old road.

The beaver ponds mark the halfway point; the trail leaves the main Pennock Creek drainage, crosses a smaller stream, and begins to climb more steeply as it leaves the streambed. The striking rock spire makes a good lunch or turnaround

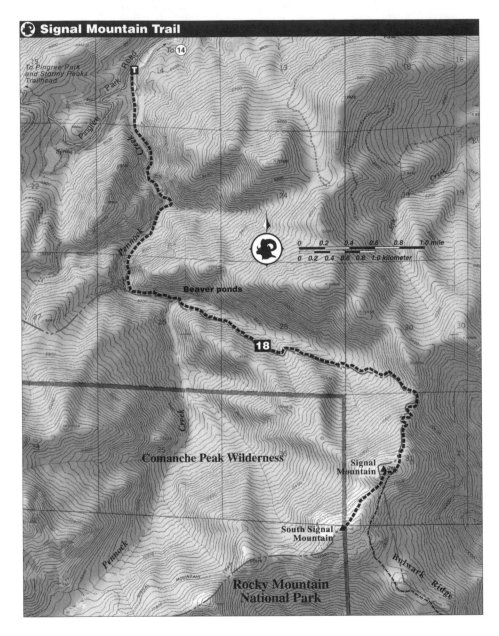

point, depending on your ambitions. After you enjoy that area, continue on the trail as it climbs to a tree-obscured saddle where you might see an old road. Pick up the faint trail on the right and continue to climb toward treeline and the North Signal Mountain summit. The South Signal Mountain summit is a short ridge walk away and is 14 feet lower than the northern summit. The view from the summit ridge is superb with a great panorama of the canyons, foothills, and plains below. You can even see Longs Peak in the distance.

TRIP 19 Stormy Peaks Trail

Distance	Up to 10.0 miles, Out-and-back
Difficulty	Varies (easy for first 2 miles, but challenging if you climb a peak)
Elevation Gain	3120 feet (starting at 9028 feet)
Trail Use	Option for kids, leashed dogs OK
Agency	Canyon Lakes Ranger District, Roosevelt National Forest
Map	Trails Illustrated *Poudre River & Cameron Pass*

HIGHLIGHTS Enjoy the impressive mountain backdrop of Comanche Peak and Fall Mountain as you traverse and then climb above the valley, gradually making your way above treeline. The trail has very rocky sections and can be wet in the early spring. The stark beauty of the burn area dominates the start, but then healthy lodgepole pine, fir, and spruce trees grace the trail.

DIRECTIONS Take U.S. Highway 287 north to State Highway 14. Then drive 26 miles west from Ted's Place to the Pingree Park Road. Drive 18 miles to the end of the Pingree Park Road and park in the last parking area on the left.

The Pingree Park fire swept through the area in 1994 destroying the Colorado State University (CSU) area facilities. The beginning of the trail has the stark beauty of the darkened timber and remnants of the fire. The trail starts off in tree cover and then takes a short set of switchbacks toward the top of the low ridgeline. The CSU campus and most of the Pingree Park area are visible from the ridgeline. Though you cannot see Emmaline Lake, you can see the top of the rocky cirque above the valley to the northwest. Watch for tree blazes that mark the trail since

it can be hard to follow, especially in the burned area; stay on the west side of the ridge. The burned trees contrast dramatically with the sky.

As you travel southwest, the 12,000-foot Fall Mountain and Comanche Peak massif is a constant and impressive backdrop. You enter a tree tunnel after the first mile that obscures the view but allows you to relish the flora for more than 0.5 mile until you reach the Comanche Peak Wilderness Boundary. A series of steep switchbacks and several rocky sections requires you, in early spring, to negotiate

View from the Stormy Peaks Trail through the stark, burned forest

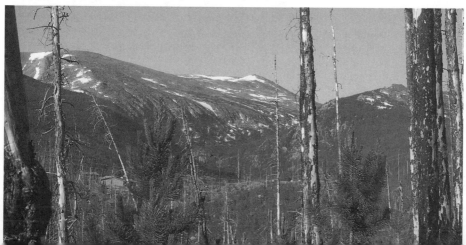

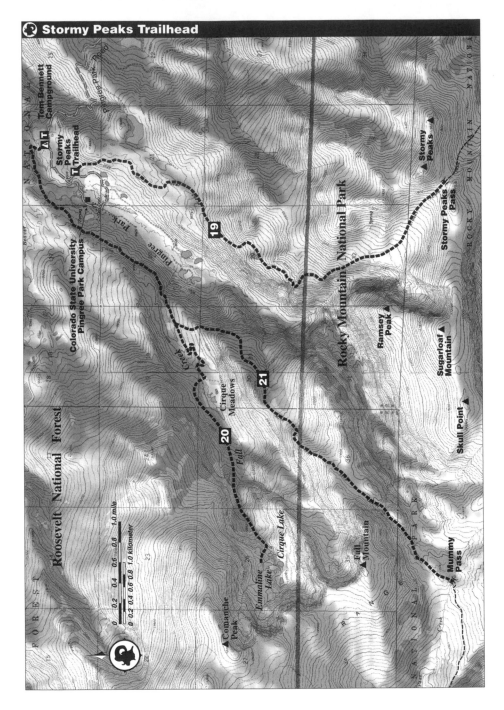

Stormy Peaks Trailhead

wet or muddy spots. The boundary is approximately 2 miles from the trailhead, and you enjoy a nice view as the trees thin with your best view yet of Comanche Peak, Emmaline Lake, Mummy Pass, and Wyoming off to the north. This is a good place for a snack, water, and photos before you start climbing again.

Once you enter the wilderness area, the trail gets considerably steeper with lots of large rocks and several small stream crossings. Hopefully, most of the rocks will be tame and all of the streams will be dry; they should be unless you are attempting an early-season trek. Look for tree blazes (slashes in the tree bark), keeping in mind that wilderness trails are not well marked. Good route-finding skills are necessary once you reach the boundary, but once you reach the major drainage and drop off there is only one way to go: sharply left (southeast) and uphill whether or not you are on a trail.

It is well worth the minor aggravation of negotiating a few wet spots and rocks because in about 0.5 mile you are treated to a superb view of the U-shaped glacier-carved "park" of Pingree in the canyon below Ramsey Peak (11,582 feet) and Sugarloaf Mountain (12,101 feet). You pay for this view, however, by gaining another 200 feet of elevation. At 3.0 miles the trail crosses into Rocky Mountain National Park, and you enjoy more views

> **Great for Kids**
>
> If you're having a family outing, you may want to rest and enjoy the views from the wilderness boundary and then turn around and retrace your steps to the trailhead.

of the glacier-carved box canyon below and get a good view of the Stormy Peaks above for the first time. This is another good break spot for water, snacks, or photos.

From here the trail veers due south and continues uphill poorly marked because of disuse. Stay parallel to the Stormy Peaks drainage, and frequently check the landscape against your map and compass so you can orient your direction. After 0.25 mile from the RMNP boundary you should see a sign for one of the RMNP Stormy Peaks campsites.

Just when you think you'll never reach treeline, you emerge into a wonderland of high mountain tundra, windswept meadows festooned with wildflowers, and dramatic rock outcroppings of the Stormy Peaks at 11,500 feet. If you feel up to it, mounting the pass or even climbing the Stormy Peaks is worthwhile, but keep watch for the namesake storm clouds so that you don't have to do a lightning dance on the way out.

Poudre Canyon & Cameron Pass Areas

TRIP 20 Emmaline Lake Trail

Distance	Up to 10.0 miles, Out-and-back
Difficulty	Varies (easy to Cirque Meadows, but moderate-plus to Emmaline Lake)
Elevation Gain	2100 feet (starting at 8900 feet)
Trail Use	Backpacking, mountain biking to wilderness or Rocky Mountain National Park boundary only, leashed dogs OK
Agency	Canyon Lakes Ranger District, Roosevelt National Forest
Map	Trails Illustrated *Poudre River & Cameron Pass*
Facilities	Restrooms at Tom Bennett Campground

HIGHLIGHTS Think pristine high mountain lake and dramatic glacier-carved cirque and your mind's eye will have the vision you are trekking toward. This is a trail that offers nice views of the Stormy Peaks and then the dramatic backdrop of Fall Mountain and the Comanche Peak massif framing the high mountain lake surrounded by the rocky, craggy cirque. After an open, sunny, and warm beginning, the cool shade of the thickly forested trail will protect you from sun and wind until just before you emerge onto the tundra and rock for the final steep ascent to enjoy the beauty of the lake.

DIRECTIONS Take State Highway 14 about 27 miles west to the Pingree Park Road turnoff. Take the road most of the way to the Pingree campus and look for the right turn for Tom Bennett Campground. Go another 0.25 mile beyond that turnoff, around a sharp left hairpin turn, staying straight when the road turns right uphill toward Sky Ranch. Park where you see a sign for Cirque Meadows; it's actually the Emmaline Lake/Cirque Meadows Trailhead.

This interesting trail is rewarding regardless of the distance you travel on it. The first mile of the trail makes a nice family out-and-back trip, while going all the way to Emmaline Lake makes for a moderate almost all-day hike for an acclimated hiker. Cirque Meadows is a magnificent intermediate stop along the way. One possible variation, since the road can be a bit tiresome on the way out, is to bike to the wilderness boundary and then hike the rest of the way to the lake. You then have a pleasant downhill ride to look forward to rather than slogging along the road at the end of a 10-mile trek.

The first 1.5 miles of the trail is out in the open on an old logging road, Cirque Meadows Road, and travels through the burn area. It is exposed to sun and wind and can be very warm or very chilly, depending on the season. Once you reach the thick tree cover, you are protected from the wind and sun. Cross Fall Creek on a footbridge.

At the intersection with Mummy Pass Trail, continue right (southwest) to Emmaline Lake. The trail enters the trees, which should provide good sun protection and cooler temperatures. The trail winds, rolls, and switchbacks through a long tree tunnel with occasional glimpses of the valley below. Pass the backcountry campground nestled in the trees and then the trail climbs steeply until you break free at Cirque Meadows. Cirque Meadows is a superb setting with the backdrop of the Fall Mountain's glacier-carved cirque and the vibrant colors of the vegetation swaying out of the wetlands.

After the wet meadows, cross a footbridge and follow the old logging road until it becomes a trail, reentering the trees and paralleling the stream. The trail zigzags through a lovely, tree-sheltered, undeveloped camping area with an active mosquito population and then climbs steeply until it breaks out of the trees. The final scrambling switchbacks take you over rocks and through tundra to the magic of Emmaline Lake and its surroundings with the Comanche Peak and Fall Mountain massif towering above.

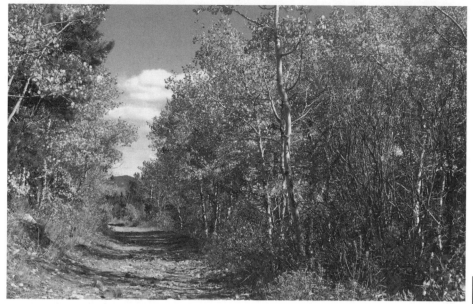

A tree-lined route in Pingree Park

Joe Grim

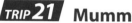 **Mummy Pass Trail**

see
map on
p. 68

Distance	Up to 14.0 miles, Out-and-back
Difficulty	Moderate-plus
Elevation Gain	2500 feet (starting at 8900 feet)
Trail Use	Mountain biking to wilderness or Rocky Mountain National Park boundary only, option for kids, leashed dogs OK
Agency	Canyon Lakes Ranger District, Roosevelt National Forest
Map	Trails Illustrated *Poudre River & Cameron Pass*
Facilities	Restrooms at Tom Bennett Campground

HIGHLIGHTS This is the most spectacular option in the area other than climbing Comanche Peak. It evolves into an open climb above treeline on tundra up a mountainside, offering splendid views of Pingree Park's superb surroundings of summits, rivers, trees, and wetlands. This awe-inspiring perch lets you see the soaring granite cirque that is part of the Comanche Peak massif and cradles Emmaline Lake. The access point for this trail that goes into RMNP, is the same as the Emmaline Lake Trail. In terms of difficulty and elevation gain, it is longer and involves slightly more elevation gain.

DIRECTIONS Take U.S. Highway 287 north to State Highway 14. Take State Highway 14 about 27 miles west to the Pingree Park Road turnoff. Take the road most of the way to the Pingree campus and look for the right turn for Tom Bennett Campground. Go another 0.25 mile beyond that turnoff, around a sharp left hairpin turn, staying straight when the road turns right uphill toward Sky Ranch. Park where you see a sign for Cirque Meadows; it's actually the Emmaline Lake/Cirque Meadows Trailhead.

The first 1.5 miles of the trail is out in the open on an old logging road, Cirque Meadows Road, and travels through the burn area. It is exposed to sun and wind and can be very warm or very chilly, depending on the season. Once you reach the thick tree cover, you are protected from the wind and sun. Cross Fall Creek on a footbridge.

As you are walking down closed Cirque Meadows Road, you have a good view of the Pingree Park campus, and its beautiful high mountain setting. In about 0.5 mile a side trail on the right heads 1.25 miles to Surprise Pond and Beaver Falls. The trail then parallels Bennett Creek, with small waterfalls and the sounds of the stream below. After approximately 1.25 miles cross Bennett Creek on a small footbridge and disregard a side trail on the left. In another 0.25 mile (about 2.0 miles from the trailhead), turn left at signed Mummy Pass Trail. The signs at the intersection list distances of 5 miles to Mummy Pass and 3 miles to the RMNP boundary.

After the intersection, the trail goes steeply uphill on one of the rockiest sections of trail. In 0.25 mile you reach the wilderness boundary beyond which mountain biking is prohibited. The trail mellows and the rocks thin after 0.75 mile. You emerge from the trees in another 0.25 mile and enter a spectacular panorama.

The switchbacks begin, and are steady, well marked, and broad as you gain another 1000 feet; pace yourself if you aren't fleet of foot and lung. The view of

---

Great for Kids

If you have weary people, have a snack and enjoy the great panorama when you reach treeline and then wander back to the trailhead. If you want to go just a bit farther (0.3 mile), try to make it to the prominent rock outcrops after the next set of switchbacks. It is an even better rest stop with superb views of the Fall Mountain and Comanche Peak massif and rocks to clamber around on.

Pingree Park is 180 degrees of wow, with the Stormy Peaks to the east, the Comanche Peak and Fall Mountain massif to the west, and the top of the cirque that frames Emmaline Lake coming into sight. After you reach a pile of shapely rocks that are a good place for an even better view (see "Great for Kids" above) the next 0.3 mile of uphill is worth the even better view of Comanche Peak. The trail levels somewhat as it goes up and over the ridgeline where you will finally top out around 11,400 feet. This area has some low willow bushes to protect you from the wind and is a good spot for a snack or lunch break. From there the trail descends 200 feet and then rolls up and over another high spot, regaining and then losing a bit of the altitude. The Mummy Range comes into view and looks like a scene out of Patagonia if there is any snowcap left when you're hiking. You will descend once again before the final ascent, circumventing the Mummy's head, and finally arriving at Mummy Pass.

Chapter 4

Colorado State Forest

This spectacular and lesser-known Colorado state park is a wonderful weekend destination with an abundant variety of hiking and biking trails, as well as lake and stream fishing and good camping and backpacking. It takes a minimum of 2 hours to reach the forest from Fort Collins (probably more like 2½ hours with summer traffic) and about 1½ hours from Grandby.

Seven Utes & Mahler Mountains

If you want panoramic views of Mount Richthofen, the Diamond Peaks, as well as a unique view of the Never Summer Range, the Zirkels, and the Medicine Bow mountain ranges, then Seven Utes and Mahler peaks are a must. Attempt this duo if you have good route-finding skills since there are few formal trails once you reach Seven Utes. A lot of the informal trails are old logging roads that can be used for mountain biking. The trail to the peaks beyond the first overlook is too narrow and covered by fallen timber to be biked, but there are lots of alternatives for intermediate to advanced bikers. The many roads can cause confusion on the way up too.

Families with young children can enjoy the great views of the peaks by following the first mile of the route and turning around. The only downside is that you might encounter all-terrain vehicles on the approach. Neither of these nontechnical peaks should be attempted without good rain gear and other equipment since the summits are far from the road.

Camping on the Pass

There is good overnight, rustic backpacking off of the Thunder Pass/American Lakes Trail, even if you are a beginner. A state park daily pass is required but there is no camping fee. It is important that you let someone know exactly where you are going and when you plan to return. I recommend picking a cozy site in some healthy trees in case the wind kicks up, which often happens. The area is good for beginners because when the sun goes down you feel like you are in the wilderness even though you are only a couple of miles from the road, giving you a margin of safety. Needless to say, a major weather event can erase that margin in a very short period of time. The Nokhu Hut and the Colorado State Forest Yurt System, or Michigan Reservoir cabins are less demanding alternatives for overnights in this high mountain paradise.

Colorado State Forest Cabins & Never Summer Yurts

There are two good, inexpensive options for staying overnight in the Colorado State Forest. The Colorado State

Park system rents several rustic cabins in the Gould area on North Michigan Lake, while Never Summer Yurts has a system of yurts available. The Lake Agnes Nokhu Hut is the latest addition to the Never Summer Yurt system. The settings for the yurts and cabins are dramatic with the Medicine Bow Mountains Rawah Range forming an enormous and majestic backdrop to the east and north, and there are nice easy trails in and around the huts with nonstop views in every direction. The North Michigan Reservoir cabins are heated by either wood-burning stoves or propane. Water is available nearby. The cabins have vault toilets within walking distance, sleep 6 to 10 people in bunk beds, and are no more than 400 feet from parking places. The yurts also vary in size and sleep 6 to 10 people. They are heated with wood-burning stoves and have a variety of bunks and beds. Dancing Moose and Grassy Hut are 0.25 and 0.6 mile from the road, respectively, while the others are farther. Two websites (http://parks.state.co.us/Parks/StateForest/CabinsandYurts and www.neversummernordic.com) include complete descriptions, pictures, and prices.

TRIP 1 Michigan Ditch Trail to Thunder Pass Trail

Distance	2.0 to 12.0 miles, Out-and-back and point-to-point options
Elevation Gain	Varies, depending on distance hiked (starting at 10,200 feet)
Difficulty	Varies, depending on distance hiked
Trail Use	Mountain biking, option for kids, backpacking, leashed dogs OK
Agency	Colorado State Forest
Map	Trails Illustrated *Poudre River & Cameron Pass*
Note	This fee area ($6 at the time of this writing) has parking and toilets on the northwest side of the highway.

HIGHLIGHTS One of the most popular trails in the Cameron Pass area, it has something for everyone. It is an almost level trail at the outset and is an excellent entrance to Thunder Pass and the Never Summer Mountains of Rocky Mountain National Park. It offers spectacular views of the Never Summer Range and Nokhu Crags across the Michigan River drainage, Diamond Peaks, and North Park off in the distance. It also features a gentle roll at the start and can be used for either hiking or biking because it is a wide service road for the Michigan Ditch, part of the Transmountain/Transcontinental Divide water storage system that funnels water from the western slope of the Continental Divide to the thirsty eastern slope cities. It can be used for short and easy family jaunts or backcountry adventure for those who want to spend the night and surmount Thunder Pass and sneak in the back door of Rocky Mountain National Park.

DIRECTIONS Take State Highway 14 to the top of Cameron Pass. Parking and toilet facilities are on the west side of the highway. The well-marked, gated trail is on the east side of Highway 14 (left side if you are driving south/west). The trail is actually a closed four-wheel-drive road used to maintain the Michigan Ditch.

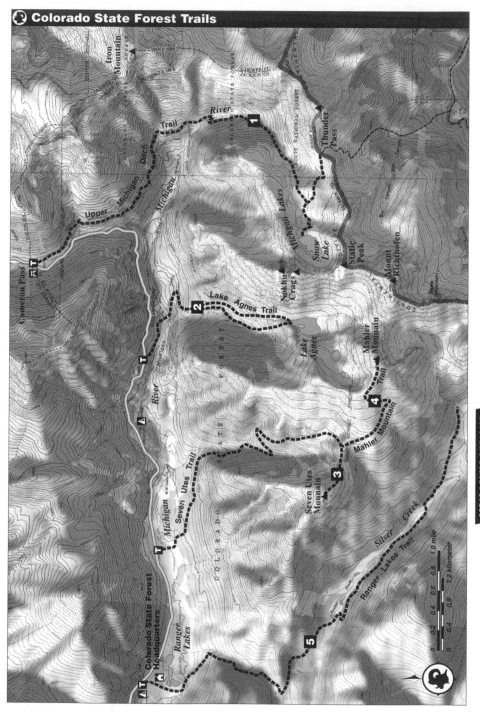

Colorado State Forest Trails

The first 1.5 miles is a flat, highly scenic trail. It is an ideal family out-and-back trip. For more adventure, continue on the winding road for another 0.5 mile until the trail intersects the Thunder Pass and American Lakes Trail. At that point either continue to follow the road around the bottom of the ridgeline and cross to the other side of the drainage to the south (if there is no snow or avalanche danger) or take the Thunder Pass and American Lakes Trail left and climb steadily toward the rocky panorama above treeline at 11,000 feet. The former is an easy, short trek on a flat trail; the latter a more challenging, longer route above treeline. If you decide to take the latter, you find a constantly climbing, but rolling trail. There are some very steep stretches but also some moderate to easy sections too. Go as far as you wish; any length is a treat.

The upper reaches of this trail offer very impressive views of the northern edge of the Never Summer Range including the summit of Richtofen, LuLu, and Mahler Peaks and the Nokhu Crags. If you make it to the top of Thunder Pass,

> **Great for Kids**
>
> If you want an easy out-and-back for small children, this is it. The first 1.5 miles follow the road. If you are taking a novice or family expedition, then take an almost flat trek and turn around at the group of cabins that are about 1 mile one-way.

you can see down into the Colorado River drainage of Rocky Mountain National Park. Continue down the west side of the pass, over the ditch road, and into Box Canyon in RMNP. You could even plan to backpack this or take a very long and challenging dayhike and arrange a car shuttle to pick you up after you emerge on the west side of Trail Ridge Road near Grand Lake. How long it takes to reach the summit of Thunder Pass is very much an individual measure. It should only be attempted as an all-day adventure by the fit and well prepared. It is a moderate-to-challenging dayhike or easy backpack on an easy-to-find trail at high altitude with very striking scenery.

American Lakes from Thunder Pass   *Joe Grim*

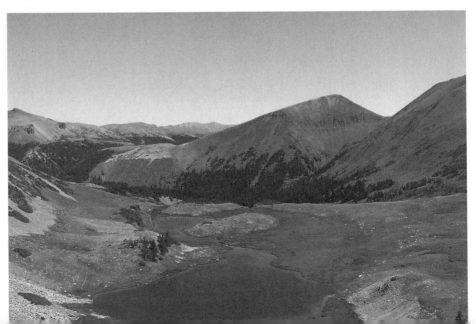

TRIP 2 Lake Agnes Trail

see map on p. 75

Distance	1.6 miles, Semiloop
Elevation Gain	500 feet (starting at 10,000 feet)
Difficulty	Easy
Trail Use	Fishing, great for kids, leashed dogs OK
Agency	Colorado State Forest
Map	Trails Illustrated *Poudre River & Cameron Pass, Rocky Mountain National Park*
Facilities	Restrooms, campground, and a yurt and cabin (yurt and cabin available for winter use only)

HIGHLIGHTS This popular and very scenic trail heads to a high mountain lake surrounded by a cirque of the Never Summer Range. The scenic drama is high, with the soaring summits and ridgelines of the Diamond Peaks, Nokhu Crags, and Mount Richthofen in view as you climb to, and circumnavigate the lake. It is a much shorter and easier route in the summer than in the winter; so take advantage of it.

DIRECTIONS The trailhead is 2.5 miles west of the summit of Cameron Pass on the left or south side of the road if you are driving west. Follow the, at first, smooth road to the bottom of the hill and turn right; Crags Campground is straight. Drive 1 mile uphill on the steep, rough, but passable road to the small parking lot.

You immediately enjoy panoramic views of the Nokhu Crags and the west side of Cameron Pass. The summer parking lot is next to the cabin used by skiers and snowshoers in the winter months but closed in the summer. Take the trail right of the restrooms uphill into the trees. The trail starts out steep but flattens on top of the short hill. The view of the Nokhu Crags is worth the price of admission. After 0.3 mile you come to an intersection. Left goes across the drainage to the American Lakes and Crags Campground Trail. Bear right and uphill for Lake Agnes. At the next intersection there are short, roughly equal trails to the lake: one in the treeless drainage, the other through trees.

When you reach the lake, there are trails going around both sides of the lake If you want to circumnavigate the lake, you can alternate your routes out and back for variety. Go left to walk on the edge of a drainage and then along scree to get to the other side. Go right to wander through trees and then emerge onto the narrow trail around the edge. After 0.25 mile the trail goes back uphill into the trees and winds back to a pretty corner. From there it goes downhill and around to the other side. Once you trek around to the far side of the lake, you can access the trail to the top of the scree heap known as Mount Richthofen. (Mount Mahler and Seven Utes Peak are much more enjoyable climbs.)

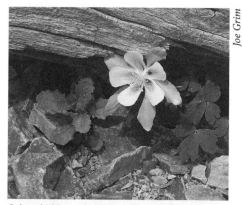

Joe Grim

Colorado blue columbine

Colorado State Forest

TRIP 3 Seven Utes Trail

see map on p. 75

Distance	2.0 to 8.0 miles, Out-and-back
Difficulty	Moderate
Elevation Gain	2000 feet (starting at 9400 feet)
Trail Use	Mountain biking (first mile only), option for kids, leashed dogs OK
Agency	Colorado State Forest
Map	Trails Illustrated *Poudre River & Cameron Pass, Rocky Mountain National Park*

HIGHLIGHTS The easier, much lower summit of neighboring peaks, Seven Utes is probably considered to be a barely significant subpeak of Mahler Mountain by grumpy geographers, but it is a truly enjoyable climb in a somewhat lesser but still magnificent panorama that includes the Diamonds and Crags.

DIRECTIONS Continue west on State Highway 14 over Cameron Pass. When you are approximately 3.8 miles past the summit of Cameron Pass and almost at the bottom of the incline, look for a partially paved drive with a green gate on the left (south) side of the road angling to the southeast. It is the former Seven Utes Lodge entrance. Park either at the partially paved closed road or park about another 0.25 mile down in the turnout on the same side and hike back on the other side of the fence lining the road. The State Forest Moose Visitors Center, which opens at 9 AM, is 2 miles west of the trailhead on State Highway 14; they can help you with advice and directions. If you reach the Ranger Lakes Campground, you have gone too far west on Highway 14 and are about 1 mile west of the trailhead.

As with most of the trails described in this book, a good time can be had by all by attempting the entire round-trip if you are a fit hiker or a much smaller segment if you are less ambitious. From the summit of Mahler, you can see Mount Richthofen, the Crags shoulder, and the tail end of the Never Summer Range, including Static Peak and Teepee Mountain. You can also glimpse the edge of North Park. Even 1 or 2 miles uphill on this gradually steepening trail gives you views, and the closer you get to Seven Utes, the more impressive they are.

Graced with stately, tall pine trees, the trailhead is at the old Seven Utes Lodge site driveway; the lodge is long gone and there are no longer any signs or markers for it. Just beyond the green gate, take either of the trails you see on the right. When you are at the trailhead, orient yourself by looking at your topographic map and then at the ridge of Seven Utes and the drainage to the southeast you want to end up in. Once you are in the trees and encountering lots of logging roads, it is easy to get disoriented. Go downhill gradually, and then go steeply uphill east and southeast on an old road. Don't take the trail going left (east) before the road steepens. There are no trail markers, but it is easier if you keep in mind the general direction you are traveling in toward the drainage.

When the trail gets steeper, it merges with another, wide, old logging road used by all-terrain vehicles and that can be mountain biked. Go to the left or east uphill on the road, and follow the trail on the left as you round the very first hard right turn—it is not well marked so look carefully for it, remembering which drainage you want to end up in. Mountain bikers can stay on the road, which will take them steeply uphill to Michigan Ditch in a roundabout way. The trail up Seven Utes is too narrow and steep and features lots of fallen trees that make biking impossible; it is not an old road and has thick vegetation and a 30- to 40-foot dropoff on your left. Behind you to the northeast is a spectacular view of the Diamond Peaks.

The trail goes downhill and to the other side of the drainage, crossing a

stream that can be difficult in early spring. Uphill back into the trees, east and south, you go as the trail steepens considerably. Dodge trees as you climb to treeline next to the drainage. Dead ahead you see the ridge that goes right (west) toward the base of Seven Utes. Keep to the right at intersecting trails. As you traverse the short ridge, you see Seven Utes to the southwest (right) and Mahler Peak to the northeast (left). You must decide which peak to climb—Seven Utes or Mahler Mountain. Add 2 hours if you choose Mahler. The trail going to the right (west) across the top of the drainage cirque is your route over to Seven Utes. Cross the top of the cirque and pick your route up to the summit. A 360-degree panoramic view of the northern edge of the Never Summer Range and the southern tip of the Rawah range of the Medicine Bow Mountains greets you.

Great for Kids

Once you crest the hill, and veer off of the old logging road and on to the trail, you will find a good spot for a photo and snack break—a good turnaround point for the inexperienced. If you continue on the narrow trail, it drops down into a drainage, and then climbs steeply uphill toward the Seven Utes saddle.

TRIP 4 Mahler Mountain Trail

see map on p. 75

Distance	10.0 miles, Out-and-back
Difficulty	Moderate to challenging
Elevation Gain	3000 feet (starting at 9400 feet)
Trail Use	Leashed dogs OK
Agency	Colorado State Forest
Map	Trails Illustrated *Poudre River & Cameron Pass, Rocky Mountain National Park*

HIGHLIGHTS Although higher and more challenging than Seven Utes, Mahler Mountain affords you panoramic views of Mount Richthofen and the Diamond Peaks, as well as a unique view of the Never Summer Range, the Zirkels, and the Medicine Bow mountain ranges. It is a real mountain while Seven Utes is just an impressive subpeak—the extra effort is worth the additional panorama.

DIRECTIONS Continue west on State Highway 14 over Cameron Pass. When you are approximately 3.8 miles past the summit of Cameron Pass and almost at the bottom of the incline, look for a partially paved drive with a green gate on the left (south) side of the road angling to the southeast. It is the former Seven Utes Lodge entrance. Park either at the partially paved closed road or another 0.25 mile down in the turnout on the same side and hike back on the other side of the fence lining the road. The State Forest Moose

Visitors Center, which opens at 9 AM, is 2 miles west of the trailhead on State Highway 14; they can help you with advice and directions. If you reach the Ranger Lakes Campground, you have gone too far west on Highway 14 and are about 1 mile west of the trailhead.

From the summit of Mahler, you can see Mount Richthofen, the Crags shoulder, and the end of the Never Summer Range, including Static Peak and Teepee Mountain, and can glimpse the edge of North Park. Graced with stately, tall pine trees, the trailhead is at the old Seven Utes Lodge site driveway; the lodge is long gone and there are no longer any signs or markers for it. Just beyond the green gate, take either of the trails you see on the right. When you are at the trailhead, orient yourself by looking at your topographic map and then at the ridge of Seven Utes and the drainage to the southeast you want to end up in. Once you are in the trees and encountering lots of logging roads, it is easy to get disoriented. Go downhill gradually, and then go steeply uphill east and southeast on an old road. Don't take the trail going left (east) before the road steepens. There are no trail markers, but it is easier if you keep in mind the general direction you are traveling in toward the drainage.

When the trail gets steeper, it merges with another, wide, old logging road used by all-terrain vehicles and that can be mountain biked. Go to the left or east uphill on the road, and follow the trail on the left as you round the first hard right turn—it is not well marked so look carefully for it, remembering which drainage you want to end up in. Mountain bikers can stay on the road, which will take them steeply uphill to Michigan Ditch in a roundabout way. The trail up Seven Utes is too narrow and steep and

features lots of fallen trees that make biking impossible; it is not an old road and has thick vegetation and a 30- to 40-foot dropoff on your left. Behind you to the northeast is a spectacular view of the Diamond Peaks.

The trail goes downhill and to the other side of the drainage, crossing a stream that can be difficult in early spring. Uphill back into the trees, east and south, you go as the trail steepens considerably. Dodge trees as you climb to treeline next to the drainage. Dead ahead you see the ridge that goes right (west) toward the base of Seven Utes. Keep to the right at intersecting trails. As you traverse the short ridge, you see Seven Utes to the southwest (right) and Mahler Mountain to the northeast (left). You must decide which peak to climb—Seven Utes or Mahler Mountain. Add 2 hours if you choose Mahler.

For Mahler Mountain bear northeast (left) and don't take the trail across the top of the cirque to your right. Instead continue uphill but bear straight and then left, making your way toward the right (southwest) side of the mountain. Avoid the steep climbs on the west-facing slopes. Make your way around to the southwest side of the mountain for a more gradual, enjoyable climb. The southwest ridge is a steady, less direct ascent. Make your way to the southwest flank of the mountain and carefully pick your way up to the top of the ridge saddle and then right (south) to the summit. It is a terrific view in all directions on top.

TRIP 5 Ranger Lakes Trail

see map on p. 75

Distance	Up to 10.0 miles (8.8 miles to the first crossing of Silver Creek), Out-and-back
Difficulty	Easy
Elevation Gain	610 feet (starting at 9280 feet)
Trail Use	Mountain biking, motorized recreation, leashed dogs OK
Agency	Colorado State Forest
Map	Trails Illustrated *Poudre River & Cameron Pass, Rocky Mountain National Park*
Facilities	Restrooms in campground

HIGHLIGHTS This trail starts behind the Ranger Lakes Campground and is easy to find. Enjoy a 2-mile round-trip jaunt to see the views in the next valley, and continue on if you want more of a workout. The parking lot at the trailhead offers great views of the riparian area, and Seven Utes Mountain. The first mile is a moderate climb in a tree tunnel until you make it over the top of the hill and things open up into a beautiful high mountain valley.

DIRECTIONS It is approximately 5.8 to 6.0 miles from the summit of Cameron Pass to the campground on the left (south) side of the road. There is a recreational area parking lot another 0.8 mile west of the Ranger Lakes Campground.

To find the trailhead drive past the campground loop road to a dead end in the day-use parking area. The trails on the left head to the lakes if you want a short side trip. The trail covered here goes straight ahead slightly downhill from the parking lot and emerges from the trees to give you a very nice view of the ridgeline of the Never Summer Mountains and Seven Utes and Mahler mountains in particular. Cross the Michigan River on a small bridge. The trail then reenters the trees and climbs uphill for over 1 mile before cresting and then descending into the Silver Creek drainage. Though the trail is a tree tunnel

View of Seven Utes Mountain from the Ranger Lakes Trailhead

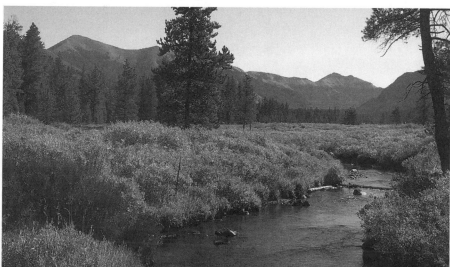

Colorado State Forest

except for a few glimpses at the hillcrest and on the descent, it is indeed a beautiful and peaceful forest.

At approximately 1.5 miles you see a trail labeled Silver Creek (which is also still Ranger Lakes Trail), bear right and stay on the main trail toward Illinois Pass. In another 0.25 mile you reach the high point of the trail with limited views. You might encounter an occasional off-highway vehicle though I neither saw nor heard any the day I was on this trail. In fact I saw no one on the trail the entire time—a rare experience. If you want to enjoy the Silver Creek Meadows, add another 2 miles to your round-trip distance, but it is well worth it. At around the 2-mile mark, go left at the trail intersection. Reach the Silver Creek drainage at just under 2.5 miles and either have a snack or lunch and reverse course or roll over more meadows and ascend higher into the foothills of the Never Summer Range.

TRIP 6 Grass Creek Yurt Trail

Distance	5.3 miles (Loop), 10.0 miles (Out-and-back)
Difficulty	Easy to moderate
Elevation Gain	400 feet (starting at 9000 feet)
Trail Use	Mountain biking, yurting, leashed dogs OK
Agency	Colorado State Forest
Map	Trails Illustrated *Poudre River & Cameron Pass*
Facilities	None other than the yurt

HIGHLIGHTS The backdrop of the Rawah Range of the Medicine Bow Mountains is the highlight of this rolling trail through a pretty valley. You can take a short, easy, loop hike or a much longer trek as high and far as your heart desires.

DIRECTIONS Take State Highway 14 over Cameron Pass west/south 10 miles to Gould. Watch for signs on the left (north) side of the highway for the State Forest Campground and the KOA, and turn right and then left to enter the campground. The entrance station includes a map. Follow the dirt road approximately 4 miles until you see the parking area for Grass Creek Yurt on the left side of the road. After you pass the North Michigan Reservoir, cross the road to find the trailhead.

View of Clark Peak and the Rawah Range from the Grass Creek Trail

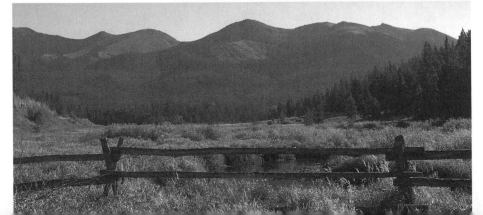

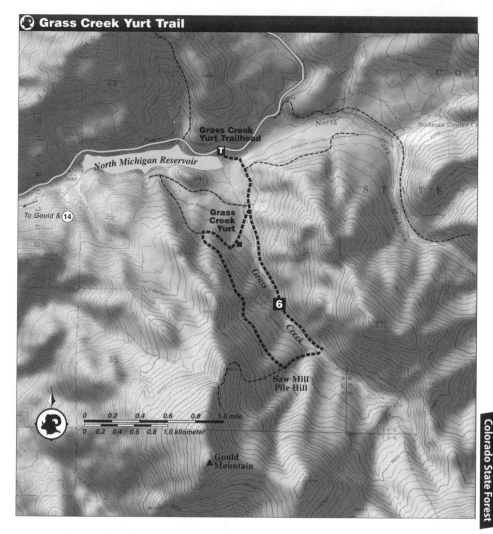

Grass Creek Yurt Trail

Grass Creek
Yurt Trailhead

North Michigan Reservoir

To Gould & (14)

Grass
Creek
Yurt

Grass

6

Creek

Saw Mill
Pile Hill

0   0.2   0.4   0.6   0.8   1.0 mile
0   0.2   0.4   0.6   0.8   1.0 kilometer

Gould
Mountain

Bockman Lumber Co.

North

S T A T E

From the trailhead you travel south toward the yurt. When you come to the trail junction, bear right to go directly past the yurt or left to travel the double track, and then single-track, trail that affords a nice view of the yurt without passing too closely. If you take the left branch, you gradually climb up the drainage. You can then either turn back on the loop to the right about 2.25 miles from the trailhead or continue straight ahead up Saw Mill Pile Hill and beyond to the end of the trail.

The right branch goes past the hut and climbs more steeply up on top of a small ridge. After approximately 2.5 miles the two branches meet again to complete the loop.

Chapter 5
Fort Collins Area

Fort Collins had the foresight to preserve and create a superb variety of city parks. It is a relatively recent arrival to the natural area and open space arena, thanks to a dedicated group of local open space advocates. While Boulder was the first arrival to the open space altar, Fort Collins and Larimer County have done an outstanding job of acquisition, and their trails and natural areas are second to none.

Fort Collins Trail System

The City of Fort Collins is surrounded by some of the best recreational trails in the nation. What started off as a modest effort turned into a network of superb urban trails, thanks to former Mayor Kelly Ohlson and friends, that make you feel like you have escaped to the rivers, foothills, parks, and pastures of rural America. The trails essentially circle the city and provide not only recreation but transportation opportunities that are far more pleasant than climbing behind the wheel of a car and negotiating your way through overzealous drivers. My favorite part of the trail system is the section that runs along the Poudre River, though every section of the trail offers something to enjoy. The northwest section of the Poudre River Trail is accessible near the town of LaPorte, and the southeast Spring Creek or Poudre River Trails are

accessible at east Prospect Road (east of Timberline), at the Edora Pool and Ice Center (EPIC), or at the Environmental Learning Center at the east end of Drake Road. Several city parks offer access; in addition to Edora, the trail system can be accessed at Rolland Moore and Lee Martinez and Lion's parks. At about 4950 feet, Fort Collins is a little lower in elevation than Boulder and Denver, both of which are over 5000 feet; Colorado Springs is around 6000 feet. The trails on the west side of town are a bit higher, and the trails around the reservoir, including Centennial Drive, are between 5500 and 6000 feet high. So altitude isn't a major factor, unless you have just arrived from sea level.

I go out of my way to commute on my bike and incorporate as much of the trail system into my commutes and errands as possible. By using bike routes and the trail system, you can create some very pleasant commutes and avoid traffic. The City of Fort Collins can be commended for providing this great system that gives a real small town community feel to the big city Fort Collins is becoming, and the city is still building the system. In 2005 the city acquired the Soapstone Natural Area approximately 40 minutes north of Fort Collins and adjacent to the also magnificent Red Mountain Natural Area purchased by Larimer County in 2005.

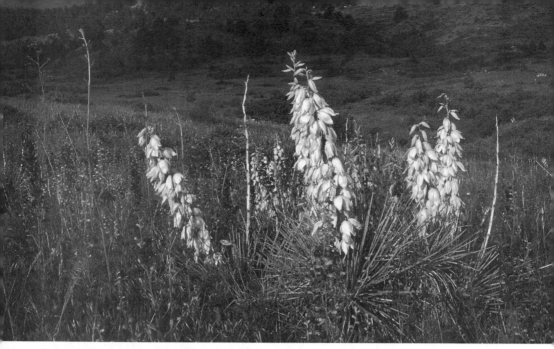

Soapweed yucca at Lory State Park

Joe Grim

Trails are being designed and developed and both areas should be open to the public no later than 2009. Check the city's website (www.ci.fort-collins.co.us) for updates and details. There is now a map available that shows the proposed trails. It looks to be a wonderful area for hikers of all ages and ambitions. Short hikes to archaeological sites, as well as longer options for hiking, biking, and horseback riding will be available.

Lory State Park

One of the gems of the state park system, this once lightly used park has been discovered. Its easy access from Fort Collins (30 to 45 minutes) makes it even more attractive; this multiuse park is relished by hikers, mountain bikers, and horseback riders and has scenic trails for everyone. There are easy, intermediate, and challenging trails, highlighted on the east by the serrated rocks of the hogback hills and blue water of the Horsetooth Reservoir. The steep foothills to the west are topped by dramatic Arthur's Rock and its craggy neighbors. There are a lot of nice picnic spots and even some overnight campsites accessible to backpackers (reservations are required). The most striking feature of this state park is Arthur's Rock, a multifaceted summit of rock outcrops that is prominent from the eastside trails and involves a 1200-foot moderate hike and rock scramble to enjoy its commanding 360-degree panorama.

Larimer County

Larimer County has also added significantly to its collection of beautiful open spaces and natural areas, with acquisitions such as Devil's Backbone and Blue Sky trail system and Eagle's Nest. There are others interspersed throughout this chapter, some of which overlap with city trails. The county recently acquired a magnificent piece of the foothills ecosystem called Red Mountain, 30 to 40 minutes north of Fort Collins (adjacent to the Soapstone property acquired by the City of Fort Collins) and another real gem. Trails are being developed in that area and should be open to the public by 2009. Together they will rival the finest foothills natural areas and parks anywhere in the world. Check the county's website (www. co.larimer.co.us) for updates and details.

The 16-mile Devil's Backbone and Blue Sky trail system rivals anything in the state for variety and scenery. It is a roller-coaster trail with an overall elevation change of 500 feet in, on, and around the unique environment of the Rocky Mountain foothills. Part of it is a technical mountain biking route though there are sections that are easy to moderate. If you want to hike the entire trail in a single day, you'll need to arrange a car shuttle unless you are an ultramarathoner in training. The three primary access points to this slice of paradise are: from the north, Horsetooth Mountain Park or Inlet Bay west of Fort Collins, in the middle from Coyote Ridge southwest of Fort Collins, and from the south the Devil's Backbone Trail outside of Loveland.

Horsetooth Mountain Park

Horsetooth Mountain and Rock are very prominent features of the skyline west of Fort Collins. A landmark visible from remarkable distances, Horsetooth Rock visually morphs into shapes not resembling teeth from the south and west, making it an interesting geological feature. Horsetooth Mountain Park offers a very large network of trails, some that connect to Lory State Park in the north and others that connect to the Blue Sky Trail in the south. The trail to the top of Horsetooth Rock is one of the most popular because of the 360-degree views that include 14,000-foot Longs Peak to the southwest and unfolding foothills and the sprawling plains to the east. It is a favorite hike for sunrise, sunset, and full-moon rambles.

Glen Haven Trails

The Glen Haven Trails are on the way to Rocky Mountain National Park (RMNP) and Estes Park and offer access to beautiful areas near RMNP and are less known and less busy than some areas of the park. These foothills trails offer mountain vistas and gorgeous riparian areas. The North Fork Trail is a little-known backpacking access area to RMNP's Lost Lake. Glen Haven and Drake are very small towns just east of Estes Park, west of Loveland, that consist of small stores, restaurants, and several houses visible from the road. The trails offer unique foothills experiences as a dramatic transition zone between the plains and the very high mountains.

TRIP 1 Poudre River Trail

Distance	16.8 miles, Out-and-back
Difficulty	Easy
Elevation Gain	Negligible
Trail Use	Road and mountain biking, running, horseback riding (on some sections), leashed dogs OK
Agency	City of Fort Collins
Map	City of Fort Collins *Poudre River Trail*
Facilities	Restrooms, picnic areas, playground, and ball fields at Lee Martinez Park

Poudre River Trail

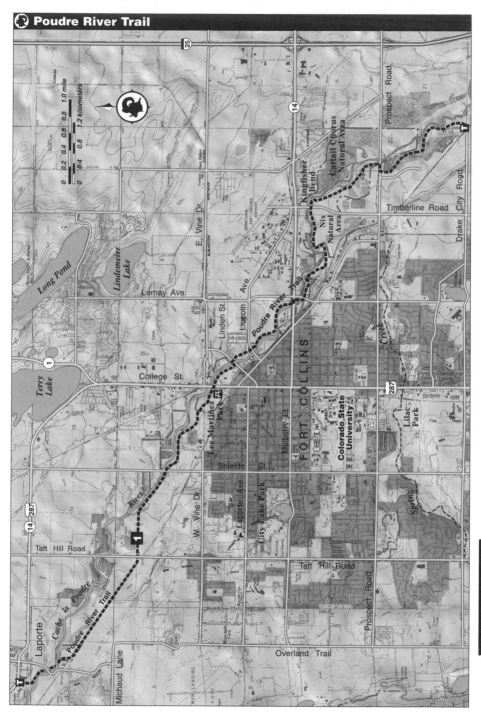

HIGHLIGHTS This delightful trail runs near the river as it winds from North West Fort Collins and Laporte, past lovely Lee Martinez Park, through old town, and past River Bend Ponds, a large open space area, to East Prospect Road. Along the way you can enjoy the sparkling river's waters and the ever-changing surroundings as you go from rural to urban and back again. It is suitable for biking or hiking.

DIRECTIONS Fort Collins is 1 to 1½ hours from Denver and Boulder, depending on traffic. You can access the trail from either end of course (the east end at East Prospect Road or the west end at Cache La Poudre Elementary and Junior High Schools) or the middle at Lee Martinez Park. The description below starts at the west end. If school isn't in session, you can park there and enjoy the small disc golf course before you start. (There is also a well-known source for cinnamon rolls nearby called Vern's.) The trail is next to the entryway for the school on the southwest side of the Old Highway 287.

From there travel south and east around the school's ball fields and join up with the river after 0.5 mile of winding, tree-lined trail. When you reach Lion's Park, a more reliable place to park when school is in session and a good place for picnics, stop briefly and enjoy a beautiful view of the river bend and foothills. From Lion's Park the trail goes under Overland Trail Road and then crosses one of the best designed footbridges in Colorado. A walking loop from Lion's Park to the school and then to the bridge lets you enjoy the river's beauty.

If you want to make a bike ride a little more challenging, take Overland Trail south over the river and turn west to climb Bingham Hill. This little loop won't add more than 3 miles to your journey but is guaranteed to pump up your heart rate to target levels. Catch your breath at the top of the hill, take a good look at the great view of the pastoral Belleview valley, and return downhill to the trail.

After crossing the Cache La Poudre River on the footbridge, the trail bends east and rolls under power lines, giving you a view of gravel mining operations with its resultant ponds and some nice pastures. A soft path next to the bike trail is designated for hiking and running. In approximately 1 mile the trail crosses Taft Hill Road; signal lights warn motorists but don't stop them, so cross carefully. On the other side are a parking lot, picnic table, and solar-powered air hose for bikes.

The next stretch of trail is even prettier with two large ponds on both sides of the trail in the first 0.5 mile, and then the trail veers closer to the river. Hikers and mountain bikers can use the soft path that is a bit closer to the shore. Another mile takes you to Shields Street and an underpass. Now the tree-lined trail has interesting and varied soft path options for snack and water breaks next to the water. You pass a bridge across the river to the north in about 0.5 mile. There are nice hiking and mountain biking options on the other side around two more nice ponds left by gravel mining that now have good vegetation for waterfowl and people.

At the next trail intersection, Lee Martinez Park, visible south of the trail, has good recreational options and open restrooms during nonfreezing months. Continuing east, cross under North College Avenue; soft surface options are more limited, and the trail is better for biking than hiking unless you like to run or hike on hard surfaces. You go quite close to the river and then see the Northside Atzlan Center to the southwest, which has restrooms, basketball courts, and a weight room and charges an entry fee. When the trail dead-ends into Linden Street, turn left (north) and cross the river to pick up the trail on the northeast side of the bridge. The next mile follows the river and passes a golf course and then goes under Mulberry Street and to street level at the intersection of Mulberry and Lemay Avenue.

Go right (south) and cross the river again to pick up the bike trail on the right (west) side of bridge. Cross under the Lemay Avenue river bridge, and continue your trek east. The winding path is lined with trees for the first 0.5 mile, climbs a small hill, and then makes a sharp turn downhill back toward the river. You pass River Bend Ponds Open Space and are away from the river until you go under Timberline Road. Enjoy a beautiful stretch of river and then pond views all the way to Prospect Road. The trail goes downhill past one of the ponds and turns south.

At the next trail intersection go left (south) rather than straight to follow the river and go under Prospect Road. When you emerge on the south side of Prospect, turn left (south) and travel between some office buildings and a couple nice ponds that often host Blue Herons and other impressive winged creatures. Turn left (east) to follow a dirt path between the ponds, which merges back into the paved path a little farther along. Go east and continue to the terminus of the trail at the Environmental Learning Center where there are restrooms. If you arrange for a car shuttle, have it fetch you here; otherwise, return to your starting point. If you prefer, you can retrace your route back under Prospect Road and then turn west until you join the Spring Creek Trail toward Edora Park, with a pool and an ice skating rink.

Starting at Lee Martinez Park and traveling west on the trail also makes for a nice out-and-back; turn around wherever you like, but reaching the bridge across the Poudre River is well worth the effort. Starting at the Environmental Learning Center or from East Prospect Road (use the office building parking lots) makes for a great out-and-back journey along the river; turn around at the intersection at Lemay Avenue where the trail crosses under the road.

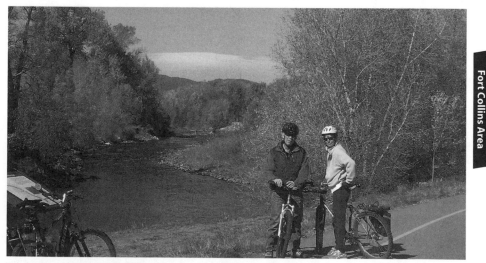

Bikers enjoy the Poudre River Trail.

TRIP 2 Spring Creek Trail

Distance	Up to 13.1 miles, Point-to-point
Difficulty	Easy
Elevation Gain	200 feet (starting at 4940 feet and heading west)
Trail Use	Road biking, running, option for kids, leashed dogs OK
Agency	City of Fort Collins
Map	City of Fort Collins *Spring Creek Trail*
Facilities	Restrooms, picnic areas, playgrounds, and ball fields

HIGHLIGHTS The Spring Creek Trail offers a wide variety of scenery, parks, ponds, meadows, and foothills. This trail follows Spring Creek through several parks in the middle of Fort Collins. It currently extends from West Taft Hill Road to the confluence of Spring Creek and the Poudre River, where it joins the Poudre River Trail. The Spring Creek Trail extends through an underpass of Taft Hill Road. This highly popular trail segment goes to Southwest Community Park and the Foothills Natural Areas. This trail segment offers its own beautiful brand of urban and suburban scenery near the foothills and through Rolland Moore and Edora parks.

DIRECTIONS Fort Collins is 1 to 1½ hours from Denver and Boulder, depending on traffic. Take Interstate 25 north to the Prospect Road exit, and then drive west to Lemay Avenue. Turn left (south) to reach the Edora Pool and Ice Rink parking lot.

From the parking lot travel west under Lemay Avenue, passing through some pretty meadows or wetlands with a good chance to see lots of birds and geese and other wildlife. You then travel along Spring Creek, go past Spring Creek Park and fire station, join a sidewalk, and go west under College Avenue and through another small park. After proceeding under the railroad tracks through a tunnel, cross a gravel road and weave around an open area before going under Centre Avenue. The community garden to the south is worth a stop. Continuing on the trail, go uphill past a nice pond populated with lots of ducks and geese and then go under Shields Street and reach Rolland Moore Park.

If you still have lots of get up and go, continue through the park, pass the tennis

> **Great for Kids**
>
> Rolland Moore Park is a good place for a picnic and playground stop if you have children along. The trail beyond this point is another 1.5 miles uphill to the foothills so you might want to enjoy a snack and water break at the park and then head back to Edora Park.

courts and the natural area, bear right, and go under Drake Road and then Taft Hill Road next to nice meadows. In another mile you reach the Cottonwood Glen Park next to the foothills and options described in the Pineridge Natural Area (Trip 4) just over the ridge. Before you reach the park, you can turn left (south) at a trail intersection toward Cathy Fromme Prairie Natural Area (Trip 3).

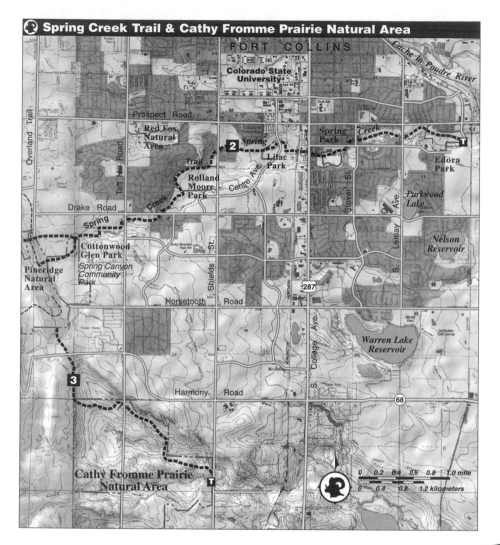

⊙ Spring Creek Trail & Cathy Fromme Prairie Natural Area

TRIP 3 Cathy Fromme Prairie Natural Area

Distance	4.6 miles, Point-to-point
Difficulty	Easy
Elevation Gain	100 feet
Trail Use	Road biking, running, option for kids, leashed dogs OK
Agency	City of Fort Collins
Map	City of Fort Collins *Cathy Fromme Prairie Natural Area*
Facilities	Restrooms and parking on Shields and Taft Hill south of Harmony Road

HIGHLIGHTS One of the earliest acquisitions to the natural areas program, this beautiful example of a short grass prairie is named for a former Fort Collins City Councilmember

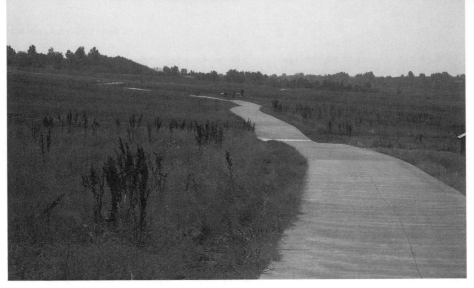

Cathy Fromme Prairie

who was an enthusiastic supporter of the program and died young of breast cancer. This paved trail offers foothills and prairie views and is popular with families with bikes and strollers. The western end of the trail offers a roundabout connection to the Foothills and Spring Creek Trails.

DIRECTIONS Fort Collins is 1 to 1 ½ hours from Denver and Boulder, depending on traffic. The parking lot for the area is approximately 0.75 mile south of the intersection of Harmony Road and Shields Street, on the west side of Shields. There is also parking on Taft Hill Road, approximately 1 mile south of the Harmony Road intersection.

From the parking lot head southwest for 0.25 mile and visit the raptor observation bunker where, if you're lucky, you'll see hawks or eagles nesting. Please stay on the trail and hide in the shelter to increase your chances of seeing the birds. When you've enjoyed this area, turn around and go north and west for the main trail. The initial 0.3 mile is a gradual uphill west along the drainage and then goes more sharply northwest and then north as the trail meanders and rolls through the generally dry creek bed. In less than 0.5 mile a side trail connects to the Dusty Sage Loop, a street in a residential area to Harmony Road through the neighborhood. In another 0.3 mile the trail crosses under Taft Hill Road and a little more steeply uphill into a foothills subdivision.

In 0.3 mile a side trail connects to Plymouth Road and continues west-northwest uphill and then more directly north, paralleling Red Fox Road to (County Road 38E). Turn right (east) for 0.25 mile, and turn left (north) onto Windom Street. Turn left on Baxter and right onto Platte to Horsetooth Road and the new Spring Canyon Community Park. You can take a bike path through the park to the north,

---

Great for Kids

Taft Hill Road is a good point for people with small children to turn around. After crossing under Taft Hill the trail climbs uphill, and ends in a neighborhood. Only continue if you want to add another mile of out and back with somewhat steep up- and downhill.

on either the east or west side of the park, to connect to the Spring Creek Trail or go west on Horsetooth Road until it ends at the trailhead.

The biking and hiking trail goes downhill into the trees and then uphill toward the Pineridge Natural Area where you connect with easy trails (see Trip 4 for more information) after going up and over the steep ridgeline trail that is straight ahead. If you go left (west) when you intersect the Pine Ridge Trail, you are traveling north on a trail with very rocky and steep downhill sections that brings you to the Dixon Dam parking lot. If you go right (north), you'll reach the small east ridge boundary of Pine Ridge. If you've chosen the latter option, look for the second trail on the left, beyond the dog park, that heads over the ridge and down the other side; it intersects with the Spring Creek Trail and ends in Cottonwood Glen Park.

TRIP 4 Foothills Trail: Pineridge Natural Area

Distance	Up to 5.0 miles, Point-to-point
Difficulty	Easy
Elevation Gain	Negligible
Trail Use	Mountain biking, running, great for kids, leashed dogs OK
Agency	City of Fort Collins
Map	City of Fort Collins *Foothills Trail: Pineridge Natural Area*
Facilities	Restrooms near parking lot

HIGHLIGHTS The Foothills Trail travels through three city natural areas as well as county recreation areas along Horsetooth Reservoir and features a wide variety of foothills topography with ponds, hills, valleys, climbs, and descents and great reservoir, city, and mountain views. It is an intermediate mountain biking trail but is easy to negotiate on foot. Making the entire round-trip on foot would be challenging; enjoying pieces of the trail is more fun.

This open space area in the foothills features some easy loop trails, a pretty foothills pond known as Dixon Reservoir, and some short hill options with nice views, and you may

Mountain biker in Pineridge Natural Area

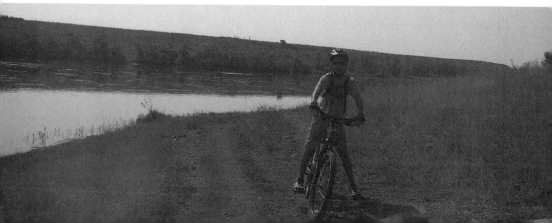

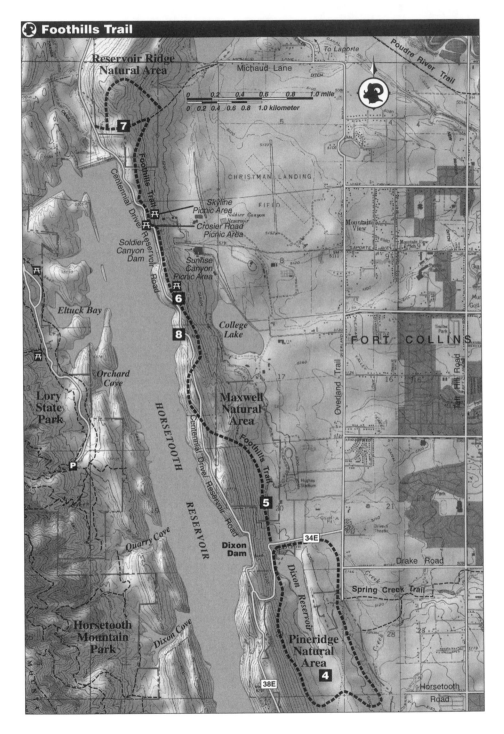

Foothills Trail

even see some prairie dogs. Adjoining a city park and a dog park, it is also the beginning of the Foothills Trail that travels north across County Road 42C.

DIRECTIONS Fort Collins is 1 to 1½ hours from Denver and Boulder, depending on traffic. There are two formal parking lots for accessing this mini-trail system—one on the road to Horsetooth Reservoir's Dixon Dam just south of Sonny Lubick Stadium on CR 42C, which is off of South Overland Trail Road, and the other at the south end of the Overland Trail Road where it dead-ends into a small city park. The Spring Creek Trail also enters Pineridge from the east.

From Dixon Dam Parking Lot

Go either north or south onto the trail that circles Dixon Reservoir and the open space. If you head north, you will go downhill, enter trees, and immediately circle the north end of Dixon Reservoir. The trail travels east and then south about 2 miles to the south end of the natural area. As you go south, you pass three options to go up the ridge on the east side of the natural area. The first, most northerly trail is much too steep, and the third, most southerly option is also steep, but the second option is a gradual switchback and the best choice to mount the eastside ridge.

When you reach the south end of the open space, the trail goes west uphill and skirts the foothills as it rolls north with some very rocky sections that can challenge novice bikers. This section of the trail tends to be wet in late spring and early summer; avoid the mud and help prevent trail erosion.

If you head immediately south from the parking lot, you also go downhill and then immediately uphill as the trail veers to the west, away from the water and then skirts the edge of the foothills and trees as it rolls south. When the trail reaches the south end, it swings east and then north for a couple of miles.

On the east side of the natural area, the two previously mentioned trails that go up and over the ridge take you either into the dog park area on the south or the small city park on the north. In both cases

the trails are moderately fast, fun downhill trails with a few twists and turns; add them to your loop if you want.

If you want to take a longer walk or ride to the east side of the trail, pick up the Spring Creek Trail in the city park. It travels several miles east all the way to Edora Pool and Ice Rink or the Environmental Learning Center and Poudre River Trails on the east side of Fort Collins. If you feel compulsive and want to cover all of the Foothills Trail in one swoop from south to north, start at the Dixon Dam parking lot. It is 1.4 miles to the Maxwell Natural Area from there and another 0.8 mile to the top where the road intersects.

From the East End of Horsetooth Road

Park where the road dead-ends and then take the footbridge across to the trailhead. You can do a short loop by going straight uphill approximately 0.5 mile to the top of the ridge and then downhill to circle the open space, for a total of approximately 5 miles. If you want a shorter hike or bike, turn north (right) on the ridge top and go about 0.25 mile to the trail that descends to the northeast and the small city park and small extension of Overland Trail Road. When you reach the bottom of the hill, turn south (right) and follow the dirt path back to your starting point next to the dog park.

TRIP 5 Foothills Trail: Maxwell Natural Area

see map on p. 94

Distance	Up to 4 miles, Out-and-back
Difficulty	Easy to moderate
Trail Use	Running, mountain biking, leashed dogs OK
Agency	City of Fort Collins
Map	City of Fort Collins *Foothills Trail: Maxwell Natural Area*
Facilities	Restrooms at top of the trail in county picnic area and parking lot on Reservoir Road

HIGHLIGHTS The Foothills Trail travels through three city natural areas, as well as county recreation areas along Horsetooth Reservoir, and features a wide variety of foothills topography with ponds, hills, valleys, climbs, and descents and great reservoir, city, and mountain views. It is an intermediate mountain biking trail but is easy to negotiate on foot. Making the entire round-trip on foot would be challenging; enjoying pieces of the trail is more fun.

This foothills open space area is west of Lubick Stadium and offers nice Fort Collins and foothills views on moderate trails. You can climb to the top of the first foothill ridgeline above the famous Aggies A or up to Reservoir Road for a view. You can also start at the Dixon Dam parking lot and then take the Foothills Trail that edges the southwest stadium parking lot to access the area.

DIRECTIONS Fort Collins is 1 to 1½ hours from Denver and Boulder, depending on traffic. You can access the trails in the area either for County Road 42C, just north of Pineridge Natural Area at the new trailhead just west of Colorado State University's Stadium parking lot or from the end of Prospect Road where it enters the Two Ponds subdivision.

The new trailhead on CR 42C is 1 mile west of the Overland Trail Road intersection, west of the stadium's south side parking lot. From the new Maxwell Open Space trailhead, the trail goes north, along a wide, level dirt road. The trail eventually turns west onto a trail and then north and intersects the trail coming in from the Two Ponds subdivision up the hill from the east and also coming downhill from the west at around the 0.5-mile mark. Turn west to go uphill past the water storage tank and switchback steeply uphill for 0.25 mile gaining another 100 feet. The trail levels as it turns west and then south. When you reach an intersection in 0.25 mile, you can continue south on the trail that goes up gradually and then steeply for a short stretch above the famous Aggies A or turn right and go

up a shorter steep hill to Reservoir Road and a nice view of the human-made lake. Once you cross Centennial Drive, also known as Reservoir Road, you enter a county fee area ($6 at the time of this writing) called Rotary Park; the trail continues to downhill to the north along the edge of the reservoir. See the description of Centennial Drive in Trip 6.

If you access the natural area from the Two Ponds subdivision, take Prospect Road until it enters the subdivision by crossing Overland Trail Road. Take the first left and park, and the trail will be on right (west) side of the street. Take the trail straight uphill for about 0.5 mile to where it intersects the trail coming from the south. Then continue straight west until the trail starts to switchback to the north past the water tank. Another 0.5

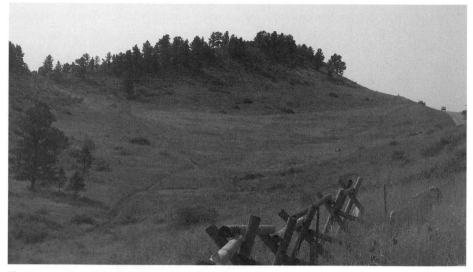

The top meadow of Maxwell Natural Area from Reservoir Road

mile leaves you near the top of the switch-backs with good views. If you continue west, the trail levels and enters a nice foothills grassy meadow area. Once you top the hill, 0.8 mile from the bottom, the trail levels and you can continue down-hill right (north) and then left (south) to reach the top of the ridge above the A, or cross the road and enter the county's

Rotary Park picnic area. The first two options are free while using the county trail will cost you ($6 at the time of this writing). It goes downhill all the way to the reservoir and then continues north for several scenic miles, passing near the Sunrise and Skyline picnic areas, which also require the county fee.

TRIP 6 Foothills Trail: Centennial Drive

see map on p. 94

Distance	4.4 to 8.0 miles, Point-to-point
Difficulty	Moderate
Elevation Gain	200 feet (hiking/biking trail); 600 feet (biking road)
Trail Use	Running, mountain biking, leashed dogs OK
Agency	City of Fort Collins (east side), Larimer County (west side)
Maps	City of Fort Collins *Foothills Trail*
Facilities	Restrooms in the Larimer County picnic and parking area
Note	County annual or day pass required for trail along east side of Horsetooth Reservoir

Fort Collins Area

HIGHLIGHTS The Foothills Trail travels through three city natural areas as well as county recreation areas along Horsetooth Reservoir and features a wide variety of foothills topography with ponds, hills, valleys, climbs, and descents and great reservoir, city, and mountain views. It is an intermediate mountain biking trail but is easy to negotiate on foot. The entire round-trip on foot makes a good running route; for hiking, enjoying pieces of the trail is more fun.

An intermediate mountain bike trail that's easy to negotiate on foot, this trail travels along the eastern shoreline of Horsetooth Reservoir. Enjoy the beauty of the sparkling water, the impressive foothills backdrop, and the richly colored rocks of hogback on this hilly trail that runs along the eastern edge of the reservoir, north of Dixon Dam. You can hike or mountain bike the fee trail or ride on the paved road (Centennial Drive) free. There are many picnic spots with sweeping views of the water and hills.

DIRECTIONS Fort Collins is 1 to 1½ hours from Denver and Boulder, depending on traffic. This trail can be accessed either through the Maxwell Open Space at no charge or from the various parking and picnic areas along the east side of the reservoir. If you want a longer hike with a significant hill climb, start at the bottom of Maxwell and follow the directions above. If you want a shorter trek with easier rolling hills along the reservoir, drive up County Road 42C and climb uphill until it intersects with Reservoir Road. Then turn north (right) and cross Dixon Dam. Climb a very steep hill to the parking area (which charges a fee) on the left (west) side of the road. You get bonus points if you bike up.

From the parking area closest to Dixon Dam (Rotary Park Picnic Area), walk north to the trailhead. You have immediate, commanding views of the water and the hills that surround it, including Arthur's Rock on the ridgeline to the west. The trail goes gradually and then more steeply downhill for about 0.25 mile where it reaches a Y-junction. Turn left (west) and go down the wide stone steps toward the reservoir for the main trail. After the steep section, the trail turns north and continues to descend more gradually, eventually leveling fairly close to the lake.

Feel free to take a side trip to the lakeshore. When the water level is low, enjoy some Colorado beachfront with some sand and bonus rocks and clay. If it is hot enough, you might take a quick dip to cool off. Since it is created by water that started as snowmelt, however, the reservoir doesn't ever get truly warm (68–70°F is tops midsummer); so if it's not hot, your stay in the water will be refreshing but brief.

The trail continues for a 0.5-mile level stretch until it nears the Sunrise Picnic Area, where it climbs a small hill to reach 0.8 mile. An informal trail then descends back to the edge of the reservoir and ends at the dam face. Simply retracing your steps is a great 2-mile round-trip with views of the water.

At 1.5 miles, the Foothills Trail goes over the top of the small ridge and continues on the east side of the ridge above the Colorado State University research campus. The trail winds down 300 feet and then back up and enters Reservoir Ridge Natural Area in 0.8 mile from the road crossing.

Great for Kids

The only steep section of this trail is the first 0.25 mile. Taking a short jaunt down to the lakeshore and beach can be a fun, short family excursion. The reservoir level does vary. At high, early summer levels, the beach can disappear; while later in the summer, as the reservoir level drops, it gets wider and wider. Stroll along the trail and enjoy the views before or after visiting the beach.

TRIP 7 Foothills Trail: Reservoir Ridge Natural Area

Distance	5 miles, Loop
Difficulty	Easy
Elevation Gain	300 feet
Trail Use	Running, mountain biking, horseback riding, leashed dogs OK
Agency	City of Fort Collins
Map	City of Fort Collins *Reservoir Ridge Natural Area*

see map on p. 94

HIGHLIGHTS The Foothills Trail travels through three city natural areas, as well as county recreation areas along Horsetooth Reservoir, and features a wide variety of foothills topography with ponds, hills, valleys, climbs, and descents and great reservoir, city, and mountain views. It is an intermediate mountain biking trail but is easy to negotiate on foot. Making the entire round-trip on foot would be challenging; enjoying pieces of the trail is more fun.

This trail segment can be accessed from either the east or west, but the most popular access is east from Michaud Lane and features a gradual climb with water and plains views with a loop trail on top. It is a very visually rewarding and popular multiuse trail. The west side of the trail overlooks the north end of Horsetooth Reservoir while the east side features good foothills scenery and views. There is very little shade, so start early, or be prepared for summer heat. This trail is usable almost year-round.

DIRECTIONS Fort Collins is 1 to 1 ½ hours from Denver and Boulder on Interstate 25, or U.S. Highway 287, depending on traffic. From either highway, take Prospect Road west to Overland Trail Road. Take Overland Trail Road north to Michaud Lane and turn west to where the road ends in a parking lot. There is also a parking lot on the west side of the Reservoir Ridge Natural Area, just below the northernmost dam of Horsetooth Reservoir. To reach it, take Centennial Drive north from the Maxwell and Pineridge natural areas, or go south from Bellevue on County Road 23 approximately 2 miles; the parking lot will be on the left (east) side of the road.

The east side of Reservoir Ridge Natural Area

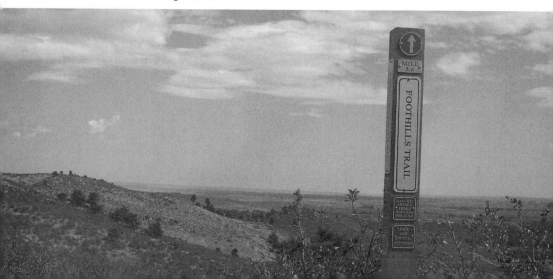

The trail climbs very gradually for the first 0.5 mile and then climbs more steeply. Another 0.25 mile takes you to the loop trail intersection. You can take the enjoyable and scenic loop around in either direction; straight ahead/bear left (south) or take a sharp right (north). The loop trail is steeper uphill to the northwest (right), mellower to the left (south) at the start. The trail to the left (south) climbs approximately 0.5 mile where it levels and reaches another intersection. If you go uphill to the west, you can hike all the way to the west edge of the area in 0.25 mile and then turn south to cross the road to the Foothills Trail, which travels along the east side of Horsetooth Reser-

voir. You can also follow the trail south another 0.5 mile to the Foothills Campus of Colorado State University and a dam.

If you choose the northwest loop, the trail climbs steeply on a rocky, scenic trail for 0.5 mile until it levels with nice views to the east and west. The trail then continues to the west 0.25 mile, before turning south, and going gradually downhill along the western boundary of the natural area. The downhill stretch goes for 0.5 mile where you see the parking lot on the west side of Reservoir Ridge. The next 0.5 mile goes back uphill, switchbacks, crosses over the ridge, and meets up with the other side of the loop.

TRIP 8 Reservoir Road/Centennial Drive

see map on p. 94

Distance	Up to 8 miles, Loop
Difficulty	Challenging
Elevation Gain	600 feet
Trail Use	Road biking, leashed dogs OK
Agency	City of Fort Collins, Larimer County
Maps	*City of Fort Collins, Larimer County*

HIGHLIGHTS This roller-coaster road or mountain biking ride on the paved county road that follows the ridgeline above the eastern edge of Horsetooth Reservoir. Commonly known as Reservoir Road, its formal name is Centennial Drive (County Road 23). It offers the sparkling scenery of reservoir water and foothills greenery that you can enjoy if you

The route looking south from Skyline Picnic Area

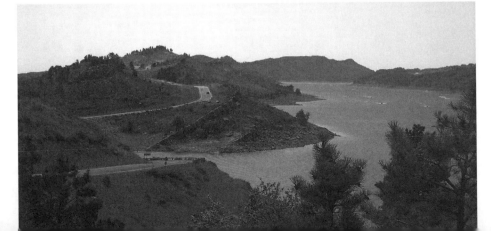

are strong of lung and loin. If you aren't, it is more fun at a leisurely pace on foot on the Foothills Trail, rather than the road.

DIRECTIONS Fort Collins is 1 to 1 ½ hours from Denver and Boulder, depending on traffic. This trip is near the Maxwell Natural Area, where you can park. You can access the Reservoir Road from County Road 42C, just north of Pineridge Natural Area past the Colorado State University Stadium. If you want a longer ride, access the road from County Road 38E, farther south on Taft Hill Road, at the intersection with Harmony Road. Turn west at that intersection, and you will be on CR 38E. If you start there, you will have to climb very steep Heartbreak Hill as you ride north.

After a warm up of your choice, go up the steep CR 42C hill to Reservoir Road, which is also a very good warm up, in and of itself, at slow speeds. (A dandelion bouquet for those who can sprint up this hill.) Go right (north) at the intersection, and continue (likely gasping) uphill another 100 yards. Then enjoy a short downhill onto the top of Dixon Dam and a flat 0.25 mile. Enjoy the view of Fort Collins, and catch your breath because you are about to encounter the steepest hill of the ride. Keep your momentum purring and your legs twirling at 90 revolutions per minute for as long as you can. Stay seated as long as you can and shift those gears down, as your bike begs you to stand on the pedals. Ask yourself why your lungs don't hold more air and perhaps think about how you should have sprung for the more expensive bike. Keep pedaling and hope a foul diesel truck doesn't pass you. Finally crest the hill and take in the magnificent view as you cruise downhill.

Take a break at the picnic area or enjoy cruising downhill. Beware of the cattle guard about 0.5 mile downhill, and take the alternate route. Savor your downhill because it will only last about 1 mile. Then climb the first of three much easier summits with some sporadic downhill sections. The last steep downhill takes you past the final dam at 40 miles per hour and the turnoff for Lory State Park (see Trips 9 and 10 for ideas if you want to take an all-day adventure detour), or turn around and reverse the ride.

If you continue, you have another 2 miles to go once you pass the north end of the reservoir, until you turn right (east) and climb the double hills of Bingham Hill Road to begin your return route. It is another 0.7 mile to the top of this significant climb. Maintain your speed on the downhill to make it over the second hill. Turn right (south) on Overland Trail Road and ride the easy rolling hills back to the stadium and your vehicle.

TRIP 9 Arthur's Rock Trail

Distance	3.4 miles, Loop and out-and-back options
Difficulty	Moderate
Elevation Gain	1280 feet (starting at 5500 feet)
Trail Use	Option for kids, leashed dogs OK
Agency	Lory State Park
Map	*Lory State Park*
Facilities	Restrooms at trailhead, backcountry campsites

HIGHLIGHTS The most popular trail in the park is a moderate climb to the bottom of the sky on top of the rugged, rocky ridgeline that is the western backdrop of Lory State Park. It is a relatively short hike with great viewpoints all the way, so shorter pieces of the hike can be very enjoyable and easily negotiated with kids of all ages. The final mile features switchbacks, and the summit requires a short, steep, rocky scramble, providing a good artery-clearing workout. Several trails go to the summit; I cover the most popular, short trail first and then some alternate trails afterward.

DIRECTIONS From Interstate 25, take the Prospect Road exit west. Take Prospect Road west, turn right (north) on Overland Trail Road to Bingham Hill Road, and turn west. Turn next left (south) at the next T-junction, turn right (west) at the next intersection, and follow the road to the turnoff for Lory State Park on the left where the paved road ends. Drive to the end of the road to the southernmost parking lot in Lory.

This is the shortest, and therefore, easiest route to the top, though it is steep. It is also the busiest trail in the park. The trail begins on the west side of the parking lot. Be aware that the restroom next to the parking lot is the only one you will encounter. This parking lot is also the departure point for trails going east to the cool water of the reservoir and south to Horsetooth Mountain Park, as well as the East and West Valley Trails that go back to the north. A display at the trailhead includes an informative overview of the flora and fauna you might encounter and people-eating creatures like mountain lions that you are unlikely to ever see. It includes hints on how to protect yourself from the asocial lions that generally prefer to feast on less contentious and tastier critters than *Homo sapiens*. Ticks aren't mentioned but are generally the only creatures that will really bother you.

Walk due west from the parking lot, passing the restroom and kiosk. When you reach the south terminus of the West Valley Trail in about 50 yards on the right (north), bear left (west). The trail enters a small arroyo that features a picturesque babbling brook and seasonal frogs. It winds through a rocky beginning that tests slick-soled footwear as it climbs in and around the rocks that can be wet in the spring and frosty in the late fall. After

> **Great for Kids**
>
> If you want an easy family outing for small children, linger along the way and enjoy the brook and abundant spring and early summer wildflowers or fall colors. Stop at the waterfall; then climb the short, steeper hill that switchbacks up, offers a view of the reservoir, and goes over the waterfall on a narrow, rocky section of trail. The Mill Creek Trail then veers to the southwest to a beautiful meadow and prominent rock outcrop before returning to the parking lot.

approximately 0.25 mile the trail turns sharply to the south and then east and switchbacks more steeply uphill. If you continue straight, you will see a pretty waterfall in the spring or early summer.

When you reach the meadow, you will see a trail that goes north as a very steep alternate route toward the visible Arthur's Rock—not a good option for small children. The standard trail turns left, switchbacks, and then crosses the south edge of the meadow, leveling before beginning the next climb. On the left (south) side the Mill Creek Link Trail heading into Horsetooth Mountain Park intersects your route. It is a nice easy alternate loop back to the southeast across the adjoining

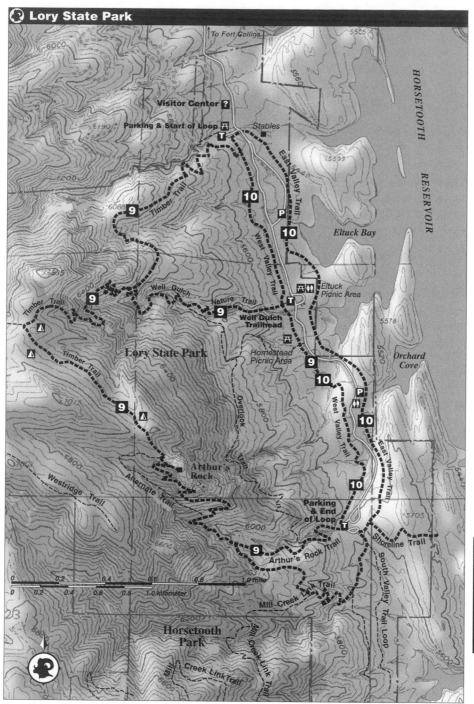

Lory State Park

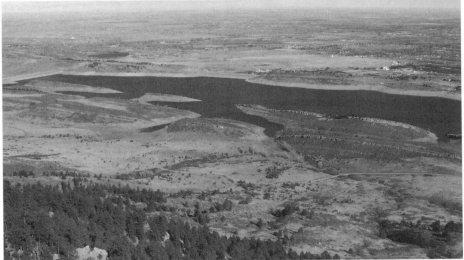

Joe Grim

The north end of Horsetooth Reservoir from the top of Arthur's Rock

meadow. It crests at the top of the short hill at the intersection. Turn left (southeast) and return to the parking lot, enjoying nice views to the south across the expansive meadows and rolling hills that lead to Horsetooth Mountain Park.

At the junction with Mill Creek Link Trail, the Arthur's Rock Trail continues straight west and climbs a little more before leveling. The trees are a nice, shady break spot. The trail narrows, and the thick tree cover can be a welcome break on a hot day. After about 0.25 mile from the junction with Mill Creek Link Trail the trail turns north, crosses the usually dry drainage, and starts to climb in earnest—beginning the steepest part of the hike. As the trail climbs it also opens up to the sun and the views. On the left (west) side of the trail is the steep, shortcut to the rock for those who want to make their hearts race and test their quad and calf muscles. The standard route goes through several sweeping switchbacks as the steepness increases. You top the first ridge in another 0.25 mile, reaching a 180-degree viewpoint from the large rock

to the right (east) from the trail, a popular turnaround for many.

From here it is another 0.5 mile to the top up the steep, rocky path that climbs into the trees and then switchbacks to the north and east until it reaches the intersection with the Timber Trail. Bear straight/right and downhill to find and mount the final scramble to the summit that is actually on the left after a short downhill. The final 25 yards of rock scrambling requires some nonslip shoes and a bit of handiwork and good lungs. At the top of the chute turn left (north), west, and then northwest to reach the actual summit rock. Enjoy the 360-degree panorama that includes all of Fort Collins and its surroundings and north to the Wyoming border. There's even an unimpressive view of Horsetooth Rock on the southwest distant ridgeline.

Timber Trail & Well Gulch Nature Trail Loop

After climbing Arthur's Rock, you can enjoy a nice moderate-plus loop hike, with or without a car shuttle, by continuing north on the Timber Trail to its intersection with the Well Gulch Nature Trail. Coming down from the summit, turn right (north), then right (north) again at the trail intersection, and climb up a short hill before leveling out. Then descend on a wide double-track trail. Pass a small meadow, enter tree cover, and then climb again to the Westridge Trail intersection. The Westridge Trail goes left (west-southwest), while the Timber Trail goes downhill to the right (north) and then northeast, where you will see a sign for campsites.

The Timber Trail continues east-southeast, switchbacking downhill, getting steeper as it goes along, offering nice views, and then narrowing into a gulley that can be wet. It veers to the northeast and opens up to a nice 180-degree view

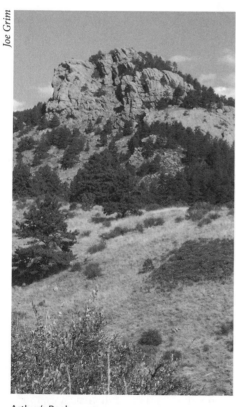

Joe Grim

Arthur's Rock

of the state park, reservoir, and points beyond. It turns south and east, jumps a few rocks, levels a bit, and then climbs as it reenters tree cover, which is welcome on hot, sunny days. It switchbacks downhill and ends up going northeast for at least 0.25 mile, traveling out into the open and more steeply down and then switchbacks on a steep slope where it is easy to end up off-trail—watch your feet closely to make sure you aren't hopping over rocks into closed trail sections. Also look out for poison ivy. The trail continues to switchback until it levels and intersects with the Well Gulch Nature Trail. The Timber Trail goes straight east and then turns north to the Timber Group Picnic Area. It will climb up gradually to a nice viewpoint and then descend slowly for more than 1 mile.

Bear right and follow the Well Gulch Nature Trail that switchbacks west and then south before turning east where it winds its way east through a small, rock-lined arroyo for about 0.5 mile east where it will intersect the park road and the West Valley Trail. Turn right (south) on the West Valley Trail for 1 mile and climb back up to where you started the hike.

Timber Trail

Another longer variation for climbing Arthur's Rock, with far fewer people, is to start at the Timber Group Picnic Area and take the Timber Trail south to the Well Gulch Nature and Westridge trails. Be careful to not mistakenly take the West Valley Trail that goes east and then south from the picnic area. Once you climb the steep stretch from the picnic area onto the Timber Trail, it is a gently climbing trail with great views of the reservoir and hogback. Since it is completely exposed to the sun, it is better to enjoy the trail before the heat of midday. When you reach Well Gulch in about 1 mile,

Fort Collins Area

Great for Kids

The Timber Trail is a very pleasant and easy out-and-back family hike with low population density. Just turn around when you reach the Well Gulch intersection. You could also continue down the Well Gulch Nature Trail and then take the West Valley Trail back to the picnic area.

---

turn right (west) and take the Westridge Trail south to the summit. You enter tree cover in a little less than 0.5 mile from the Well Gulch intersection, but the steep uphill warms you until you take a water and snack break.

The Well Gulch Trail is another possible starting point for a longer, less pop-ulous climb of Arthur's Rock or is a treat as a short family jaunt, especially in the spring and fall, to see wildflowers and changing colors, respectively. In the spring there are often a few frogs in the small stream that dries up later in the year. The beginning of the trail twists uphill through the rocky arroyo but the first 0.5 mile is an easy climb if you go slowly. The trail wanders over rocks, through nice tree cover, and across a small meadow. It eventually breaks into the open and goes more steeply uphill to the north to intersect with the Westridge and Timber trails. The latter takes you to the Arthur's Rock summit. From the Well Gulch it is a steep climb to the ridge top.

TRIP 10 East & West Valley Trails

see map on p. 103

Distance	7.0 miles, Loop
Difficulty	Easy
Elevation Gain	300 feet (starting at 5200 feet)
Trail Use	Mountain biking, running (occasionally snowshoeing and cross-country skiing), leashed dogs OK
Agency	Lory State Park
Map	*Lory State Park*
Facilities	Restrooms at both trailheads

HIGHLIGHTS Easy, rolling, gradually climbing trails on both sides of the pretty valley that is the eastern edge of Lory State Park. Enjoy the panorama of the hogback rocks on the east, the Arthur's Rock foothills ridgeline on the west, and all of the high-desert foothills flora and fauna in-between. This trail can be enjoyed year-round with appropriate clothing.

DIRECTIONS From Interstate 25 take the Prospect Road exit west. Take Prospect Road west, turn right (north) on Overland Trail Road to Bingham Hill Road, and turn west. Turn left at the next T-intersection and right (west) at the next intersection, and follow the road to the turnoff for Lory State Park on the left where the paved road ends.

These trails run parallel to each other on the east and west edges of the valley floor. They form a nice loop together or can be used independently for same-side out-and-back treks. You can start your adventure from either the north or south end of the park. If you want to drive less, take the first right just past the visitors center into the Timber Group Picnic Area and Park. The West Valley Trail starts with a short uphill section that goes south. Be careful not to accidentally end up on the Timber Trail that goes more steeply uphill to the southwest. You also pass the Well Gulch Nature Trail as you travel south and a nice picnic area for a snack or water break.

When you reach the high point, you are at the south end of the park road and can take a restroom or water break, cross

the parking lot to the east, and take the East Valley Trail back to your starting point. You will pass a picnic area and restrooms near the Well Gulch Nature Trail. You can also detour to the bay areas for picnic or snack breaks with water views.

TRIP 11 Eagle's Nest Natural Area

Distance	Up to 5.0 miles, Semiloop
Difficulty	Easy
Elevation Gain	200 feet (starting at 6000 feet)
Trail Use	Running, horsing around, option for kids, leashed dogs OK
Agency	Larimer County
Map	*Larimer County*
Facilities	Restrooms at trailhead

HIGHLIGHTS This area makes up in beauty what it lacks in size—towering rock formations, access to the north fork of the Poudre River, a pretty riparian bottom land, an easy rolling trail, and sweeping views almost all the way to Wyoming. The trail has no shade and so is best on cool days or with an early start on hot ones. The area features two loops (the Three-Bar and the OT trails) connected in a figure-eight. The trails are named after former ranching brands. The sweeping views of the soaring rock formations that hide the eagle's nest and the sparkling trickle that is the north fork of the Poudre River make this a worthwhile, hilly trek.

DIRECTIONS From the Denver or Fort Collins areas, take State Highway 287 north to Livermore and turn left (west) past the Forks store, turn left (southwest) 0.25 mile from Highway 287; and look out for the sign on the right that points out the dirt road on the left. Drive 1 mile uphill to the parking area.

The only restroom is in the parking lot. Hiking both loops adds up to approximately 5 miles. The Three-Bar Trail loop, which you reach first, rolls away along the foothills and features sweeping views to the north and east. At the trailhead, either proceed straight downhill north on the road for the first loop, or bear left (west), which is what I recommend for somewhat better out-and-back scenery. You have outstanding 180-degree views from the outset. This lovely wildflower stroll roller coasters along to a nice view of Eagle's Nest Rock. The trail then takes a bit of a plunge downhill, goes through

a livestock fence, and continues down to the bottom of the drainage.

At the intersection with a ranch road, approximately 1 mile out, you will see a sign saying that there is no public access to the road, either east or west. Cross the drainage and go north uphill to another road crossing; the west is not accessible, but the Three-Bar Trail loop continues to the right (east). Look south and enjoy the band of cliffs, several folds of rock climbing the ridge. In another 0.25 mile you reach the second road crossing. The trail descends past a metal trail marker and drops into a pretty draw at around 1.5 miles. Pass through two more stock

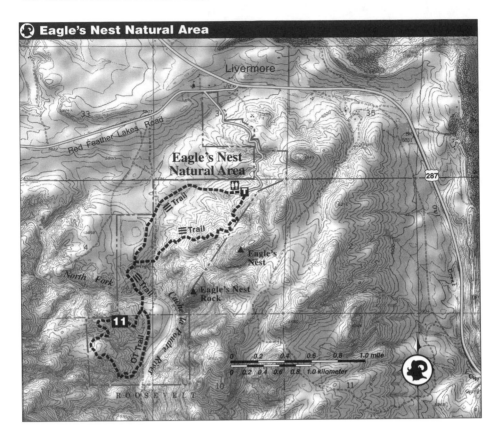

Eagle's Nest Natural Area

fences in the next 0.3 mile before reaching the river crossing and the OT Trail. When you reach the bottom of the hill, go left toward a small opening in the fence that leads into a grassy open meadow that can be used for picnics (but is usually closed from February 1 through July 15 because of the golden eagle's nesting area). If that's closed, veer to the right side of the bridge next to the river, and take a water or snack break while sitting on a friendly fallen tree.

If you don't want a break and want to walk another 2 miles before returning, continue straight past the metal OT Trail marker and cross the river bridge. Go uphill about 100 yards to reach the beginning of the OT Trail loop, next to another metal OT Trail post. I suggest bearing right (north) uphill, where the

> **Great for Kids**
>
> The area where the trail crosses the Poudre River is a good turnaround point for people with small children or who are looking for an easier journey. You can picnic along the river, and enjoy the view of the cliffs.

nonstop views begin in about 200 yards. The riparian river valley opens to the west, and cliffs soar on the south, and a tumble of foothills parapets to the north. After rounding a corner of the loop you see another cactus-speckled arroyo. The trail then rolls across the hills, with ever changing, highly satisfying scenery as the beautiful riparian river valley opens up before you. You can see some fire-scorched trees in the distance. There is a

0.5-mile downhill section that ends with some short switchbacks.

At the bottom of the hill you intersect a ranch road inaccessible to the public; take a sharp left and begin your return trek. The next flat mile is surrounded by pastureland, and you might see some longhorn steers grazing; don't excite the bulls. Cross back over the river bridge and go back uphill to the Three-Bar Trail loop, the way you came. Approximately 0.25 mile uphill from the first livestock fence, you reach a ranch road. Turn left at the metal trail post to take the other side of the Three-Bar Trail loop back to the parking area if you want some variety. Somewhat less steep than the other side of the loop, it is a two-track dirt road. If you look carefully, you can see Red Mountain just over the top; doing its Monument Valley imitation. The 1-mile trek features a steeper section for the last 0.25 mile.

TRIP 12 Horsetooth Rock Trail

Distance	7.0 miles, Out-and-back
Difficulty	Moderate
Elevation Gain	1500 feet (starting at 5700 feet)
Trail Use	Mountain biking, running, option for kids, leashed dogs OK
Agency	Larimer County
Map	*Larimer County Parks, Horsetooth Mountain Park*
Facilities	Restrooms and picnic area at trailhead
Note	This Larimer County fee area had a $6 fee at the time of this writing.

HIGHLIGHTS Hiking any part of this trail is a treat, and summiting the rock requires a rocky scramble that adds to the thrill. Just hiking to the base of the rock gives you nice views of the plains and reservoir and the impressive east side of Horsetooth Rock. The Audra Culver Trail option offers a view of Longs Peak's snowy summit.

DIRECTIONS The park is 30 minutes from Fort Collins. From South Taft Hill Road turn west onto County Road 38E. It travels west and then switchbacks south up to Horsetooth Reservoir. Bear left and continue south and then west around the reservoir. The road climbs over a ridge, drops into the South Inlet Bay area, and then turns west and uphill again where you see the parking lot on the right (north) side of the road.

When leaving the parking area, either go straight (north) on the Horsetooth Rock/Soderberg Trail or left (west) to the service road. The trail winds over and around the hills and provides more interesting scenery. The service road is as steep as but much wider than the trail. They meet back up at an intersection and continue north for 100 yards. At that point you once again have the option of using either the road or trail. The road switchbacks up the hill to the left (southwest), and the Horsetooth Rock/Soderberg Trail continues straight. The service road is a much easier route for mountain bikers because of its width and offers peak views that you won't see on the narrower, rockier trail. For variety, you could go up the road and down the Horsetooth

Rock Trail or vice versa; they intersect at the top of the ridge.

Go left (southwest) uphill on the service road, signed as the Audra Culver Trail and switchback steeply for the first 0.25 mile with nice views to the west and south. On a clear day you will see Longs Peak in the distance. The trail travels north along the top of a ridge, goes into a small arroyo, and then swings a little east. A route on the left, the actual, narrow Audra Culver Trail goes straight up toward the south summit, edging along the west side of the ridgeline. If you go straight on the service road, it switchbacks once before intersecting with the Horsetooth Rock Trail.

If you stayed on the Horsetooth Rock Trail at the first intersection, it continues straight and comes to an intersection with the Horsetooth Falls Trail in about 0.25 mile. Turn sharply left (west) uphill to continue on to the rock. Go straight if you want to take the short easy jaunt to

Horsetooth Falls (see the rest of the route description below). You can also continue past the turnoff for the falls and hike all the way north into Lory State Park. The Horsetooth Rock Trail narrows and becomes steep and rocky. The shade on this trail is very welcome on hot, sunny days. It climbs approximately 0.5 mile to the top of the ridge, where you will see the Audra Culver Trail on the left coming in from the south. Bear right and go slightly downhill through the trees. The trail levels briefly before climbing again, scrambling over some rocks and veering west as it does so. In a little more than a 0.25 mile you emerge from the trees to a good view of Horsetooth Rock.

At this point, the trail travels due west and you can either climb the half of the rock on the south or that on the north. The south side, though shorter, is a bit trickier and not frequently climbed. Only try the south side if you are a creative, confident rock scrambler. For the north half of Horsetooth Rock, the most frequently climbed "standard" trail, continue straight (north) as the trail traverses and edges through rocks, descends slightly, and then climbs steeply over more rocks and dirt before leveling for 25 yards, traversing south to north at the base of Horsetooth Rock. The steep dirt trail then climbs into the trees and veers steeply due west between trees next to the summit route. When the dirt trail dead-ends, the final summit scramble is on the left (south) side of the trail. Carefully pick your route to the top. There are about three safe variations that avoid drop-offs along the edge. Enjoy your well-earned arrival on the small summit and the spectacular view that goes with it.

Great for Kids

If you aren't planning to climb the rock, this is a good place to have a snack and water break and then turn around. The trail gets much steeper and rockier from here and requires intermittent rock scrambling that can be fun unless you have slippery shoes or aren't ready for the exertion and altitude gain. Most people are fine if they go at their own pace and aren't afraid of rock scrambling and heights. If anyone in your party has balance difficulties or a fear of heights, have them wait or turn around. Some people have fallen to their deaths or have been seriously injured on the standard, non-technical route.

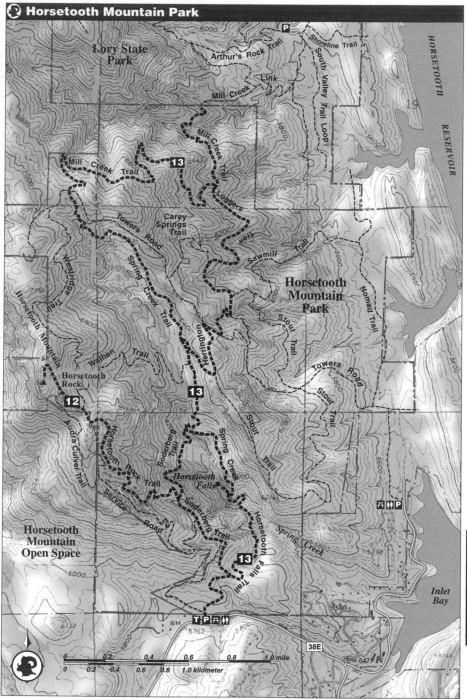

Horsetooth Mountain Park

Lory State Park

Arthur's Rock Trail

Shoreline Trail

South Valley Trail Loop

Link

Mill Creek

Mill Creek Trail

Mill Creek Trail

Loggers Trail

Mill Creek Trail

Carey Springs Trail

Towers Road

Sawmill Trail

Spring Creek Trail

Westridge Trail

Horsetooth Mountain

Walken Trail

Horsetooth Rock

Audra Culver Trail

Horsetooth Rock Trail

Soderberg Trail

Spring Creek Trail

Stout Trail

Herrington

Herrington

Stout Trail

Towers Road

Stout Trail

Nomad Trail

Horsetooth Mountain Park

Horsetooth Mountain Open Space

Service Road

Horsetooth Falls

Soderberg Trail

Horsetooth Falls Trail

Horsetooth Falls Trail

Spring Creek

Inlet Bay

HORSETOOTH RESERVOIR

BM 5762

38E

BM 547

0   0.2   0.4   0.6   0.8   1.0 mile
0   0.2   0.4   0.6   0.8   1.0 kilometer

TRIP 13 Horsetooth Falls & Connecting to Lory State Park

see map on p. 111

Distance	2.0 miles to Horsetooth Falls (Out-and-back), 9.0 miles if continuing to Lory State Park (Point-to-point)
Difficulty	Easy to Horsetooth Falls, moderate to Lory State Park
Elevation Gain	300 feet (starting at 5700 feet), another 300 feet if connecting to Lory State Park
Trail Use	Mountain biking, great for kids, leashed dogs OK
Agency	Larimer County
Map	*Larimer County Parks, Horsetooth Mountain Park, Lory State Park*
Facilities	Restrooms at the primary trailhead

HIGHLIGHTS This is an easy trek for families with small children. The first 0.25 mile is steep, but the trail mellows and offers a nice stroll to a pretty little waterfall (that sometimes dries up during the summer or fall if there is a drought). The foothills ecosystem and views are worth the trek even if the falls are a trickle.

DIRECTIONS The park is 30 minutes from Fort Collins. From South Taft Hill Road turn west onto County Road 38E. It travels west and then switchbacks south up to Horsetooth Reservoir. Bear left and continue south and then west around the reservoir. The road climbs over a ridge, drops into the South Inlet Bay area, and then turns west and uphill again where you will see the parking lot on the right (north) side of the road.

When leaving the parking area, either go straight (north) on the Horsetooth Rock/Soderberg Trail or left (west) to the service road. The trail winds over and around the hills and provides more interesting scenery. The service road is as steep as but much wider than the trail. They meet back up at an intersection and continue north for 100 yards. At that point you once again have the option of using either the road or trail. The road switchbacks up the hill to the left (southwest) and has been named the Audra Culver Trail; the Horsetooth Rock/Soderberg Trail continues straight. The Audra Culver Trail is a much easier route for mountain bikers because of its width and offers peak views that you won't see on the narrower, rockier trail. For variety, you could go up the Culver Trail and down the Horsetooth Rock Trail or vice versa; they intersect at the top of the ridge.

Go left (southwest) uphill on the Audra Culver Trail and switchback steeply for the first 0.25 mile with nice views to the west and south. On a clear day you see Longs Peak in the distance. The trail travels north along the top of a ridge, goes into a small arroyo, and then swings a little east. A route on the left goes straight up toward the south summit. If you go straight, it switchbacks once before intersecting with the Horsetooth Rock Trail.

The main trail continues straight and comes to an intersection with the Horsetooth Falls Trail in about 0.25 mile. When the Horsetooth Rock Trail turns left (west) uphill, go straight on the Soderberg/Horsetooth Falls Trail. The trail goes gradually downhill for approximately 0.5 mile; be sure to enjoy the foothill and plains views and the unique foothills fauna and flora. After the trail winds through a clump of trees and rocks, look for the spur trail that breaks off to the left (west) for the falls. After soaking in the scene, savor the mostly downhill journey back to the parking lot.

Connecting to Lory State Park

One of the most enjoyable jaunts in the area is a thru-hike with a car shuttle going from Horsetooth Mountain into Lory State Park or vice versa. It allows you to enjoy the "wilderness" in your backyard; you can make it a challenging day by including climbs of Horsetooth Rock and Arthur's Rock in Lory. You can easily mountain bike round-trip if you are an intermediate mountain biker and don't mind walking some steep advanced sections.

Where the spur trail to Horsetooth Falls branches off to the left (west), continue straight (north) uphill on the Soderberg Trail toward Lory State Park rather than turning left toward the falls, or enjoy the falls, and then continue on this trail. The trail switchbacks and gradually climbs to the top of the ridge, and intersects the Spring Creek Trail (0.6

mile from the falls), with nice views to the east. The trail roller coasters significantly as it travels north through comely meadows, and 0.8 mile from the falls passes the Wathen Trail that comes in from the left (west).

Approximately 1 mile north of the falls, you will see the Herrington Trail on the right (east) side of the trail. Use it to climb up on the ridge top. You can either stay on the ridgetop on the Towers Trail 3 miles, until it intersects the Mill Creek Trail in Lory State Park, or descend to the valley floor fairly quickly on the Herrington Trail. The Herrington Trail descends steeply to the Loggers Trail, which will also take you to the Mill Creek Trail in Lory State Park. The combination of the Herrington and Loggers trails will save you at least 0.5 mile on your jaunt to Lory Park because they are more direct. Once you reach the Mill Creek Trail, it is then a gentle roller-coaster climb over hills to the closest parking lot at the south end of Lory.

TRIP 14 Coyote Ridge Trail

Distance	3.0 to 7.0 miles, Out-and-back
Elevation Gain	500 feet (starting at 5500 feet)
Trail Use	Mountain biking, running, horseback riding, option for kids, leashed dogs OK
Difficulty	Moderate
Agency	Larimer County
Map	*Larimer County Parks, Fort Collins Natural Areas, Coyote Ridge Trail*
Facilities	Restrooms 0.75 mile west of trailhead parking lot

HIGHLIGHTS You will enjoy three geological walls of foothills rock formations stretching to the horizon and an enjoyable roller-coaster hike or bike up, along, and over the "hogback" ridgeline between rock formations and into a hidden grassy valley. The trail is most often used as a nice out-and-back but can also be used as a connector trail to the Rimrock and Blue Sky trails, for longer adventures. It is a pretty hogback and foothills area worthy of moderate out-and-back trips for novice hiking or intermediate to expert mountain biking.

DIRECTIONS This access point is 1 mile south of the Larimer County Landfill on the west side of Fort Collin's Taft Hill Road and Loveland's Wilson Road (Larimer County Road 19).

Fort Collins Area

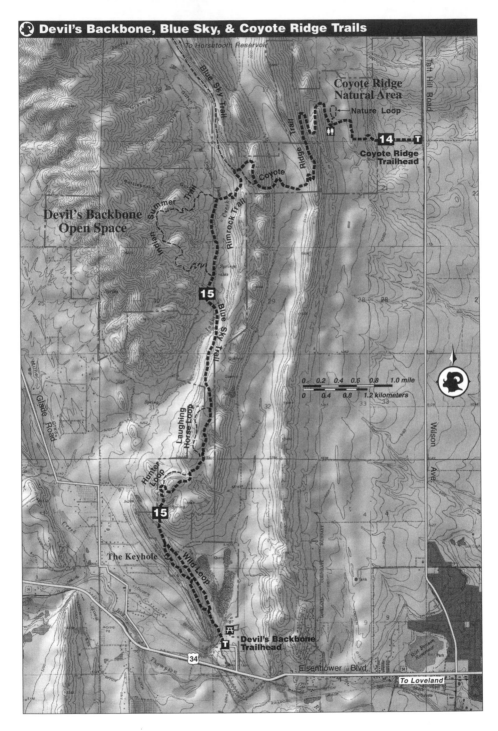

Devil's Backbone, Blue Sky, & Coyote Ridge Trails

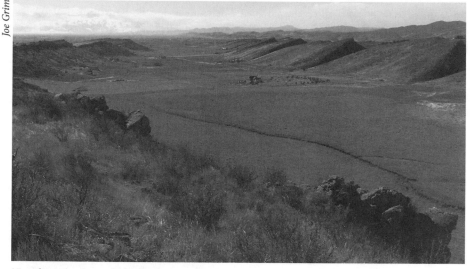

Joe Grim

View from the Coyote Ridge Trail

From the parking area the trail gradually and then more steeply climbs due west up the wide double-track trail (former road) up for 0.25 mile. It heads north along the first small ridge for 200 yards and then down steeply into the first valley interlude. From there the trail climbs 200 yards gradually up to a restroom (open year-round) and small visitors center (rarely open) that are 1 mile from the trailhead. It takes a sharp right, travels 0.25 mile north along the next foothill, sneaks to the left (west) around the hill, and then climbs more steeply for 0.25 mile southwest to an overlook with wildlife sign. You are now in the second unique foothills habitat, with a variety of cacti and wildflowers.

Climb north 0.25 mile and then south 0.25 mile to reach the top of the ridge. The trail then continues to the south 200 yards on the ridge before descending on stair steps at least 100 feet down into the hidden valley. After crossing the almost 0.5-mile meadow, the trail climbs through a notch in the next set of foothill to the top of its ridgeline where it intersects the Rimrock Trail. You have the

Great for Kids

The stretch after the overlook is steeper and longer so this might be a good turnaround point for groups with little people. If they have the energy, it is well worth the view to negotiate the next two long switchbacks that end up on top of the highest ridge in another 0.25 mile or so. The view from the ridgetop is splendid in every direction, especially to the west. This is a good place for a snack and water break and makes a nice round-trip of 3 miles.

choice of continuing south to the end of the Devil's Backbone Trail that terminates west of Loveland off of State Highway 34 going north to Horsetooth Mountain Park or Inlet Bay, or simply crossing the valley, enjoying a nice loop in the next foothill "garden" and returning to the trailhead after a solid moderate hike or bike workout. It is less than 0.5 mile of gently climbing trail to cross the valley and enter the next enchanted area. When it leaves the open fields of short prairie grass, the trail sneaks around the corner

Fort Collins Area

and climbs sharply and more narrowly uphill. About 300 yards ahead surmount this small hill and enjoy another nice view of the seemingly endless series of foothills in both directions. Before the uplift of the Rocky Mountains, they were the bottom of a vast inland sea.

These rugged, land-based waves of foothills can be thousands of feet high, on par with the Appalachian Mountains, and are covered with foothills zone vegetation. Surmounting the hill you can either go south and east on a loop to return from whence you came; or go downhill to the trail intersection and turn left, and go downhill south toward the Devil's Backbone Trail. If you go uphill to the right (north), you can trek all the way to South Inlet Bay and Horsetooth Mountain Park. The route toward the South Inlet Trailhead is easy mountain biking or hiking.

The route to Devil's Backbone is also very easy until you reach a series of steep steps that surmount a ridge. At that point the route becomes more challenging for the next 0.5 mile, as the trail narrows and becomes steep at both ends of the ridge, and many rocks appear. As you descend, you have excellent views of an arroyo and then the foothills to the west.

The steep section at the south end of the trail levels after your descent and offers some options. You can go straight up the slightly rolling valley, or bear right (west) and climb up toward the hogback where you can eventually enjoy a view through a rock window to the west. This loop is more hilly but also more scenically rewarding. The valley option is also pleasant and more mellow and wide, especially if you are on a bike.

see map on p. 114

TRIP 15 Devil's Backbone, Blue Sky, & Coyote Ridge Trails

Distance	Up to 16.0 miles, Point-to-point
Difficulty	Easy to moderate
Elevation Gain	400 feet (starting at 5500 feet)
Trail Use	Mountain biking, running, option for kids, leashed dogs OK
Agency	Larimer County
Map	*Larimer County Parks, Natural Areas, Blue Sky and Devil's Backbone Trail*
Facilities	Restrooms at trailhead

HIGHLIGHTS This very popular county trail west of the City of Loveland connects with the Coyote Ridge and Blue Sky trails. This trail weaves through the dramatic rock formations in the foothills known as the "hogback." A beautiful swath of land, Devil's Backbone Open Space was saved from development, and you can make your way north, all the way to Horsetooth Mountain Park west of Fort Collins in it. You can set up a one-way car shuttle with the Coyote Ridge access being the exit point short of South Inlet Bay and Horsetooth Mountain Park. That adventure is approximately 7 miles one-way and follows a pretty, moderate, roller-coaster trail. This trail can be used for nice out-and-back jaunts of any length; the eye candy makes it a treat regardless of your ambitions. Since there is virtually no shade on the trail, start early in the morning or early evening to avoid the blazing sun or use it in the spring, fall, or even winter when temperatures are cool.

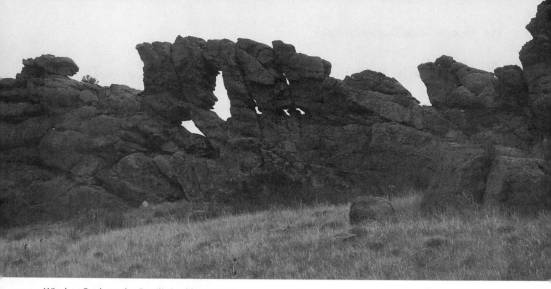

Window Rock on the Devil's Backbone Trail

DIRECTIONS From Loveland take U.S. Highway 34 west of Loveland to just past mile marker 88 (4 miles west of a Kmart). Turn right (north) onto Hidden Valley Drive just east of the old water tank. The trailhead is on your left. From Denver take Interstate 25 north to Exit 257B for U.S. Highway 34 and Loveland. Drive west through Loveland and follow directions from above. From Fort Collins take Taft Hill Road south from Fort Collins to U.S. Highway 34 (Eisenhower) and turn right (west). Proceed west on U.S. Highway 34 and follow directions from Loveland above.

The trail goes north and then west across a drainage and uphill before climbing gradually in a northerly direction. After approximately 0.5 mile the trail splits with a higher loop going left (west) up to the ridgeline for a view of the foothills through a rock window to the west. This loop is closed for part of each year because it is a nesting area for birds of prey. The trails join up again in about 1 mile. You are then traveling in a broad valley with nice rock formations on both the east and west ridgelines framing the scene. The trail rolls gently for the first mile and then crosses the drainage and climbs more steeply.

The trail up to this point is easy for biking; once it climbs onto the east ridge, however, it becomes an intermediate trail with some very rocky, steep, and narrow sections, which are great for hiking but more challenging for biking. Once you reach the top of the ridge, the trail levels and the views are a treat in every direction. Over the next 0.5 mile the trail descends gradually, evolving into steps, forcing most bikers to dismount. The trail rolls in the valley until it morphs into the Blue Sky Trail. As mentioned, the Blue Sky Trail will take you to South Inlet Bay at Horesetooth Reservoir, west of Fort Collins.

Great for Kids

Although the window rock view is worth the climb, it is also a good turnaround point for families with small children; after this point the trail switchbacks downhill for 0.5 mile, narrows, and gets steep and rocky as it climbs uphill.

TRIP 16 Bobcat Ridge Natural Area: Valley Loop Trail

Distance	Up to 4.5 miles, Loop
Difficulty	Easy
Elevation Gain	200 feet (starting at 5500 feet)
Trail Use	Mountain biking, running, horseback riding, option for kids, leashed dogs OK
Agency	City of Fort Collins
Map	*City of Fort Collins, Bobcat Ridge Natural Area*
Facilities	Restrooms and picnic area at trailhead
Note	Dogs are not permitted.

HIGHLIGHTS One of the most recent additions to the Fort Collins natural areas system, this superb slice of foothills southwest of Horsetooth Mountain Park near Masonville almost makes you feel like you are in the red rock canyon country of Utah. The soaring cliffs and foothills, pretty rolling terrain, and quiet invite reverie. Arrive early if you want solitude. It is also sun drenched with little shade and so is not a good midday summer hike but is ideal for spring and fall. It offers easy mountain biking too at least until you reach the eroded sections where the rocks pop out. The recently opened Ginny Trail loop is an advanced mountain biking adventure that is steep and rocky (see Trip 17).

DIRECTIONS Take County Road 38E to the southwest side of Horsetooth Reservoir; continue uphill past Horsetooth Mountain Park and then downhill to Masonville. Turn left on County Road 27 and then right (west) on County Road 32 in a little more than 0.5 mile.

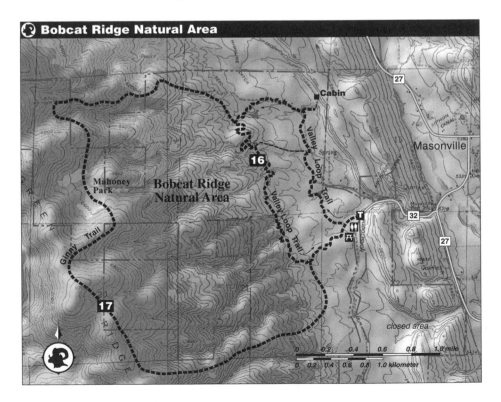

The 4.5-mile Valley Loop Trail is an easy, gently rolling trail that includes a possible side ramble to a historic cabin. It is much flatter for a longer distance if you go counterclockwise. If you want to start on the hilly section, turn left (south for a clockwise loop) after the picnic area at the sign that reads HORSES. If you want an easy out-and-back trip good for small children or less ambitious adventures, head right (north) to go in a counterclockwise direction. The trail travels north with nice views of the hogback formation and distant foothills and rolls through a couple of drainages on small footbridges. After approximately 1 mile you reach the first significant hill. Go left uphill for the loop; go right (northeast) on a side trail to see the historic cabin that was probably a ranch bunkhouse.

The trail, continuing on the loop, goes into the hills section and then rolls along the west side of the valley. Stay on the trail and off the roads the trail crosses. The trail rolls as it climbs higher and

> **Great for Kids**
>
> The ranch ruins detour is only a 0.25-mile round-trip and worth it since the city has provided excellent signage for self-guided tours. Going out-and-back to the cabin avoids any significant hills and is an easy 2-mile jaunt that could be followed by a picnic. The cabin is surrounded by old ranching equipment, the red rock and hogback views are excellent, and you'll even see an old well and a water pump.

higher and gives you ever better views of the valley and the beautiful foothills surroundings. After another 0.75 mile you can enjoy some shady spots for a water or snack break. There are also some excellent photo opportunities to the south. The trail plunges and climbs gently the entire way until it reaches the south end of the valley and goes gradually downhill back to the picnic and parking area.

TRIP 17 Bobcat Ridge Natural Area: Ginny Trail

Distance	Up to 6.0 miles, Loop or Out-and-back
Difficulty	Moderate hike, challenging mountain bike
Elevation Gain	1500 feet (starting at 5500 feet)
Trail Use	Option for kids, mountain biking, leashed dogs OK
Agency	City of Fort Collins
Map	*City of Fort Collins, Bobcat Ridge Natural Area*
Facilities	Restrooms and picnic area at trailhead
Note	Dogs are not permitted. Bikers can only travel uphill on the Powerline Trail segment, which means that mountain bikers wanting to complete the entire loop will need to do so in a counterclockwise direction.

HIGHLIGHTS One of the most recent additions to the Fort Collins natural areas system, the Bobcat Ridge Natural Area is a superb slice of foothills southwest of Horsetooth Mountain Park near Masonville that almost makes you feel like you are in the red rock canyon country of Utah. The soaring cliffs and foothills, pretty rolling terrain, and quiet invite reverie. Arrive early if you want solitude. It is also sun drenched with little shade and so is not a good midday summer hike but is ideal for cooler spring and fall days. It offers easy mountain biking too—at least until you reach the eroded sections where the rocks protrude. The recently opened Ginny Trail is a moderate hike and challenging mountain biking adventure that features steep switchbacks and lots of boulders. It could also be called the "Bobcat Ridge Fire Trail" because its journey onto the higher slopes is through the middle of the area scorched by an intense fire that burned 70 percent of the forested portion of Bobcat Ridge Natural Area in 2000. The plant life is recovering, but the experience is visceral since visitors can still smell the ashes. The stark scenery is dramatic and offers a transitional sort of beauty that reminds us that the natural world is one of constant change. The trail offers commanding views of the red rock cliffs, the west face of Horsetooth Rock, and the foothills and plains stretching out to the horizon.

DIRECTIONS Take County Road 38E to the southwest side of Horsetooth Reservoir; continue uphill past Horsetooth Mountain Park and then downhill to Masonville. Turn left on County Road 27 in Masonville, and then right (west) on County Road 32 in a little more than 0.5 mile.

You can only access the Ginny Trail by using the Valley Loop Trail as a connector. For the shortest and most direct route, go straight (southwest) from the parking area and then bear left past the picnic area, turning left where you see the horse sign. It's an easy climb for the first 0.7 mile, gaining 100 feet to the beginning of the Ginny Trail, which you will see uphill on the left. If you just want an out-and-back hike, you can then venture as far and as high as you wish on the Ginny Trail before reversing course to the trailhead.

Once you reach the Ginny Trail the fun begins. You will climb steeply, going fairly straight up a small ridge for the first 0.25 mile, and then switchbacking, gaining approximately 250 feet on the switchbacks in the first 0.6 mile. After 0.6 mile the trail levels for 0.25 mile. Enjoy the break because the next 0.6 mile is one of the steepest sections. The scenic, fire-ravaged scenery is unique and dramatic as you clamber over ridge after ridge. You start climbing again around 0.8 mile from the start of the Ginny Trail. Over the next 0.7 mile you climb around 500 feet to reach near 1.5 miles (approximately 2.2 miles from the parking area).

Great for Kids

The first mile of this trail combination is an easy out-and-back for small children or short outings. You will reach the Ginny Trail after a gradual climb of 0.7 mile on the south portion of the Valley Loop Trail. Once you reach the Ginny Trail, slowly follow the switchbacks as they wend through the burn area. The charred trees provide a stark contrast to the usually blue sky and colorful surroundings. The first 0.3 mile climbs and steepens as you gain another 150 feet. You will be startled by the outstanding panorama to the south this extra elevation affords. Have a water break and reverse your course, enjoying the great views all the way back to the picnic area where you can have a snack or beverage break.

At that point you can catch your breath and savor an almost flat mile with spectacular views all around. As a crow flies, you will be approximately 1.5 miles from the beginning of the Ginny Trail, but you probably don't have wings to rely upon for the return, so plan on more than 3 miles back to the parking area. This is a good time to decide if you want to complete the loop, continuing north and descending to Powerline Road and then the north end of the Valley Loop Trail. It is roughly equidistant, but Powerline Road is a less challenging descent. You cannot, however, descend via Powerline Road on a bike because only uphill biking is permitted on that trail.

It is much flatter for a longer distance if you go counterclockwise, but it is also much farther to reach the Ginny Trail. The trail travels north with nice views of the hogback formation and distant foothills and rolls through a drainage on a small footbridge. After approximately 0.6 mile you reach the Powerline Road "trail," turn left, and go gradually uphill on the rolling trail for 0.5 mile. As the trail gets much steeper you will intersect the western side of the Valley Loop Trail. The Powerline Trail continues you straight uphill climbing approximately 150 feet going west rather quickly, as you pass the Valley Loop Trail first on the left and then on the right. The trail flattens temporarily before starting its steady climb of more than a mile to the summit. As the trail climbs higher and higher you will, of course, have ever improving views of the valley and the beautiful foothills surroundings.

TRIP 18 Crosier Mountain Trail

Distance	Up to 10.0 miles, Out-and-back
Difficulty	Moderate
Elevation Gain	2800 feet (starting at 6500 feet)
Trail Use	Leashed dogs OK
Agency	Canyon Lakes Ranger District, Roosevelt National Forest
Map	Trails Illustrated *Cache La Poudre & Big Thompson*

HIGHLIGHTS This beautiful foothills hike is in a montane transition zone between the lower foothills and the higher mountains. It offers great views of the Glen Haven Tributary of the Big Thompson Canyon, the destruction done by the 2000 Bobcat Fire, and the snow-capped peaks of Rocky Mountain National Park.

View of Estes Park and Rocky Mountain National Park from the Crosier Mountain summit

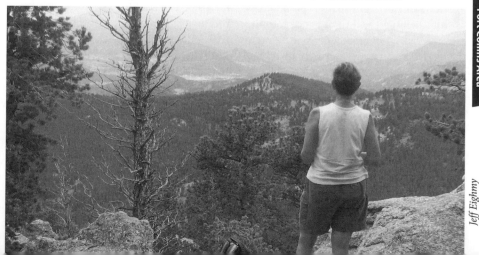

Jeff Eighmy

Fort Collins Area

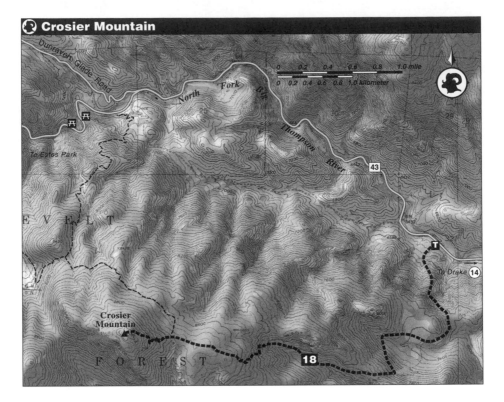

DIRECTIONS Take Interstate 25 or State Highway 287 to Loveland (from the Denver/Boulder areas) and then State Highway 34/Big Thompson Canyon Road west 14 miles to Drake. Turn right at Drake and drive 2.4 miles, watching carefully for the small turnout on the left side of the road. There is a barbed wire fence, wooden gate, and a U.S. Forest Service trailhead sign barely visible from the road about 100 feet uphill from the gate entrance. The two other accesses closer to Glen Haven require longer climbs to the summit. The one from Glen Haven is very popular with equestrians.

The trail starts gradually uphill across an open field and then winds into the evergreens. The trail steepens as it enters the trees and begins to switchback. It gets very steep for the next 0.5 mile. Just when you begin to wonder if attempting this trail was a mistake it levels out a bit in a forest primarily composed of tall fir trees. After you catch your breath for 0.25 mile, the trail starts to climb again steeply and rewards you with nice views of the canyon before reentering the trees. This is a good place for a few photos of the val-ley since the trail levels out nicely as you mount a ridgeline and travel below a large rock outcropping. As the trail goes back into the thicker trees, it steepens again but is less steep than it was previously. Signs of the Bobcat forest fire are visible on the highest cliff. That fire affected approximately 50 percent of the trees you can see but stops at a beautiful mountain meadow that stretches in front of you and is a good place for a break. This part of the hike can be wet if you are early or late in the season.

Nature's Domain

It is clear that nature owns this canyon and humans are visitors. In summer 2000 the Bobcat Fire burned out of control for more than a week before being subdued. In 1976 a flash flood scoured Glen Haven and the Big Thompson Canyon. The flood was caused by a spectacular electrical storm and downpour of 11 inches of rain that fell over the canyon and its tributaries in about four hours. The river rose 20 feet in a matter of minutes. Almost 200 people were killed as the flood carried away houses and cars and completely destroyed U.S. Highway 34. The force of the water carried debris out to Interstate 25. These chaotic ways of nature produce the dramatic scenery of cliffs and canyons you enjoy on this hike. If you do get caught in a sustained downpour and hear flash flood warnings, climb to the highest place you can in the canyon and stay there. Do not stay with your vehicle or try to outrun the flood.

After crossing the meadow, the trail is not well marked, but it runs southwest of the peak. The trail enters the trees again and climbs steadily toward the top of Crosier Mountain as it winds west and south next to a draw. The trail begins climbing steeply, turns west, switchbacks over a ridge, and then goes downhill into a gulch. You pass through a grove of aspen and around a ridge and into another more level open area. After winding around a ridge, you finally see Crosier's summit. When your crest the top of Crosier Mountain, you have a panoramic treat with views of the canyons, plains, and the snow-crested peaks of the Continental Divide.

TRIP 19 North Fork Trail

Distance	Up to 14.8 miles, Out-and-back
Difficulty	Easy to challenging, depending on distance
Elevation Gain	1800 feet (starting at 8000 feet)
Trail Use	Fishing, camping, leashed dogs OK
Agency	Canyon Lakes Ranger District, Roosevelt National Forest, Rocky Mountain National Park
Map	Trails Illustrated *Cache La Poudre & Big Thompson*, *Rocky Mountain National Park*
Facilities	Restrooms at trailhead, campsites

HIGHLIGHTS This lesser-known trail features peaceful varied topography in a riparian area. It winds through the forested broad canyon of the North Fork of the Big Thompson River with striking rock outcrops and meadows, then climbs through a backcountry campground and more broad meadows, and eventually ventures above treeline and into the stark beauty of the Lost Lake glacial cirque.

DIRECTIONS Take Interstate 25 or State Highway 287 to Loveland and then State Highway 34 (Big Thompson Canyon Road) west to State Highway 14 miles to Drake. This trail is at the end of Dunraven Glade Road, which is approximately 7 miles from Drake on the right side of County Road 43 if you are traveling west. It is another 2.4 miles down the well-maintained gravel road.

Fort Collins Area

Also known as the Dunraven and Lost Lake Trail, this trail goes through a narrow portion of the Comanche Peak Wilderness before entering Rocky Mountain National Park (RMNP) and is a great way to spend a day in a pretty mixed pine-and-aspen-forested valley. It is fairly level for a very long time after an initial rapid descent, making it a good choice for family excursions or mellow outings. If you want a challenging all-day round-trip, make the lake your goal, and you won't be disappointed with a trek through a dazzling array of sights and sounds: sparkling water, golden meadows, and chaotic ridgelines.

From the parking lot the well-marked trailhead has a display with a trail description and map. Proceed past the toilet facilities and up a slight hill at the outset. The trail then descends about 0.5 mile down to the North Fork of the Big Thompson River losing perhaps 150-plus feet of elevation. When you reach the bottom, you discover a wonderland of pretty brookside settings, tall pines, and a meandering babbling brook. The trail does have a few stream crossings on footbridges and there are a few very narrow, potentially wet spots in the first mile. The conditions can vary widely, depending on sun exposure; the first mile is likely to be dry in late spring because it is open to southern exposure.

After about 0.5 mile cross the stream on a footbridge, the first of many crossings. The trail then narrows and rolls as it parallels a horse camp across the stream from you. The trail then recrosses the stream and climbs uphill past a closed gate that notes the North Fork Trail and the horse camp. You then gradually climb and enter a high tree canopy; at which point you enjoy every variation of sunlight bouncing through the tress to dapple the trail at your feet. Though you are in a thick forest, the trees are tall and the branches high, so the ceiling is open and you have good views all the way.

Cross the stream a couple more times and leave the Comanche Peak Wilderness area to enter RMNP. Go through several golden meadows and then reach the backcountry campsites about 2 miles from the trailhead. There is a good bridge for a stream crossing to reach the sites. The trail climbs significantly before you enter RMNP but then levels again. You can decide when to turn around, depending on the conditions and your ambitions. Going all the way to Lost Lake means traveling below an impressive high ridge just beyond Lost Falls, almost 7.4 miles from the trailhead.

Other Options

This trailhead also offers access to the Signal Mountain Trail, which is at the top (north) side of the parking lot. This trail into the Comanche Peak Wilderness is a challenging, steep, rolling ridge trek to the top of Signal Mountain. The trail is above Dunraven Canyon and eventually allows hikers views of the Continental Divide, though there is fairly thick lodgepole pine tree cover for most of the route. It is a very long access route to the Pingree Park area mentioned in Chapter 3.

View from the North Fork Trail

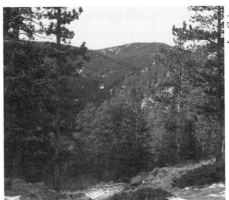

Joe Grim

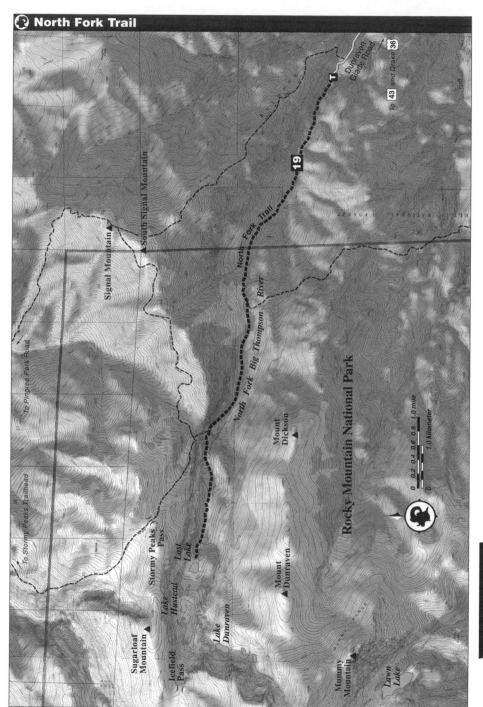

North Fork Trail

Chapter 6

Rocky Mountain National Park: East

Rocky Mountain National Park (RMNP) features some of the most spectacular scenery in North America. Each of three separate chapters cover the east, west, and south sides of the park. Most of it is within easy driving distance of the Denver, Boulder, and Fort Collins areas, making it a very popular destination for locals, as well as nature lovers from around the globe. The uplift of the ancient Rocky Mountains and the enormous glaciers that carved out characteristic U-shaped valleys and glacial moraines created the soaring cliffs and majestic peaks. The mystical beauty of this landscape can enthrall you for a lifetime. The park offers some of the best hiking and backpacking trails in North America. Backpacking does require inexpensive national park permits.

Visit during the week if you want to avoid the crush; it is still well worth the visit even if you can only visit on a weekend since most visitors don't venture more than a mile from their cars or the trailheads. You can avoid the weekend crowds by hiking the lesser-known trails that I describe in this and the following two chapters. A wide variety of ranger-led hikes, as well as nightly campfire talks during the summer months, are free to the public. Pick up the schedules at the visitors centers or campgrounds, call the visitors center, or visit the park's website, which is listed in Appendix 3, for details.

Biking in the park is possible only on the extensive paved and gravel roads. A very popular, but somewhat hazardous ride is Trail Ridge Road. It is a spectacular bike ride with steep drop-offs of several thousand feet and very narrow shoulders. It is not appropriate for beginners or children. It is also possible to bike one-way (west) on unpaved Fall River Road. Mountain bikers like to use gravel Fall River Road for the uphill to the visitors center and Trail Ridge Road for the downhill back to Estes Park. It is well worth starting at sunrise to avoid the wide motor homes that share the dizzying heights of the highest (12,000 feet) through-highway in the U.S.

Dogs are not allowed on the trails in Rocky Mountain National Park due to the millions of visitors. (Imagine the impact of millions of dogs.) They are allowed in campgrounds.

Don't feed the elk, moose, bears, mountain goats, deer, or birds any time of the year. They become addicted to treats and become pests with bad habits that sometimes have to be relocated or destroyed to protect humans. Don't approach any wild animals—it is against park rules and also very dangerous, especially if they have their young with them. Though they might look docile, they are wild animals

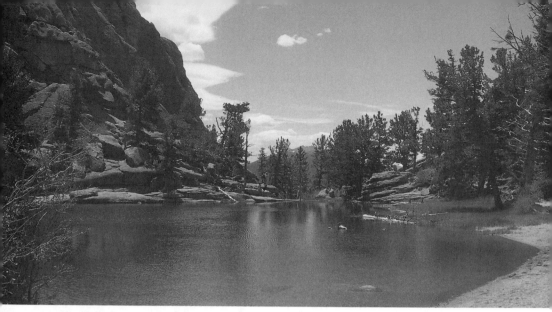

Sparkling Gem Lake at McGregor Ranch (Trip 1)

that have been known to pursue and even forcefully evict tourists from their turf. You will likely see elk herds on the east side of the Continental Divide and moose on the west. They sometimes wander into the town of Estes Park, much to the dismay of the town's residents. Hundreds of elk can be seen in the Moraine Park area in the fall during the mating season; their eerie, whistling mating call is a unique auditory nature experience. Although stopping along the park's narrow roads is frowned upon, it is hard not to gawk at these magnificent animals, and there is ample designated parking.

The east side of RMNP is 70 miles from Denver. Allow at least 2 hours to get to Estes Park from Denver or about 1½ hours from Boulder, depending on the route you choose. Plan for additional time to find the trailheads; plus, it is a scenic drive, so take your time and enjoy it. From Denver take Interstate 25 north and exit at the Loveland and Highway 34 exit. Take Highway 34 west through the spectacular Big Thompson Canyon. Alternatively, you may go through Lyons on Highway 7, past the southernmost section of the park, Wild Basin, on the way to Estes Park. From Boulder this alternate route can be accessed on State Highway 36; it intersects State Highway 34 in Estes Park. When you reach Estes Park on State Highway 34, continue to the third traffic light and you will see a sign for RMNP. Turn left at the sign and go up a hill, bear right at the stop sign, and then bear right at the intersection 0.5 mile after the next traffic light. You will see signs for the Beaver Meadows visitors center, which is worth a stop to see the overall map of the park, the fairly specific trail maps for areas such as Bear Lake, and a 3-D map graphically depicting the dramatic terrain you will be immersed in. You can also fill your water bottles there. A second visitors center at the Fall River Road entrance features a restaurant.

Moraine Park

This magnificent glacial moraine is where you will find two very popular trails—the Cub and Fern lakes trails. Moraine Park has a majestic setting, one of the most impressive in the park. The ever-changing mountain weather and light make it a magical place where large herds of elk roam freely, especially in the fall mating season. Many people know that this is *the* place to hear bull elks bugling in the fall, an eerie sound seemingly unworthy of such large masculine animals. If you want to enjoy the bugling without the crowds, come early, or snag a campsite on a full-moon weekend. Since it is relatively low (8100 feet) and stays relatively warm until the depths of winter, it's good for hiking early and late in the season. There is also a nice campground in Moraine Park open year-round.

Bear Lake

With easy accessibility, including for those in wheelchairs; a wide variety of trails; and a classic rocky mountain setting, the Bear Lake area is one of the most popular and populated areas in the park year-round. The Bear Lake area is high at 9475 feet, so visitors may have a little difficulty catching their breath if they charge uphill before becoming acclimatized. The throngs of summer can be avoided by getting a very early start. On weekends, especially by afternoon, the parking lot and the trails fill up. If you want to sleep in and have a late breakfast, plan to take the Bear Lake Shuttle; it stops in the parking lot across from Glacier Basin Campground and on Bear Lake Road to pick passengers up and is well marked with signs. Most people don't get far from the parking lot or Bear Lake, but enough do to make an early start a good idea. Remember to bring lots of warm clothing even if it is balmy in the flatlands. The mountains create their own climate, and it can be very cool and windy when it isn't at lower elevations. There are restrooms but there isn't any water.

Bear Lake is the starting point for a wide variety of trails; challenge yourself by attempting to climb 12,300-plus-foot Flattop Mountain or enjoy short and easy family trails. The Dream, Nymph, and Emerald lakes system is the easiest place to explore but very rewarding nonetheless, while the Flattop Trail is the entry point for more challenging terrain.

Glacier Gorge Trailhead

An entry point to one of the most magical parts of the park, Glacier Gorge Trailhead resembles the ethereal pictures of the Rocky Mountains painted by Albert Bierstadt in the late 19th century. Massive granite walls, waterfalls, cascading streams, and the majestic cliffs of Mt. Lady Washington and Longs Peak soar above, while views of the Mummy Range grace the horizon to the northeast. The first part of this trail is a very popular hiking destination; fortunately, the population thins out as you go deeper into the backcountry. Alberta Falls is good for beginners and family trips. The trails to Alberta Falls, the Loch, Mills Lake, Jewell Lake, and Black Lake all originate at this trailhead. You can also connect to the North Longs Peak Trail from the Glacier Gorge Trail.

Other Trails to Explore: Fall River Road

Spectacular Chapin, Chiquita, and Ypsilon mountains look daunting from Deer Ridge and Trail Ridge Road, but they are very climbable from their tame but steep, tundra-covered backsides. Although they are not described in detail in this book, you can reach the trailhead from Fall River Road and climb all three in a long day or just one while enjoying the panoramic view.

TRIP 1 McGregor Ranch

Distance	Up to 10.0 miles for the loop, 4 miles for out-and-back to Gem Lake
Difficulty	Easy to moderate
Elevation Gain	1129 feet (starting at 7728 feet)
Trail Use	Running, rock climbing, option for kids
Agency	Rocky Mountain National Park
Map	Trails Illustrated *Rocky Mountain National Park*
Facilities	Restrooms at trailhead
Note	Bikes are allowed on roads, not trails, in Rocky Mountain National Park.

HIGHLIGHTS The ranch is in a unique setting on the northeast edge of Estes Park. It is a working ranch with the dual backdrops of the rock climbers' paradise of lofty Lumpy Ridge on the north, and views of majestic Longs Peak and the Rocky Mountain National Park massif in the distance to the southwest and west. Most of the trails are easy and

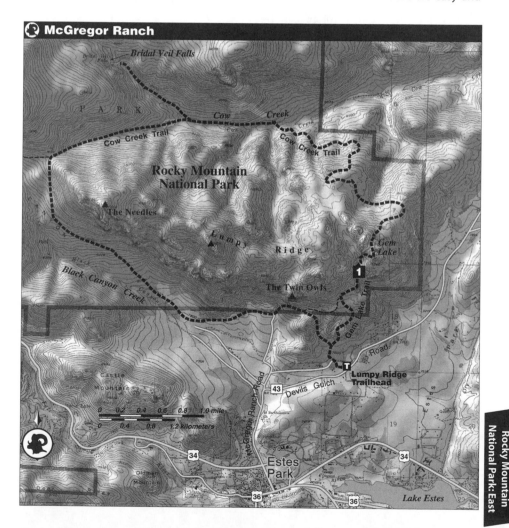

can be hiked year-round because of the ranch's relatively low elevation. Enjoy gorgeous meadows with grazing stock, soaring monolithic granite cliffs, and rolling easy to moderate trails with hidden lakes tucked away on the north side of the ridge. If you're daring and fleet of foot, you can watch the spectacle of lightning storms reaching across Estes Valley, as the usual afternoon parade of thunderstorms roll off the high mountain ridges, and you can run to shelter before they reach the ranch.

DIRECTIONS From State Highway 34 turn right at the first light in Estes Park, and go uphill past the Stanley Hotel. At the next intersection turn right on to Devil's Gulch/Glen Haven Road (County Road 43) northeast from Estes Park. There is now a large new parking lot on the north side of Devil's Gulch Road, 0.5 mile from the ranch's front gate. Many of the trails are sun drenched and can get quite warm in the midday sun, so getting an early start is a good idea.

Once you reach the parking lot, you have two choices. The very large loop that circles Lumpy Ridge can be a very nice all-day, moderate hike that visits part of the Cow Creek Trail in McGraw Ranch, and Gem Lake—the long way around. (There is no adequate parking at McGraw Ranch so this is the only recommended access to the Cow Creek Trail.) It is easier but just as enjoyable to savor smaller chunks of the loop by either going left (roughly northwest) or right (roughly east and then north). The route to the left is a much easier and more gradual, rolling climb than the straight uphill route to the right (east). If you don't want to see Gem Lake and would rather stay on the southwest side of Lumpy Ridge, the latter is the way to go; it's an enjoyable out-and-back trek that you can approach with a leisurely pace with nice views and no steep sections. If you want to see Gem Lake, go right (east) straight uphill; for this route see the latter part of this trail description.

Great for Kids

If you want an easy out-and-back trek, go to the left (west), the recommended route for families with young children. The trail travels uphill gradually from the parking lot, and actually then goes gradually downhill for the first 0.5 mile. At the bottom of the hill you cross the former, closed parking lot to get to the trailhead. It is back up a short hill. You will pass the Twin Owls Trail on the right (north) side of the trail on the way.

At the trailhead, go downhill to the left, uphill to the right is a rock climbers' side trail that goes straight and then veers north. Stay on the main trail, bear left, and go downhill to follow the gently rolling trail. Enjoy the views to the south and west and take photos as soon as you can before the afternoon thunderstorm clouds roll in and the sun travels to the west, making good pictures difficult. As you walk, study the rock faces to the right (north) side of the trail. You will likely see rock climbers dangling high and defying gravity on the granite ridges.

When the trail begins to climb steeply, enjoy a picnic and turn around unless you want to follow the trail as it evolves into a moderate, though shady climb through the captivating ponderosa pine forest. When your legs have had enough, reverse course and call it good.

You can imagine the vistas on Twin Owls while strolling below, but don't attempt the routes unless you are a skilled technical rock climber and have the necessary equipment with you—even the lower routes can be deceiving and deadly. Excellent guide services in Estes Park can safely teach you the necessary skills and accompany you on the climb. Pass through several gates, being sure to fasten them behind you to prevent cattle from roaming onto your return path. The trail rolls along for almost 1.5 miles before it enters trees and begins to climb in earnest.

In another 0.5 mile round the end of Lumpy Ridge and track around to the north side and the edge of Black Canyon, intersecting Cow Creek Trail in McGraw Ranch. You traverse the backside of the ridge on a narrower trail and enjoy obstructed views through thick tree cover and rock outcrops as the trail descends into the valley. Once you have accomplished that, you still face a moderate trek that ends with a nice rock garden, sweeping views, a steep uphill,

and then downhill back to the parking lot. Turn around and retrace your steps if you've had enough; if you're just getting warmed up, however, and don't hear or see thunderstorms, plunge ahead. Stop for a nice long break and study Gem Lake's unique rock-carved setting. The rest of the trail is a stroll through a granite sculpture garden that winds its way east and then southeast, gradually rolling over and around the east end of Lumpy Ridge. Don't take the trail that branches north and then east to McGraw Ranch. Once you have rounded the ridge, take the first trail that heads down to the new parking lot, or you will have a longer loop on the Twin Owls Trail back to the lot.

Shorter Route to Gem Lake

If your primary goal is to see lovely Gem Lake, then start up the right (east) trail from the parking lot and travel straight uphill. Though the trail starts very steep, it mellows considerably after the first 0.75 mile. The first mile features a magnificent rock garden that is worth the trip for even a short, strenuous out-and-back hike that

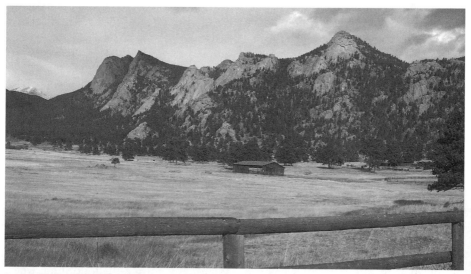

Lumpy Ridge in McGregor Ranch

doesn't include the whole trek to the pond. After the trail levels temporarily, it travels more northerly and rounds the east end of Lumpy Ridge as you climb lots of steep steps. In another long mile, you reach Gem Lake where you can enjoy a nice break before your return. Your total round-trip will be around 4 miles with a gain of 1000 feet. If you'd like to make the

10-mile loop from this end, continue on the trail and complete the loop by rounding the west end of Lumpy Ridge. As you travel into the thicker tree cover, you get glimpses of the McGraw Ranch valley 800 feet below. To complete the loop, you descend 800 feet into the valley and then climb back out at the other end from Black Canyon around 500 feet.

TRIP 2 Horseshoe Park

Distance	2.0 miles, Semiloop
Difficulty	Easy
Elevation Gain	100 feet (starting at 8600 feet)
Trail Use	Great for kids
Agency	Rocky Mountain National Park
Map	Trails Illustrated *Rocky Mountain National Park*
Note	Bikes are allowed on roads, not trails, in Rocky Mountain National Park.

HIGHLIGHTS This short and easy walk is at most a 2-mile round-trip suitable for families or someone out for a nice, easy workout. It can be turned into a more challenging trek by continuing up to Deer Mountain. Early in the season you will encounter a fair amount of moisture on the trail.

DIRECTIONS When you reach Estes Park on State Highway 34, continue to the third traffic light and you will see a sign for RMNP. Turn left at the sign and go up a hill, bear right at the stop sign, and then bear right at the intersection 0.5 mile after the next traffic light. You will see signs for the Beaver Meadows visitors center, which is worth a stop to see the overall map of the park, the fairly specific trail maps for areas such as Bear Lake, and a 3-D map graphically depicting the dramatic terrain you will be immersed in. You can also fill your water bottles there. A second visitors center at the Fall River Road entrance features a restaurant. From the Beaver Meadows entrance drive toward Trail Ridge Road and climb the long hill to the Deer Junction and the Deer Mountain trailhead. Just after Deer Junction turn right (north) toward Fall River Road. At the bottom of the hill, Horseshoe Park Trailhead parking lot is on the right (east). The trailhead is on the right back toward Deer Mountain.

From the Fall River entrance follow the signs toward Trail Ridge Road; it is closed in the winter, as is the western extension of Fall River Road. Pass the turnoff on the right (west) for Fall River Road; the trailhead is the next parking lot on the left (east) side of the road.

The trees on the trail are a colorful mixture of pine, fir, and aspen; the trail's

proximity to the road is not a problem because of the thick cover. The trail starts to climb gently after about 0.5 mile and never gets steep, leveling out several times along the way. Bear right at the trail intersection to go up to the closed Horseshoe Park Lodge. The trail levels and then heads down a slight downhill when you reach the group campground and old

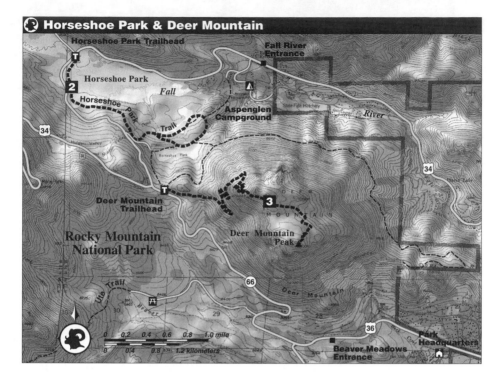

Horseshoe Park & Deer Mountain

lodge. There are picnic tables. The lodge is a good place to enjoy a snack, water, or photo break. Before turning around walk downhill into the beautiful meadow that gives the horseshoe-shaped park its name.

You can circle the meadow and walk up toward Deer Mountain or just turn around. If you go into the meadow and turn left, you will see the loop trail on the left. If you see it around the end of the hill (it will eventually intersect the trail you came in on), you can take it as an alternate route back to the parking lot. If it isn't obvious, retrace your steps to the trailhead.

TRIP 3 Deer Mountain

Distance	2.0 to 6.0 miles, Out-and-back
Difficulty	Easy to moderate
Elevation Gain	1075 feet (starting at 9908 feet)
Trail Use	Great for kids
Agency	Rocky Mountain National Park
Map	Trails Illustrated *Rocky Mountain National Park*
Note	Bikes are allowed on roads, not trails, in Rocky Mountain National Park.

HIGHLIGHTS The Continental Divide and Longs Peak are the magnificent backdrop for this trail when you fix your gaze on the southwest horizon. To the northwest is the Mummy

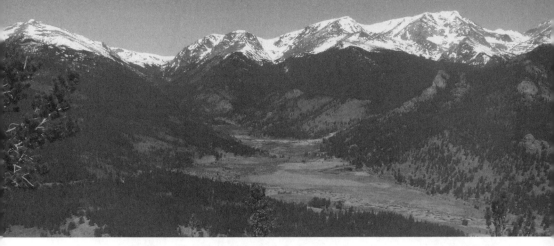

View from Deer Mountain of Chapin, Chiquita, and Ypsilon moutains   *Joe Grim*

Range with the soaring massif of Chapin, Chiquita, and Ypsilon mountains. Best of all, the views are immediate. Wander only 100 yards from the trailhead to enjoy the spectacle, making this ideal for flatland visitors and for families with young children looking for short excursions. Hiking all the way to the top is a nice moderate climb for more ambitious hikers.

DIRECTIONS When you reach Estes Park on State Highway 34, continue to the third traffic light and you will see a sign for RMNP. Turn left at the sign and go up a hill, bear right at the stop sign, and then bear right at the intersection 0.5 mile after the next traffic light. You will see signs for the visitors center, which is worth a stop to see the overall map of the park, the fairly specific trail maps for areas such as Bear Lake, and a 3-D map graphically depicting the dramatic terrain you will be immersed in. You can also fill your water bottles there. A second visitors center at the Fall River Road entrance features a restaurant. From park headquarters near the Beaver Meadows entrance, disregard the Bear Lake Road turnoff on the left and drive 4.5 miles to Deer Ridge Junction. There is parking on both sides of the road. From the Fall River entrance follow the signs toward Trail Ridge Road. Pass the turnoff on the right for Fall River Road. When you reach the intersection at the top of the hill, turn left (east) and park immediately at Deer Trail Junction and the trailhead for Deer Mountain.

The trail starts up some stone steps; slightly hidden from view on the left is a great view of the Chapin, Chiquita, and Ypsilon mountain massif. Find your way through the ponderosa pines and on to the rocks and dig out your camera to prepare for the upcoming magnificent views; in another 0.25 mile you'll have a superb view of Longs Peak and the Continental Divide. The trail climbs, goes downhill for a short stretch, turns east, and begins to climb more steeply. Enjoy the beautiful aspen, lodgepole pine, and limber pine trees as you climb the ridge, where there are some good viewpoints on the right. You'll likely see some chipmunks too. The view continues until you enter trees and the switchbacks begin after the first 0.5 mile. There is good shade from the hot sun on summer days if you didn't get up early, or chilly winds to keep you cool if it is spring or fall. Broad, gradual switchbacks are the heart of the climb. You gain a wide ridge around the 2-mile mark. In another 0.8 mile you come to the side trail on the right that takes you to the top where you will enjoy a superb panorama.

TRIP 4 Cub Lake

see map on p. 136

Distance	Up to 4.6 miles, Out-and-back
Difficulty	Easy
Elevation Gain	550 feet (starting at 8100 feet)
Agency	Rocky Mountain National Park
Map	Trails Illustrated *Rocky Mountain National Park*
Note	Bikes are allowed on roads, not trails, in Rocky Mountain National Park.

HIGHLIGHTS This trail is very popular year-round. In fall large herds of bugling elk are exceeded only by flocks of people there to hear them dueling for romance. The height of the elk bugling is in the beautiful fall season (mid-September through early October), which is also often warm but can feature a chilly breeze. The route can be hiked as a loop, with your return on the Fern Lake Trail, but you will end up 1 mile short of the Cub Lake Trailhead, with 1 mile of walking along the road to get back to your car at the Cub Lake Trailhead. To intersect the Fern Lake Trail, walk past Cub Lake and follow the trail as it climbs the ridgeline on the north side of the trail up about 200 feet to meet the Fern Lake Trail.

DIRECTIONS When you reach Estes Park on State Highway 34, continue to the third traffic light and you will see a sign for RMNP. Turn left at the sign and go up a hill, bear right at the stop sign, and then bear right at the intersection 0.5 mile after the next traffic light. You will see signs for the visitors center, which is worth a stop to see the overall map of the park, the fairly specific trail maps for areas such as Bear Lake, and a 3-D map graphically depicting the dramatic terrain you will be immersed in. You can also fill your water bottles there. A second visitors center at the Fall River Road entrance features a restaurant. After going through the Beaver Meadows entrance take the first left onto Bear Lake Road. After a hairpin S turn, pass the sign for Moraine Park, take the next right, and then turn left at the sign for the Cub Lake and Fern Lake trailheads. Continuing straight takes you into the Moraine Park Campground, which remains open in the winter.

The trail immediately crosses two streams on wooden bridges. The first mile or so borders the open expanses of Moraine Park and offers nice views back to the east and south and is the most likely section for elk or moose. Clamber over some very large rocks in about 0.5 mile. The trail rolls over more rock formations while bordering the willow-highlighted riparian area. The trail climbs gradually through colorful wetlands with a variety of eye candy—magnificent ponderosa pines, rock formations, reeds, willows, water, and distant peaks. Eventually the trail climbs more steeply (not for long though) under thicker tree cover to the edge of the lake. Once you reach the lake, climb over to Fern Lake for the return, veer south and hike through Hollowell Park to Bierstadt and Bear lakes, or simply return to the trailhead.

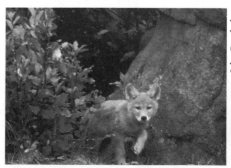

Coyote pup in Rocky Mountain National Park

John Bartholow

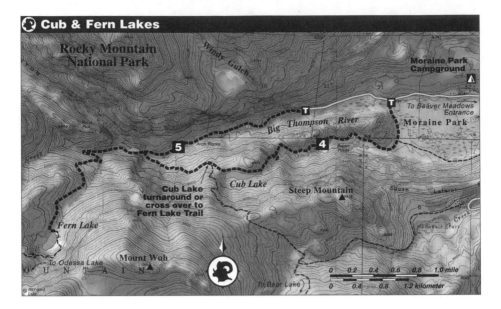

Cub & Fern Lakes

TRIP 5 Fern Lake

Distance	Up to 7.6 miles, Out-and-back
Difficulty	Moderate
Elevation Gain	1380 feet (starting at 8120 feet)
Trail Use	Option for kids
Agency	Rocky Mountain National Park
Map	Trails Illustrated *Rocky Mountain National Park*
Note	Bikes are allowed on roads, not trails, in Rocky Mountain National Park.

HIGHLIGHTS This trail can be used for a short, easy hike just to the featured lake or a major adventure by starting at Moraine Park and finishing at Bear Lake. If you do that, start early to avoid storms, and use a car shuttle or the park shuttle. You can also use this trailhead to climb all the way up to Odessa Lake another 500 feet in elevation and 0.6 mile beyond Fern Lake. That part of the trail is very steep and makes the trek a moderate to challenging hike if you then go all the way to or return from Bear Lake.

DIRECTIONS When you reach Estes Park on State Highway 34, continue to the third traffic light and you will see a sign for RMNP. Turn left at the sign and go up a hill, bear right at the stop sign, and then bear right at the intersection 0.5 mile after the next traffic light. You will see signs for the Beaver Meadows visitors center, which is worth a stop to see the overall map of the park, the fairly specific trail maps for areas such as Bear Lake, and a 3-D map graphically depicting the dramatic terrain you will be immersed in. You can also fill your water bottles there. A second visitors center at the Fall River Road entrance features a restaurant. After going through the main entrance take the first left onto Bear Lake Road. After a hairpin S turn, pass the sign for Moraine Park, take the next right, and turn left at the sign for the Cub and Fern lake trailheads. Continuing straight takes you into Moraine Park Campground, which remains open in the winter.

The trail covers terrain very similar to that of Cub Lake Trail. It starts as a very gradual climb and then steepens considerably, climbing out of the Moraine Park lowlands and surmounts a higher plateau to Fern Lake. From there, if you have the time and ambition, you can switchback high onto the ridge and gain spectacular views of the entire Moraine Park valley and climb up and over into the Glacier Gorge/Bear Lake drainage. It is one of the more spectacular jaunts you can take in the park without going up to the very highest reaches. You can also create a loop out of this and the Cub Lake Trail, which intersects this trail at approximately 1.8 miles and around 8500 feet. You climb another 1000 feet from this trail intersection to Fern Lake. The trail begins easy and rolling. At around the 0.5-mile mark you will reach a large monolithic rock. This can be your turnaround point (see sidebar.)

Great for Kids

If you're hiking with young children and want a very easy jaunt, this is a good, very short turnaround point, because the elevation gain to this point is negligible; the trail steepens, and climbs another 400 feet to the intersection with Cub Lake Trail. If your group feels up to hiking farther, continue to that intersection where there is a natural pool and footbridge that is a good picnic spot. After that intersection the trail gets much steeper and switchbacks up from the valley.

You have a commanding view of the Moraine Park valley on the way up before you enter thick tree cover. You then see two picturesque waterfalls, the second about 0.25 mile from the lake. Once you reach the lake, some impressive cliffs are visible high above, and you will likely see evidence of some very busy beavers.

TRIP 6 Mill Creek Basin

Distance	Up to 5.0 miles Cub Lake Overlook (out-and-back), 6.4 miles to Cub Lake Trailhead (point-to-point)
Difficulty	Easy to moderate
Elevation Gain	1000 feet (starting at 8200 feet)
Agency	Rocky Mountain National Park
Map	Trails Illustrated *Rocky Mountain National Park*
Facilities	Restroom at trailhead
Note	Bikes are allowed on roads, not trails, in Rocky Mountain National Park.

HIGHLIGHTS This is the next trailhead you come to on Bear Lake Road after Moraine Park. The park starts off as a magnificent high mountain meadow, ringed by ponderosa pines and aspens, with a pleasing view of the surrounding hills. It can also be used as a less busy alternate route to Cub Lake or to access Bierstadt or Bear lakes. The fairly gradual climb can be turned into an out-and-back trek of any length and offers a very nice view of Cub Lake from on high if you don't want to go the entire 6.5 miles past the lake and to the Cub Lake Trailhead.

DIRECTIONS When you reach Estes Park on State Highway 34, continue to the third traffic light and you will see a sign for RMNP. Turn left at the sign and go up a hill, bear right at the stop sign, and then bear right at the intersection 0.5 mile after the next traffic light.

You will see signs for the Beaver Meadows visitors center, which is worth a stop to see the overall map of the park, the fairly specific trail maps for areas such as Bear Lake, and a 3-D map graphically depicting the dramatic terrain you will be immersed in. You can also fill your water bottles there. A second visitors center at the Fall River Road entrance features a restaurant. From the Beaver Meadows entrance, drive 0.5 mile and turn left on Bear Lake Road. Drive approximately 3.5 miles from the Beaver Meadows entrance, traveling downhill past the Moraine Park Campground and Museum and then uphill through a pine forest adjacent to a YMCA camp. When you emerge from the trees, Hollowell Park is straight ahead. As the road reaches the turnoff and makes a hairpin turn to the left, turn right into the parking area for the trailhead.

This fairly easy and relatively short hike to an overview of Cub Lake is a fun out-and-back hike. This trailhead can also be used for a somewhat steeper 1-mile climb to Bierstadt Lake or the beginning of a loop back to the Cub Lake Trailhead. When you start your hike, read the sign about the log sluice that was used until 1907. From the trail you can see the aspen descending the mountainside where the sluice used to be. The aspen trees are the canopy for the route to Bierstadt Lake; it is magical when the leaves are resplendent in the fall.

Regardless of your destination, take the trailhead across the meadow and bear left in 0.25 mile at the first intersection. The right branch at that first intersection is a horse trail over to Moraine Park. If it isn't the height of horse season, it is a pleasant rolling stretch that parallels the road but is high enough to avoid the highway noise. It is a rather long stroll, but the Cub Lake Overlook route to the left (west) is the better choice.

If you turn left, you will cross the level meadow for 0.25 mile and then go gradually uphill into the trees. It is always fun to hike next to a cascading stream; this treat is Mill Creek. At the next intersection at approximately the 1.25-mile mark, go left again and climb a moderate mile up to Bierstadt Lake or go straight (west and northwest) for the overview of Cub Lake. Don't follow the first stream cross-ing to the left (southwest), which goes up to Bierstadt, to remain on the Cub Lake overview branch of the trail. The overview trail climbs gradually through the trees, crests, and then descends as it opens up to a pretty meadow. It then winds back into the trees, with steeper and flatter sections alternating for over a mile, until it opens up into a great view down the moraine onto Cub Lake.

The trail to Bierstadt Lake is wide, rocky in some sections, and primarily a tree tunnel (with lots of shade from quaking aspens on warm days), until you get to the ephemeral lake that does a disappearing act in dry years. Even if you encounter a dry lakebed, you will still, weather permitting, have a spectacular view of Hallet Peak.

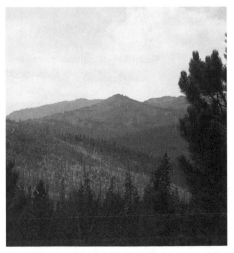

View from the Hollowell Park Trail

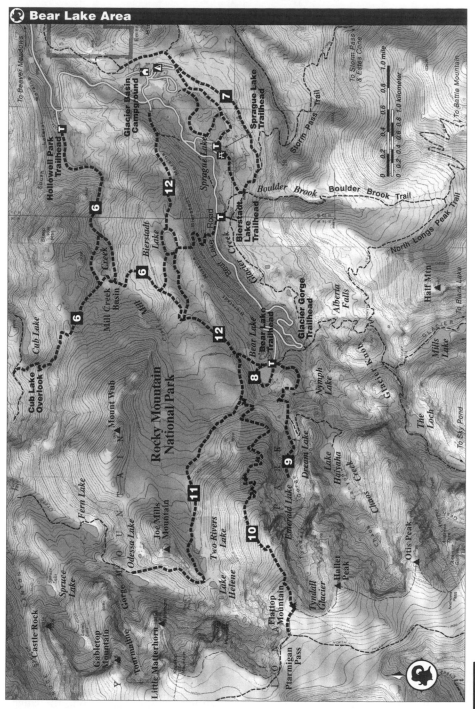

Bear Lake Area

TRIP 7 Glacier Basin & Sprague Lake

see map on p. 139

Distance	Up to 3.0 miles, Loop or semiloop
Difficulty	Easy
Elevation Gain	200 feet (starting at 8710 feet)
Trail Use	Option for kids, wheelchair accessible
Agency	Rocky Mountain National Park
Map	Trails Illustrated *Rocky Mountain National Park*
Facilities	Restrooms, picnic areas, and a horse stable
Note	Bikes are allowed on roads, not trails, in Rocky Mountain National Park.

HIGHLIGHTS The Sprague Lake area offers a couple of nice, easy loops, as well as the trailheads for more ambitious adventures such as the Boulder Brook/North Longs Peak and Storm Pass trails. The easiest trip is simply around the lake itself, only 0.5 mile with no elevation gain; it's wheelchair accessible and offers great views of the peaks on the Continental Divide—the usual suspects: Flattop, Hallet, and friends.

DIRECTIONS When you reach Estes Park on State Highway 34, continue to the third traffic light and you will see a sign for RMNP. Turn left at the sign and go up a hill, bear right at the stop sign, and then bear right at the intersection 0.5 mile after the next traffic light. You will see signs for the Beaver Meadows visitors center, which is worth a stop to see the overall map of the park, the fairly specific trail maps for areas such as Bear Lake, and a 3-D map graphically depicting the dramatic terrain you will be immersed in. You can also fill your water bottles there. Take the first left after the Beaver Meadows visitors center on to Bear Lake Road. Approximately 1 mile from Hollowell Park or 4.5 miles from the Beaver Meadows entrance. Take a left on Bear Lake Road and drive until you come to Glacier Basin Campground. Parking is on the right (west) side of road, and the trailhead is on the east side of the campground. The Sprague Lake area, and parking lot, is the next left on the south side of the road, and is approximately 0.5 mile from the Glacier Basin Campground parking lot.

The easy longer loops can be started at either Glacier Basin Campground, which is closed during winter months, or Sprague Lake. The best views are seen at Sprague Lake or at the campground with limited but nice views along the way. There is ample parking at either end of the loop with parking lots across from the campground off of Bear Lake Road or at the Sprague Lake picnic area. If you want a very easy one-way trek for small children or people who aren't acclimated to the altitude, this can be done as a two-car shuttle.

If you want a longer hike, start the entire 3-mile loop from the Sprague Lake Picnic Area across from the livery. Start by walking toward the lake, edging along the left (counterclockwise) side of the lake, and then looking for a trail connection on the left side of the lake before you come to a picnic area beside the trail. Take the trail downhill into the trees toward the campground. Take the right (uphill) fork in 0.5 mile and switchback to the top of the ridge, to the best view of the route with the Mummy Mountains in the distance along with Flattop and Hallet. You then loop back along the ridgeline toward the Storm Pass and Boulder Brook trails, passing both trails as you roller coaster southwest and then north-

Great for Kids

The easiest adventure is simply circum-navigating the flat trail 0.5 mile around the lake. There are even a few picnic spots and benches along the way. If you would like to do more, the next easiest one-way trek for families with young children is to start at the high point at Sprague Lake and walk downhill to the Glacier Basin Campground, using a car shuttle. If you want to avoid a shuttle, do a simple out-and-back adventure of any length to be determined by the participants' motivation. If you are going to go out and back, I suggest starting from Glacier Basin Campground (park across the road) since it is the flattest part of the route and you can avoid the ridge walk trail on the left entirely. Starting at Sprague Lake is doable as an out-and-back but is more challenging terrain since it is somewhat uphill on the way back. All of the options are easy.

west, looping back toward Sprague Lake. The trail descends the ridge and crosses a creek as you bear right toward the lake. Do not take the trail that is marked as a return route to the Glacier Gorge Campground.

If you prefer to go the other way around the loop, start at the picnic area next to the Sprague Lake parking lot, ascend a short (200 yard), steep hill that turns into an easy climb, and enter a lodgepole pine forest. Look for and follow the orange markers on the tree limbs. A trail entering from the left is marked Glacier Gorge/Bear Lake; take it left to climb to an intersection with the Boulder Brook and Glacier Gorge trails. Follow the sign to the left toward the Glacier Basin Campground. The trail goes downhill, over Boulder Brook twice, and rolls before another short climb. Crest the hill and intersect the Storm Pass Trail on the right. Continue downhill to the left and toward the campground. Enjoy the

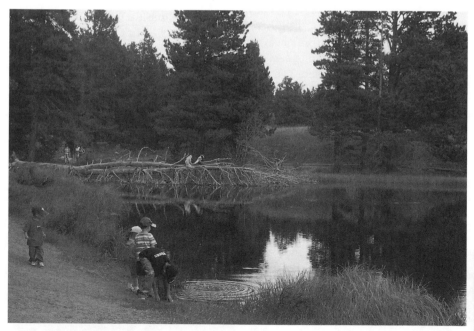

Children enjoying placid Sprague Lake

best view of the route with the Mummy Mountains in the distance and Flattop and Hallet Peaks back to the west. This is a nice place for a break. Continue straight ahead another 0.5 mile to the campground, or take the first trail on the left to Sprague Lake.

Boulder Brook & North Longs Peak Trails

If you'd like a longer trek than that described above, enjoy the nice, quiet, but steep hike from Sprague Lake up the Boulder Brook Trail all the way to the North Longs Peak Trail. Follow the directions above to where the trail intersects with the Boulder Brook Trail; instead of turning toward the campground, go straight uphill on the Boulder Brook Trail. After a gradual start, the trail becomes very steep as it follows the brook. It finally levels briefly and opens up with the sparkling brook and wildflowers providing superb entertainment. It travels through a narrow grassy area, crosses the stream twice, reenters sparser aspen trees, and goes steeply uphill. The trail is a little hard to follow at times because it isn't heavily used, but you will eventually intersect the North Longs Peak Trail. There you can travel up it left (east) toward Granite Pass or enjoy the sweeping view and return to Sprague Lake.

Sprague Lake & Storm Pass

The Storm Pass Trail can be accessed from either Sprague Lake or near Lily Lake and the Longs Peak and Estes Cone Trailhead. It is a great candidate for a car shuttle, if you want to hike only 5 miles; otherwise, it's a 10-mile out-and-back round-trip. Follow the main route description above, and when you reach the Storm Pass Trail intersection go straight or bear right (east-south-

Glaciation

Volcanoes and uplift provided the building blocks for the beautiful Bear Lake and Glacier Gorge areas. But the real artisans of nature were the glaciers that formed about 2 million years ago and slowly "walked" down the stream-cut, U-shaped valleys. In the highest valleys the deep snow compacted into blue ice and then flowed as glaciers widened the erosion—carving out the characteristic U-shaped valleys. These converging rivers of ice flowed into the lower valleys where the ice melted and dropped debris along the valley sides, known as lateral moraines. The last glaciers started about 28,000 years ago and flowed together from Odessa Lake Gorge and other tributary valleys to form a large glacier that melted into Moraine Park, which you cross on the way to Bear Lake. Terminal moraines, material left at the farthest extent of a glacier, naturally dam Bear Lake.

east) and climb the hill gradually rather than descending to Glacier Basin Campground. Climb steadily for almost 0.5 mile; the trail swings due south and gives you a nice view of the north side of Longs Peak. You then travel downhill, losing at least 100 feet, into a very pretty valley and nice meadow.

The pass is another 3 miles mostly uphill after the sign marking Wind River and Storm Pass. The trail edges the meadow and reenters the trees in about 100 yards and begins to climb at first gradually and then more steeply. It is not well marked but is used frequently enough to be visible as it winds through the trees. It alternately steepens and levels as it steadily climbs through the thick tree cover.

TRIP 8 Around Bear Lake

see map on p. 139

Distance	1.0 mile, Loop
Difficulty	Easy
Elevation Gain	Negligible (starting at 9475 feet)
Trail Use	Great for kids, wheelchair-accessible
Agency	Rocky Mountain National Park
Map	Trails Illustrated *Rocky Mountain National Park*
Facilities	Restrooms and picnic shelter
Note	Bikes are allowed on roads, not trails, in Rocky Mountain National Park.

HIGHLIGHTS This short, wheelchair-accessible stroll around Bear Lake is ideal for families with small children or people having difficulty adjusting to the altitude. The views are nonstop from soaring mountains to quaking aspen.

DIRECTIONS When you reach Estes Park on State Highway 34, continue to the third traffic light and you will see a sign for RMNP. Turn left at the sign and go up a hill, bear right at the stop sign, and then bear right at the intersection 0.5 mile after the next traffic light. You will see signs for the Beaver Meadows visitors center, which is worth a stop to see the overall map of the park, the fairly specific trail maps for areas such as Bear Lake, and a 3-D map graphically depicting the dramatic terrain you will be immersed in. You can also fill your water bottles there. Take the first left after the Beaver Meadows visitors center on to Bear Lake Road. Drive to the Bear Lake parking lot, or take the shuttle in the parking lot across from Glacier Basin campground. The Beaver Meadows entrance near RMNP head-quarters is the best entry point for access to Bear Lake Road, which is approximately 0.25 mile from the entrance station. Turn left (south) onto Bear Lake Road and follow it to its terminus at the Bear Lake parking lot, passing Moraine Park, Hollowell Park, Glacier Basin Campground, Sprague Lake, and the Glacier Gorge Trailhead along the way.

Circumnavigate in either direction with your camera out and ready. Maintain a leisurely pace and stop frequently to enjoy the magnificent setting and scenery. If you have the energy, take a short jaunt uphill toward the other smaller lakes described in Trip 9: Nymph, Dream, and Emerald.

View of Hallet Peak from Bear Lake

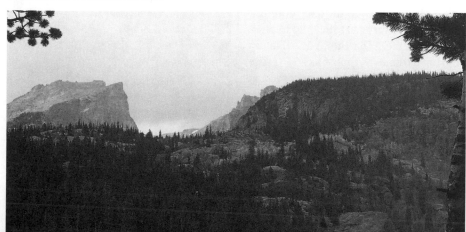

TRIP 9 Nymph, Dream, & Emerald Lakes

see map on p. 139

Distance	3.6 miles, Out-and-back
Elevation Gain	605 feet (starting at 9475 feet)
Difficulty	Easy
Trail Use	Great for kids
Agency	Rocky Mountain National Park
Map	Trails Illustrated *Rocky Mountain National Park*
Facilities	Restrooms
Note	Bikes are allowed on roads, not trails, in Rocky Mountain National Park.

HIGHLIGHTS It is easy to understand why these Bear Lake trails are among the most popular. They are relatively short and easy to navigate, and they feature some of the most beautiful scenery in the park.

DIRECTIONS When you reach Estes Park on State Highway 34, continue to the third traffic light and you will see a sign for RMNP. Turn left at the sign and go up a hill, bear right at the stop sign, and then bear right at the intersection 0.5 mile after the next traffic light. You will see signs for the Beaver Meadows visitors center, which is worth a stop to see the overall map of the park, the fairly specific trail maps for areas such as Bear Lake, and a 3-D map graphically depicting the dramatic terrain you will be immersed in. You can also fill your water bottles there. Take the first left after the Beaver Meadows visitors center on to Bear Lake Road. Drive to the Bear Lake parking lot, or take the shuttle in the parking lot across from Glacier Basin campground. The Beaver Meadows entrance near RMNP headquarters is the best entry point for access to Bear Lake Road. Bear Lake Road is approximately 0.25 mile from the entrance station. Turn left (south) onto Bear Lake Road and follow it to its terminus at the Bear Lake parking lot, passing Moraine Park, Hollowell Park, Glacier Basin Campground, Sprague Lake, and the Glacier Gorge Trailhead along the way.

It is only 0.5 mile and a 225-foot gain to Nymph Lake so it is not a difficult hike. Since the trail starts at almost 10,000 feet and is uphill, small children might find it to be quite enough. For an average, fit adult it is a stroll in the park and well worth the effort. Loop the lake around to the right in or very near the trees to enjoy views of Hallet, Thatchtop, and Flattop. Touring around Nymph Lake is a nice, short family outing and can be combined with some off-trail walking on the way back to Bear Lake, as well as a circuit of Bear Lake.

Another 0.6 mile and 200 feet get you to the sleepy shoreline of Dream Lake. The hike from Nymph to Dream lake is also a real treat ("eye candy" if you will).

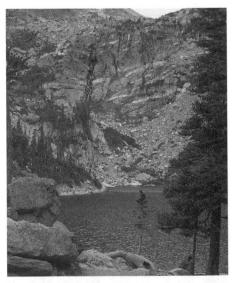

Emerald Lake

From the other side of Nymph Lake, the trail continues uphill to the left; you soon see a striking view of Longs Peak. Don't be drawn to go straight uphill to the right even though you are likely to see tracks going that way—that route leads onto a cliff. Bear left and continue at a fairly low angle, staying above the picturesque valley spreading out on the left and below the impressive rock cliffs on the right. Stately, magnificently healthy evergreens climb the mountainsides; their branches and needles seem etched in crystal because of the high-altitude atmosphere.

The various paths to the lake eventually merge at the top, with bearing to the right as the most common route. Weave your way through a few rocks and then see the stunning setting for Dream Lake, true to its name. This is a terrific photo opportunity spot because of its exquisite surroundings, towering mountains and cliffs, and scruffy wind-sculpted trees with gnarled roots.

Another 0.7 mile and 200 more feet of elevation gain get you to Emerald Lake at approximately 10,300 feet, which also has an impressive setting. The shoulder and cliffs of Flattop Mountain soar on the north, while Hallet Peak and Tyndall Glacier complete the panorama of this high mountain jewel.

TRIP 10 Flattop Mountain & Hallet Peak

see map on p. 139

Distance	8.8 miles to summit of Flattop Mountain, 10.0 miles to summit of Hallet Peak, Out-and-back
Difficulty	Moderate to challenging
Elevation Gain	2849 feet (starting at 9475 feet)
Trail Use	Option for kids
Agency	Rocky Mountain National Park
Map	Trails Illustrated *Rocky Mountain National Park*
Facilities	Restrooms at Bear Lake
Note	Bikes are allowed on roads, not trails, in Rocky Mountain National Park.

HIGHLIGHTS This moderate to challenging hike features some of the best views of the sheer, granite west side of Longs Peak and the magical, glacier sculpture of Glacier Gorge with a majestic, bird's-eye view of Bierstadt, Sprague, Bear, Dream, and Black lakes. The west side of Longs Peak and the famous Keyboard of the Wind (ridgetop rock sentinels) sweep into Black Lake, and Hallet's sharp prow becomes ever more impressive as you climb into the sky. You can enjoy these views covering part of the trail to the overlooks, without summiting Flattop.

DIRECTIONS When you reach Estes Park on State Highway 34, continue to the third traffic light and you will see a sign for RMNP. Turn left at the sign and go up a hill, bear right at the stop sign, and then bear right at the intersection 0.5 mile after the next traffic light. You will see signs for the Beaver Meadows visitors center, which is worth a stop to see the overall map of the park, the fairly specific trail maps for areas such as Bear Lake, and a 3-D map graphically depicting the dramatic terrain you will be immersed in. You can also fill your water bottles there. Take the first left after the Beaver Meadows visitors center on to Bear Lake Road. Drive to the Bear Lake parking lot, or take the shuttle in the parking lot across from Glacier Basin Campground. The Beaver Meadows entrance near RMNP headquarters is the best entry point for access to Bear Lake Road, which is approximately 0.25

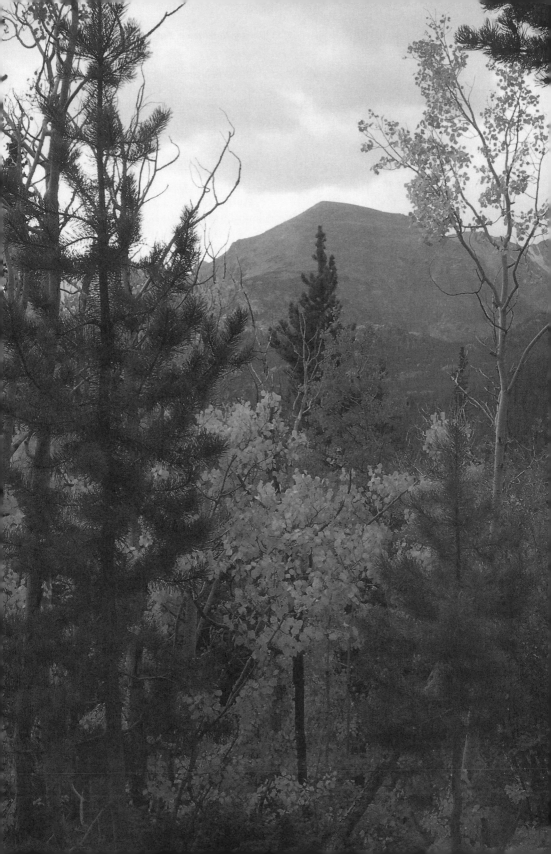

mile from the entrance station. Turn left (south) onto Bear Lake Road and follow it to its terminus at the Bear Lake parking lot, passing Moraine Park, Hollowell Park, Glacier Basin Campground, Sprague Lake, and the Glacier Gorge Trailhead along the way.

While summiting Flattop is a noteworthy achievement, hiking part of the way is also something you can thoroughly enjoy because of the panoramic views and the flora and fauna of the various alpine zones along the way. At treeline the stunted, wind-shaped krumholtz forest looks like something out of a child's fairy tale. If you get an early start and the weather holds, summiting is very doable for anyone of average fitness, as long as you allow enough time to adjust to the altitude and for water and snack breaks. If you have a compulsive, goal-oriented side that tries to convince you to ascend too quickly at the outset, restrain it; otherwise, you'll have too little energy for the steep upper slopes.

From the Bear Lake parking lot, walk right toward the lake. When you reach the shoreline, you can see the impressive massif of Hallet Peak but the summits of Flattop and Hallet are out of sight. Go to the right and watch for the signed route that takes you gradually uphill through the pretty aspens that frame the lake and Hallet Peak. At the first major switchback, at about 0.25 mile, you reach to the Bierstadt Lake Trail, a nice short hike covered in Trip 12. Go left to stay on the Flattop Mountain Trail, which climbs steeply and opens up to spectacular views to the south. The next stretch parallels Bear Lake affording you some of the best views of Longs Peak, Bear Lake, Glacier Gorge, and the glacier-carved, U-shaped valleys—a perfect place for photographs since you will soon be in the trees again, and it will be awhile before you emerge from them.

After about another 100 yards the trail levels and veers north into the shade of

> **Great for Kids**
>
> Though hiking time will vary by group, making it to the stretch that parallels Bear Lake and then circling the lake could be an hour-plus family jaunt—a good goal with very small children. There's a nice uphill stroll option switchbacking on the Bierstadt Lake and Flattop Mountain Trail, through a pretty aspen grove and some great views before returning to crowded Bear Lake.

Engelmann spruce trees and then opens up enough for you to see east into Mill Creek Basin. If you look up high straight ahead, you can see the route up Flattop and the prow of Hallet peaking over the top. The flat stretch lasts about 0.25 mile, and then you climb steadily for 0.5 mile to reach the intersection with the Flattop Mountain Trail, which switchbacks more steeply up to the left, while the Odessa Lake Trail continues to climb straight ahead. Continue to Flattop, switchbacking narrowly and then widely and climbing steadily, mostly in fir and spruce trees. In about 0.25 mile you reach a nice view of Mill Creek Basin before the trail turns sharply to the left. You can see all the way down to McGregor Ranch and Lumpy Ridge. This viewpoint is another possible family turnaround point, until you reach the Dream Lake Overlook, another steeper 0.5 mile or more. The trail bears southwest as it climbs to the edge of the cliffs and the overlook, where you once again have great views of both Longs and Hallet peaks. This popular destination is another turnaround spot for those not climbing the peak. At this point you will be approximately one-third of the way to the top in terms of overall effort.

After this, just getting to treeline can easily take another 30 to 45 minutes or more if you stop frequently for breaks and are not a runner. Treeline (usually around 11,000 feet) is approximately 2.5 miles from Bear Lake; leaving about another 2 steep miles and 1300 feet to the summit. From the overlook, the trail switchbacks widely tracking more toward the north and passing next to a small rock outcrop; some cairns along the way mark it. The trail travels almost to the northern ridge and outcrops before tracking back to the south and reaching the treeline. At this point you get good views of the Mummy Range; Chapin, Chiquita, and Ypsilon mountains; and Mummy Mountain. If you are determined and very fit and take few breaks, you can reach treeline in a little over 1 hour; most of the time you will encounter at least a nice breeze at that point. You might need an extra layer of clothing, depending on the time of the year, or a cool drink if the sun is beating down. This is a good time to have a snack and a drink and decide if discretion is the better part of valor, given the time of the day, and the clouds in the sky.

Depending on the time of the year, particularly early in the hiking season, you might need to avoid some snowfields and small streams of water. How long it takes you to hike from the treeline to the summit depends on your condition and that of the trail. I highly recommend that you turn around if it is raining or thunder is rumbling. The trail traverses and climbs steadily first northwest and then southwest to the top of the next ridgeline to a false summit; the actual summit is out of view to the west. If you're hiking on a beautiful day and have plenty of time to make the return trip, you can have a lot of fun. The views are nonstop once you reach treeline. As you near the summit, there are breathtaking views of Dream Lake's valley and both the pointy false summit and actual summit of Hallet Peak. You will also see the Tyndall Glacier. From the flat, windswept top you can see over the Continental Divide and into the west side of RMNP, the trail that goes all the way to Grand Lake, and the origin of the Colorado River.

Hallet Peak

Hallet Peak, almost 400 feet higher at 12,713 feet, is on the other side of the cirque, and Tyndall Glacier from Flattop Mountain. You don't have to summit Flattop to climb Hallet, though many people like to climb both in the same day. Once you reach the top of the last ridge on Flattop, you can see the routes up both peaks and decide if you have enough energy and good weather for both or if one summit will do. The critical issues are the likelihood of a drenching, lightning storm or the fall of darkness before you reach Bear Lake—the mountains will be there for another day.

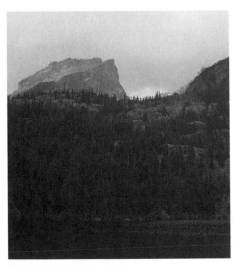

Hallet Peak from Bear Lake

TRIP **11** Odessa Lake

see map on p. 139

Distance	8.2 miles, Out-and-back
Difficulty	Moderate
Elevation Gain	1205 feet (starting at 9475 feet)
Agency	Rocky Mountain National Park
Map	Trails Illustrated *Rocky Mountain National Park*
Facilities	Restrooms at Bear Lake
Note	Bikes are allowed on roads, not trails, in Rocky Mountain National Park.

HIGHLIGHTS This traversing trail is a moderate jaunt that branches off from the Flattop Mountain Trail (Trip 10) about 1.4 miles from Bear Lake. When you emerge from the trees, you'll be enraptured by the views of Mill's Mountain and Mount Wuh, and the high mountain splendor of Odessa. If you make it to Odessa Lake, three 12,000-foot peaks and the impressive Odessa Gorge will be your reward. You can even complete a superb scenery, point-to-point trip all the way to Fern Lake and Moraine Park if you park a car there or don't mind trekking back uphill to Bear Lake.

DIRECTIONS When you reach Estes Park on State Highway 34, continue to the third traffic light and you will see a sign for RMNP. Turn left at the sign and go up a hill, bear right at the stop sign, and then bear right at the intersection 0.5 mile after the next traffic light. You will see signs for the Beaver Meadows visitors center, which is worth a stop to see the overall map of the park, the fairly specific trail maps for areas such as Bear Lake, and a 3-D map graphically depicting the dramatic terrain you will be immersed in. You can also fill your water bottles there. Take the first left after the Beaver Meadows visitors center on to Bear Lake Road. Drive to the Bear Lake parking lot, or take the shuttle in the parking lot across from Glacier Basin campground. The Beaver Meadows entrance near RMNP headquarters is the best entry point for access to Bear Lake Road, which is approximately 0.25 mile from the entrance station. Turn left (south) onto Bear Lake Road and follow it to its terminus at the Bear Lake parking lot, passing Moraine Park, Hollowell Park, Glacier Basin Campground, Sprague Lake, and the Glacier Gorge Trailhead along the way.

From Bear Lake it is a fairly steady and somewhat steep climb that eventually levels. In less than 0.5 mile the Bierstadt Lake Trail continues straight (northeast) while the Flattop Mountain and Odessa Lake Trail takes a sharp left (west) uphill. After the intersection, climb above Bear Lake and look out across the valley at Glacier Gorge and Longs Peak—a good place for photos. The trail then enters the trees, but after 100 yards the trail affords a nice view of Mill Creek Basin and the rounded, thickly forested shoulder of Mount Wuh. It travels more northwesterly, levels out, and climbs at a slower rate.

Where the Flattop Mountain Trail switchbacks sharply left (west) uphill, continue straight (northwest) on the Odessa Lake Trail. Though the trail isn't steep, the slope it is carved into is. The trail is usually well traveled and obvious but might be obscured in the trees you have to navigate through and somewhat difficult to negotiate if you are the one of the first ones on it in early spring before the snow has completely melted. It is not well marked beyond this point, but it climbs steadily to the left (northwest) and does not descend into the Mill Creek drainage toward the right (northeast) as some errant routes indicate. You can generally follow tracks another mile until you reach treeline. At that point the trail is easier to find, but you need good route-finding skills if you lose the trail and have to angle your way left (northwest) first up to Two Rivers Lake and then Odessa Lake. Look for the trail carefully when you break out of the trees; you don't want to unnecessarily climb the steep, open slopes of Mills Mountain left (west) of the trail.

From 10,000 feet the trail steadily climbs in and out of the more sporadic and wind-twisted trees for the next approximately 1.5 miles and 600-plus feet, winding past the small Two Rivers Lake and Lake Helene. The mind has a way of shortening, or lengthening, distance, depending on the body's level of exertion. You reach the impressive Odessa Lake Gorge after you round a bend to the left and are treated to the majestic, windswept visages of Notchtop (12,129 feet), Knobtop (12,331 feet), and Little Matterhorn (11,586 feet). Their majestic presence makes this casual jaunt into more of an achievement and wilderness experience.

If it is late in the day, reverse course to make sure you are below treeline before the afternoon thunderstorms start. The way back is much easier because you can often enjoy the downhill, rather than gasping your way up. If you do get off track, keep Mill Creek Basin on your left and go south until you reach the Bear Lake cliff and basin, then take another left (east) turn. If you started early and are up for the exertion, continue from Odessa Lake all the way to Fern Lake and even Moraine Park.

Bighorn Sheep

In spring you are most likely to see bighorn sheep at lower elevations. In winter you are more likely to see them in Big Thompson Canyon and at lower elevations near Horseshoe Park and Sheep Lake. You might also encounter the sheep high above Wild Basin. They are, however, very rare sights in most parts of the park. The bighorn's recovery from near extinction in the park is a remarkable conservation story.

Though they were able to exist symbiotically with Native Americans for hundreds of years, they almost didn't survive the arrival of European hunters in the late 1800s. They numbered only 200 by the end of the 19th century. Protection has revived these hardy dwellers of the highest reaches of the park and they now number more than 800. They are extremely well adapted to eating even the roughest of forage with their multiple stomach digestive tracks, and their unique hooves allow them to leap and cling to the rocky, high-mountain precipices with breathtaking ease, making them the envy of climbers and hikers. Recent research has shown the size of the herd is declining; RMNP and wildlife biologists are investigating this alarming turn of events.

TRIP 12 Bierstadt Lake

see map on p. 139

Distance	2.8 miles, Out-and-back
Difficulty	Easy
Elevation Gain	566 feet (starting at 8850 feet)
Agency	Rocky Mountain National Park
Map	Trails Illustrated *Rocky Mountain National Park*
Facilities	Restrooms at Bear Lake
Note	Bikes are allowed on roads, not trails, in Rocky Mountain National Park.

HIGHLIGHTS This nice short jaunt for families and beginners starting from Bear Lake offers great views of the entire glacier-carved valley back to Sprague Lake and up Glacier Gorge to Longs Peak. It is one of the most popular routes from Bear Lake; avoid crowds by starting early or hiking during the week.

DIRECTIONS When you reach Estes Park on State Highway 34, continue to the third traffic light and you will see a sign for RMNP. Turn left at the sign and go up a hill, bear right at the stop sign, and then bear right at the intersection 0.5 mile after the next traffic light. You will see signs for the Beaver Meadows visitors center, which is worth a stop to see the overall map of the park, the fairly specific trail maps for areas such as Bear Lake, and a 3-D map graphically depicting the dramatic terrain you will be immersed in. You can also fill your water bottles there. Take the first left after the Beaver Meadows visitors center on to Bear Lake Road. Drive to the Bear Lake parking lot, or take the shuttle in the parking lot across from Glacier Basin Campground. Though starting at Bear Lake makes it a slightly longer hike (about 0.25 mile), it is a much easier, gradual climb. Since the Bierstadt Lake Trailhead parking lot is often full early, the shuttle bus is the best option. If you want a steep, moderate, somewhat shorter climb, however, it is the way to go.

Bierstadt Lake from the Flattop Mountain Trail

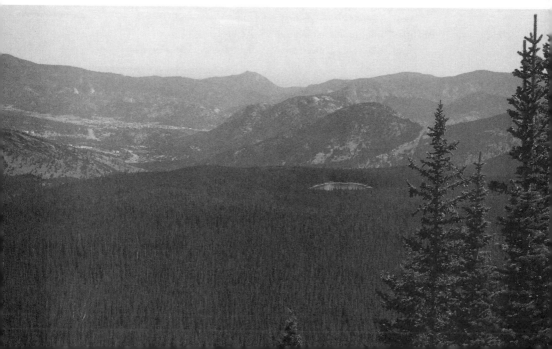

When you start at the Bierstadt Lake Trailhead, it switchbacks up the side of the moraine from the valley floor through a very nice stand of aspen trees. You have great views in all directions. Longs Peak neighbors Storm Peak and Mt. Lady Washington to the west, and Longs Peak to the south. As the trail starts to level the aspens give way to lodgepole pine. You soon intersect Bear Lake Trail coming in from the west (left). Turn right at this intersection and bear right at the next two trail junctions as well. You eventually round the southern end of the lake and end up on the lake's west side. From there reverse course to your starting point or continue downhill to Bear Lake if you have arranged a shuttle.

Wind up through the aspen and pine from Bear Lake, and when the Flattop and Odessa Trail veers left (about 0.5 mile), go right or straight toward Bierstadt Lake. The trail continues to climb gradually as the aspen give way to pine but actually goes downhill for about 0.3 mile before leveling and reaching the lake, meaning you'll have a bit of uphill on the way back to Bear Lake. The trail meanders to the west end of the lake where the trees open up a bit more so you can see the spectacular setting better. There is an even better view of the mountain backdrop from the east end of the lake. You can pick up the trail down to Mill Creek Basin from the east side of the lake; if you would like a nice downhill loop, plant a car at that trailhead.

TRIP 13 Alberta Falls

Distance	1 mile, Out-and-back
Difficulty	Easy
Elevation Gain	100 feet (starting at 9240 feet)
Trail Use	Great for kids
Agency	Rocky Mountain National Park
Map	Trails Illustrated *Rocky Mountain National Park*
Facilities	Restrooms at trailhead
Note	Bikes are allowed on roads, not trails, in Rocky Mountain National Park.

HIGHLIGHTS This is a great family or photography excursion if you have small children or people not prepared for or uninterested in long hikes or altitude. A short, easy round-trip, it can easily be extended once you've reached the falls if you want; the trail is a gateway to gorgeous Glacier Gorge.

DIRECTIONS When you reach Estes Park on State Highway 34, continue to the third traffic light and you will see a sign for RMNP. Turn left at the sign and go up a hill, bear right at the stop sign, and then bear right at the intersection 0.5

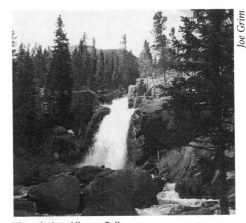

Joe Grim

Thundering Alberta Falls

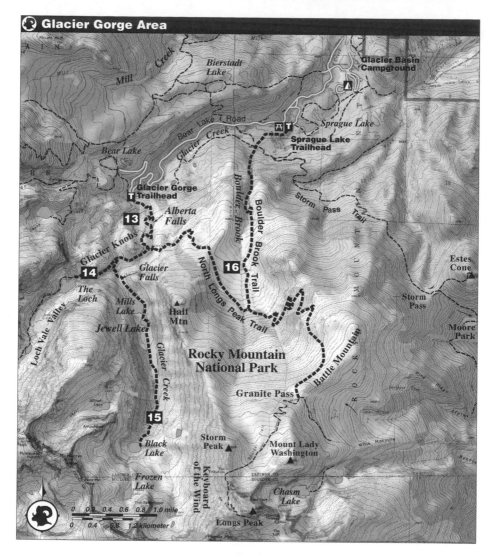

Glacier Gorge Area

mile after the next traffic light. You will see signs for the Beaver Meadows visitors center, which is worth a stop to see the overall map of the park, the fairly specific trail maps for areas such as Bear Lake, and a 3-D map graphically depicting the dramatic terrain you will be immersed in. You can also fill your water bottles there. Take the first left after the Beaver Meadows visitors center on to Bear Lake Road. Drive to the Glacier Gorge parking lot. Glacier Gorge Trailhead is easy to locate on the way to Bear Lake. The new parking lot and restrooms are a major improvement; the parking lot is approximately 1.2 miles before of the Bear Lake lot. If it is full, park in the Bear Lake lot and take the pleasant, short jaunt on the trail from the Dream Lake Trail to the Glacier Gorge Trail. If you want to sleep in and start late, using the park shuttle bus eliminates the stress you'd experience trying to park in the full lots.

The trail travels west from the parking lot, paralleling the small gorge before turning south and crossing a footbridge. It then begins a steady but not very steep climb. It eventually climbs back to the petite canyon carved by a small stream that can flow dramatically for a short time during the spring runoff. The intensity of the falls varies widely during the year, according to stream flow, and is most impressive during spring runoff as well. While the trail is usually quite safe when it's not wet and slick, it is a good idea to keep children close and away from the edge of the cliffs. If you go up the trail beyond the 0.5 mile to the falls, the views of the Mummy Range in the distance and the cliffs of the Bierstadt Moraine across Prospect Canyon improve with every step. From Alberta Falls the trail is steady but not very steep.

TRIP 14 The Loch

see map on p. 153

Distance	5.4 miles, Out-and-back
Difficulty	Moderate
Elevation Gain	940 feet (starting at 9240 feet)
Agency	Rocky Mountain National Park
Map	Trails Illustrated *Rocky Mountain National Park*
Facilities	Restrooms at trailhead
Note	Bikes are allowed on roads, not trails, in Rocky Mountain National Park.

HIGHLIGHTS One of the most rewarding in the park, this hike is also very popular. The Loch, Scottish for "lake," is in a magnificent setting, surrounded by Otis, Taylor, and Powell peaks and offers great photographic opportunities.

DIRECTIONS When you reach Estes Park on State Highway 34, continue to the third traffic light and you will see a sign for RMNP. Turn left at the sign and go up a hill, bear right at the stop sign, and then bear right at the intersection 0.5 mile after the next traffic light. You will see signs for the Beaver Meadows visitors center, which is worth a stop to see the overall map of the park, the fairly specific trail maps for areas such as Bear Lake, and a 3-D map graphically depicting the dramatic terrain you will be immersed in. You can also fill your water bottles there. Take the first left after the Beaver Meadows visitors center on to Bear Lake Road. Drive to the Glacier Gorge parking lot. Glacier Gorge Trailhead is easy to locate on the way to Bear Lake. The new parking lot and restrooms are a major improvement; the parking lot is approximately 1.2 miles before the Bear Lake lot. If it is full, you will have to park in the Bear Lake lot and take the pleasant, short jaunt from the Dream Lake Trail to the Glacier Gorge Trail. If you want to sleep in and start late, using the park shuttle bus eliminates the stress you'd experience trying to park in the full lots.

The hike starts at the same trailhead as all other destinations in Glacier Gorge. After passing Alberta Falls (Trip 13), the trail climbs steadily through loose switchbacks to the intersection with the North Longs Peak Trail. Go right at this intersection. The trail then climbs around Glacier Knob with interesting parapets all around. It continues up on the north side of the Icy Brook drainage that wends

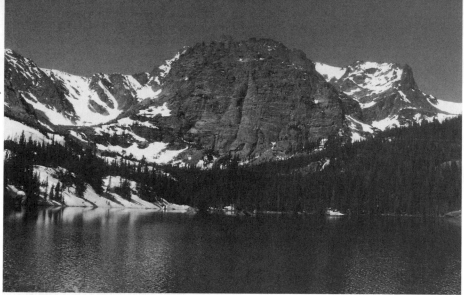

The Loch with Powell and Taylor mountains

its way through the rock. After the intersection the trail narrows and scenery is rewarding as you near the entrance of the Loch Vale Valley. The switchbacks level out and you continue between impressive steep canyon walls. After winding through the canyon, the trail opens up and climbs again with switchbacks virtually all the way to the lake.

If you want a longer, more challenging, and bracing wilderness hike, this is one of the better ones in the park that is easily accessible. It takes you below the west side of Longs Peak and the aptly named Keyboard of the Wind, rock sentinels that whistle and moan in the frequent high winds. The glacier-sculpted valley of rock art has some amazing sites; as with many of the destinations in RMNP, the farther you go, the more enchanting it becomes.

TRIP 15 Jewell & Black Lakes

see map on p. 153

Distance	10 miles, Out-and-back
Difficulty	Moderate
Elevation Gain	1400 feet (starting at 9200 feet)
Trail Use	Backpacking
Agency	Rocky Mountain National Park
Map	Trails Illustrated *Rocky Mountain National Park*
Facilities	Restrooms at trailhead
Note	Bikes are allowed on roads, not trails, in Rocky Mountain National Park.

HIGHLIGHTS If you want a longer, more challenging, and bracing wilderness hike, this is one of the better ones in the park that is easily accessible. It takes you below the west side of Longs Peak and the aptly named Keyboard of the Wind, rock sentinels that whistle and moan in the frequent high winds; you're likely to see some amazing sites in this glacier-sculpted valley of rock art. As with many of these destinations, the farther you go, the more enchanting it becomes. If you want to visit three lakes in magnificent settings, this trek is for you. The journey to the first two can be nice daytrips in and of themselves. Black Lake is a moderate to challenging hike, depending on conditions. On a calm summer's day it is delightful; fall and spring offer ice and windchill that keep you on your toes. Hearing high winds approaching from the Keyboard of the Wind on Longs Peak on an unsettled day is an experience you won't want to miss.

DIRECTIONS When you reach Estes Park on State Highway 34, continue to the third traffic light and you will see a sign for RMNP. Turn left at the sign and go up a hill, bear right at the stop sign, and then bear right at the intersection 0.5 mile after the next traffic light. You will see signs for the Beaver Meadows visitors center, which is worth a stop to see the overall map of the park, the fairly specific trail maps for areas such as Bear Lake, and a 3-D map graphically depicting the dramatic terrain you will be immersed in. You can also fill your water bottles there. Take the first left after the Beaver Meadows visitors center on to Bear Lake Road. Drive to the Glacier Gorge parking lot. Glacier Gorge Trailhead is easy to locate on the way to Bear Lake. The new parking lot and restrooms are a major improvement; the parking lot is approximately 1.2 miles before of the Bear Lake lot. If it is full, you will have to park in the Bear Lake lot and take the pleasant, short jaunt from the Dream Lake Trail to the Glacier Gorge Trail. If you want to sleep in and start late, using the park shuttle bus eliminates the stress you'd experience trying to park in the full lots.

A dayhike to any of the lakes is quite enjoyable because of the great scenery you see in all directions. Once you get beyond Alberta Falls, you continue to wind back and forth over Glacier Creek next to the small gorge that gives you more than one overlook and photo opportunity. Eventually the gorge opens up with cliffs soaring above on both sides of the trail.

The first trail junction you come to is the North Longs Peak Trail that splits to the left and goes toward Granite Pass (high on the flank of Longs Peak), Boulder Brook, and the infamous boulder field on Longs Peak. Take the right branch toward Mills Lake and Loch Vale. The trail steepens but you are treated to views of Arrowhead and Chief's Head peaks in the distance ahead with the gorge on your left and Glacier Gorge Canyon an inviting entry point to this majestic topography.

The trail goes downhill for a short distance and eventually goes back into the trees. You then reach the next major intersection. To the left is the Black Lake Trail (the lake is 2.8 miles from here);

to the right is the trail to Loch Vale, also known as the Loch (Trip 14). You encounter a second stream crossing in a relatively short distance that features wooden steps and rocks. You see some cairns as well as wooden steps for route-finding.

There are at least two good routes to Mills Lake from here—surmounting the rocks or taking a more circuitous route through the trees if you don't like scrambling. You are very close to the lake so it is well worth the trouble. Once you reach the lakeshore, you are treated to stunning views of Mt. Lady Washington and can see the Keyboard of the Wind on the southwest side of Longs Peak. This is a great place for photos or a snack or lunch break, but you might have to find a wind-sheltered spot to enjoy it. On a warm summer's day though the cool breeze is welcome.

Once you reach Mills you have walked 2.8 miles from the Glacier Gorge Trailhead and are 2.2 miles from Black Lake. There is a campground about 0.25 mile ahead, but you need a permit from

Ribbon Falls near Black Lake, with a backdrop of McHenry's Peak
Joe Grim

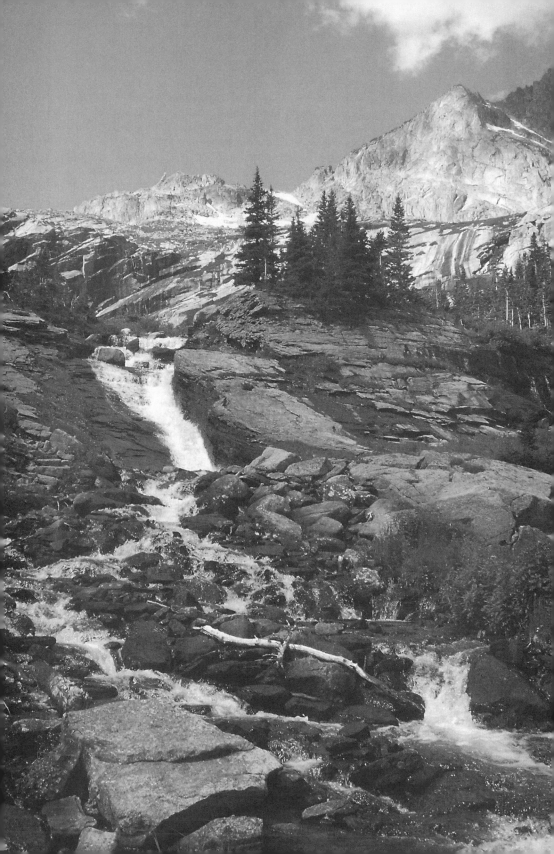

A Black Lake Overnight

Warm weather in the flatlands or even at the beginning of a trip means nothing in the rapidly changing and very localized weather of the higher reaches of the Rockies. It was a delightful winter's day in Boulder, a quite tolerable 49°F, balmy for mid-January, and my companions and I were sure that our venture to Black Lake for a mid-winter camping trip would be blessed with unseasonably sultry weather. When we arrived at the trailhead, we were greeted by 30-mile-per-hour gusts that felt tolerable at 40°F. When we arrived at Mills Lake hours later, we had enough snow to put on our snowshoes half the time. The winds had increased and were pushing us around in what we estimated at gusts of about 50 miles per hour and the temperature was about 20°F. The lake surface was several inches of thick ice. A protracted hour-long struggle took us another mile to Jewell Lake as the winter sun sank very low on the horizon.

At that point the wind was performing a sound and light show of its own. It was like watching huge surf rolling in off of the Pacific. We could see the wind hit the ridgeline of Mt. Lady Washington 2000 feet above and drive spindrift high into the beams of golden sunlight through the wispy cloud cover. The wind went through our down jackets and drove snow onto our necks; the winds were later clocked at just under 100 miles per hour in RMNP, and the temperature sank to minus 25°F that night. It was a long night with only a single-burner stove to produce heat; so much for our sultry winter sojourn at Black Lake.

RMNP to spend the night. This is a good place to turn around if you are hiking it in the early spring, find the mixture of rocks and mud annoying, and don't want to encounter more of the same. One of the interesting aspects of more challenging and remote trails is that they require more flexibility and creativity than just marching down an easy path.

If you keep going, the trail winds around the east edge of the lake with lots of interesting options over, under, and around large outcroppings and towering trees. Eventually the main trail wanders rather far to the east away from the lakeshore. You also eventually reach an open meadow area with great views of Stone Man Pass and Arrowhead, Chief's Head, and McHenry's peaks. You are then only about 200 yards from the very steep stretch that takes you up to the edge of Black Lake. At the south end of the lake is pretty Ribbon Falls. The standard trail is to the left (east) side of the falls.

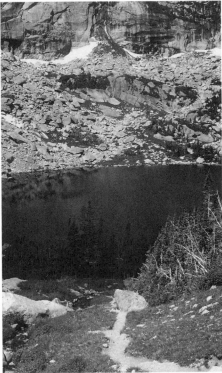

Joe Grim

Black Lake

TRIP 16 North Longs Peak Trail

see map on p. 153

Distance	13.6 miles to Granite Pass, Out-and-back
Difficulty	Varies, depending on the distance hiked
Elevation Gain	2840 feet (starting at 9240 feet)
Trail Use	Backpacking, rock climbing
Agency	Rocky Mountain National Park
Map	Trails Illustrated *Rocky Mountain National Park*
Note	Bikes are allowed on roads, not trails, in Rocky Mountain National Park.

HIGHLIGHTS This trail is lightly used, a surprise given the unique terrain and beautiful views. The first mile or so to the Boulder Brook Trail intersection offers superb views of Glacier Gorge, Flattop and Hallet peaks, the Mummies, and the entire valley on the return. This trail can also be used for climbs of Storm Peak, Mt. Lady Washington, and even Longs Peak if you want to avoid the crowds of the main Longs Peak Trail and don't mind the extra distance.

DIRECTIONS When you reach Estes Park on State Highway 34, continue to the third traffic light and you will see a sign for RMNP. Turn left at the sign and go up a hill, bear right at the stop sign, and then bear right at the intersection 0.5 mile after the next traffic light. You will see signs for the Beaver Meadows visitors center, which is worth a stop to see the overall map of the park, the fairly specific trail maps for areas such as Bear Lake, and a 3-D map graphically depicting the dramatic terrain you will be immersed in. You can also fill your water bottles there. Take the first left after the Beaver Meadows visitors center on to Bear Lake Road. Drive to the Glacier Gorge parking lot. Glacier Gorge Trailhead is easy to locate on the way to Bear Lake. The new parking lot and restrooms are a major improvement; the parking lot is approximately 1.2 miles before the Bear Lake lot. If it is full, park in the Bear Lake lot and take the pleasant, short jaunt from Dream Lake Trail to Glacier Gorge Trail. If you want to sleep in and start late, using the park shuttle bus eliminates the stress you'd experience trying to park in the full lots.

From the starting point at the Glacier Gorge Trailhead, the trail climbs 400 feet gradually to the intersection with the North Longs Peak Trail at 0.75 mile. From there it is a little less than 2 miles to the Boulder Brook Trail intersection. This alone makes a great round-trip trek of approximately 5.5 miles. If you continue, it's another 4 miles one-way from the intersection, or a total of 6.8 miles one-way to Granite Pass at 12,080 feet, an ambitious but spectacular round-trip.

The trail goes downhill from the intersection for approximately 100 to 200 feet, immediately greeting you with great views of the Mummy Range and valley as well as Glacier Gorge. This part of the trail is very open to sun and wind, but don't be dismayed if it is a hot day because you will soon be on a north-facing and tree-shaded section of the trail. Climb back out of the draw after a small stream crossing. It then levels out and enters a short new growth forest of lodgepole and spruce. After another 0.5 mile or so round the bend into the Boulder Brook drainage for an impressive view of the summit of Longs Peak. You can also see the north shoulder of the mountain's massif soaring above and daring you to make the climb above treeline to Granite Pass.

About 4 miles from the trailhead you enter a more mature forest of taller trees. This is a reasonable turnaround point since views are obscured from here until you near treeline; plus, the trail tops out at this point at approximately 10,000 feet giving you a 1000-foot gain for the day. If you want to continue, going above treeline is a great climb; the trail is easy to follow and switchbacks widely across the mountainside before sprinting steeply next to some rock outcrops where you enjoy panoramic views as Mt. Lady Washington and Storm Peak come into view. Reaching Granite Pass is always a thrill since it is part of the summit route on Longs Peak. In early spring the trail to the boulder field can virtually be a running stream, so wear waterproof boots if you're hiking the top of this trail in late spring or early summer. Storm Peak is another 1.25 miles (one-way) and 1300 feet of vertical if you have the irresistible urge to summit a peak.

Sprague Lake Access

For a route with far fewer people than the Glacier Gorge Trail and a more subtle beauty to accompany the solitude, start at the Sprague Lake Picnic Area across from the livery. When you enter the Sprague Lake parking area, follow a one-way spur to the right to the small picnic area and the trailhead. After ascending a short (200 yards), somewhat steep hill the trail levels out to an easy climb in the lodgepole pine forest. The trail is marked with orange markers on tree limbs. After about 0.5 mile turn left onto a trail signed GLACIER GORGE/BEAR LAKE and continue to climb to an intersection with the Boulder Brook and Glacier Gorge Trails. Bear straight (south) onto Boulder Brook Trail.

This trail starts gradually for more than 0.3 mile or so and then begins to climb more steeply, eventually narrowing above Boulder Brook. It is a beautiful riparian area and tree-covered glade; the steep trail is a little difficult to follow when you leave the stream. It leaves the stream and wanders between two separate streams before finally intersecting the North Longs Peak Trail. It is impossible to not intersect this trail, but how efficiently you do so depends on your route-finding skills. If you lose the faint trail, continue south until you intersect it. Once you reach the North Longs Peak Trail, turn east (left) to continue to Granite Pass.

Chapter 7
Rocky Mountain National Park: West

West of the Continental Divide and over Trail Ridge Road lays another part of the magical kingdom of Rocky Mountain National Park. It features the aptly named and majestic Never Summer mountain range; the headwaters of the mighty Colorado River, which is no more than a sparkling stream at this point; the lush, glacier-created Kawuneeche River Valley; and the delights of adjacent Grand Lake, Shadow Mountain Reservoir, Lake Granby, and Monarch Lake. This part of the park is popular but not as crowded as the heavily used eastern slope and has cooler temperatures and more frequent rain showers. It is most easily accessible from Memorial Day to mid-October while Trail Ridge Road is open, and it closes when the snows make it too dangerous to navigate.

Trail Ridge Road

Trail Ridge Road is the highest continuous road in the U.S., topping out at more than 12,000 feet, and is one of the most spectacular rides on the planet. It is a very worthwhile drive, in spite of the slow traffic and crowds. Some prefer to experience the ride on a bike. Get an early start to avoid the afternoon thunderstorms and the heavy motor home and trailer traffic, as well as the fumes and hazards that come with them. There are also some short high-altitude hikes on top near the visitors center for those who can tolerate altitude. Driving the entire route, taking short family jaunts, enjoying the viewpoints, and stopping in at the visitors center can take up most of a day. You'll need warm clothing since the temperatures rarely exceed the 60s

The author hiking the Ute Trail on a misty, magical day

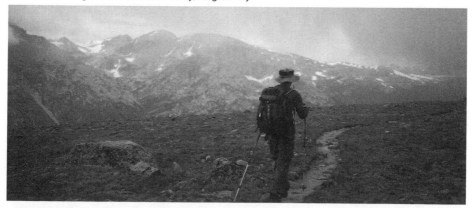

and the breeze is usually chilly, regardless of the season. The temperature is usually at least 20 degrees cooler than Estes Park or Grand Lake, especially early in the morning or late in the afternoon or evening. The road can close suddenly (temporarily) at any time if it is hit by a hail or snowstorm—not unusual during any month of the year. When you see the lack of guardrails and the thousands of feet you would plummet if you drove off the road, you will understand that it cannot be navigated when it's slick. The road usually opens Memorial Day weekend and closes for the winter by late October or early November.

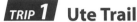 **Ute Trail**

Distance	Up to 8.0 miles, Out-and-back and Point-to-point options
Difficulty	Easy to challenging
Elevation Gain	300 feet (starting at 11,500 feet), 3000 feet (starting at 8400 feet)
Trail Use	Option for kids
Agency	Rocky Mountain National Park
Map	Trails Illustrated *Rocky Mountain National Park*
Facilities	Restrooms at Upper Beaver Meadows
Note	Bikes are allowed on roads, not trails, in Rocky Mountain National Park.

HIGHLIGHTS This first trail you reach as you crest Trail Ridge Road is above treeline through the tundra and so has sensational views of Forest Canyon and one of the more amazing alpine massifs in the world. The parking lot is tiny so carpooling and an early start are necessary to beat fellow hikers and the common lightning and thunderstorms that often start around 11 AM. You can also climb up from the Lower Beaver Meadows Trailhead, where there is ample parking.

DIRECTIONS When you reach Estes Park on State Highway 34, continue to the third traffic light and you will see a sign for RMNP. Turn left at the sign and go up a hill, bear right at the stop sign, and then bear right at the intersection 0.5 mile after the next traffic light. You will see signs for the Beaver Meadows visitors center, which is worth a stop to see the overall map of the park, the fairly specific trail maps for areas such as Bear Lake, and a 3-D map graphically depicting the dramatic terrain you will be immersed in. You can also fill your water bottles there. One trailhead for this route is on Trail Ridge Road, 13.5 miles west of Beavers Meadows and approximately 5 miles east of the Trail Ridge Road Visitors Center. The parking is limited to only about three vehicles, but there is space for another three about 0.5 mile west. The other trailhead is at the bottom of Trail Ridge Road, 0.8 mile from the Beaver Meadows entrance; turn left and drive less than a mile up the dirt road to the Upper Beaver Meadows Trailhead. The Upper Beaver Meadows Trailhead takes you to the Ute Trail.

A very easy and breathtaking jaunt above treeline with very little elevation gain or loss, this route will have you walking on the clouds. Or you can take a challenging car-shuttle hike downhill 3000 feet to Upper Beaver Meadows or uphill 3000 feet from Upper Beaver Meadows to the trailhead on top of Trail Ridge. If you want, you can do a simple out-and-back trip for up to 3 miles and only have to climb about 100 feet; this option takes you uphill 100 feet for the

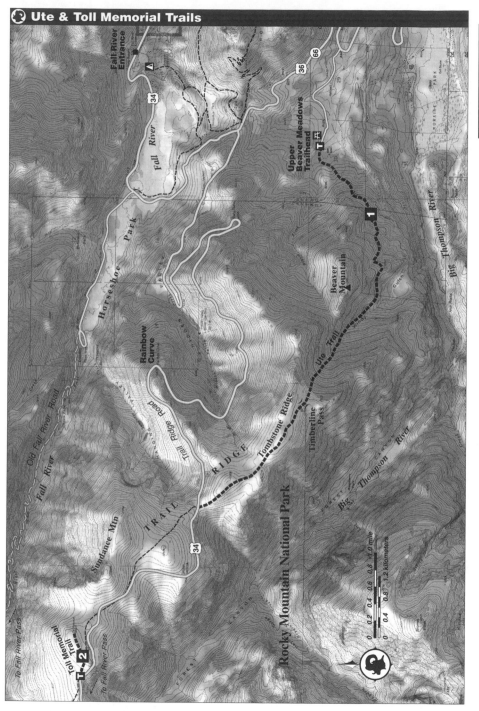

Ute & Toll Memorial Trails

first 0.25 mile from the parking area. You enjoy immediate and continuous exciting views and are surrounded by a marvelous rock garden. When you catch your breath, you have 0.25 mile of level trail before descending about 80 feet over the next 0.5 mile.

Great for Kids

At the 1-mile mark you are only 0.5 mile from getting an impressive peek at Tombstone Ridge. If you have had enough and want to avoid additional climbing at high altitude, have a snack or some water and turn around. But if you and your party are, however, feeling well at altitude, climb up a little to a high point around 11,600 feet, and enjoy Tombstone Ridge before reversing course.

The trail climbs to top out around 11,600 with a nice view of nature's rock sculpture on Tombstone Ridge and then descends 100 feet past the ridge and reaches Timberline Pass in about 0.75 mile, 2 miles from the upper trailhead. There you can enjoy the view of Beaver Mountain before it plunges 2000 feet over the next 2 miles into Windy Gulch and then traverses around Beaver Mountain with great views of the Longs Peak and the Continental Divide massif. As you descend, you see the artistically twisted krumholtz trees that have been stunted by the severe environment. Descend another 1000 feet, more gradually, over the next 2.5 miles into Beaver Meadows.

In case you're interested, the Ute Trail also has a segment from the Trail Ridge Road Visitors Center that parallels the road downhill to Milner Pass.

 Toll Memorial Trail

see map on p. 163

Distance	1.0 mile, Out-and-back
Difficulty	Easy
Elevation Gain	260 feet (starting at 12,110 feet)
Trail Use	Great for kids
Agency	Rocky Mountain National Park
Map	Trails Illustrated *Rocky Mountain National Park*
Facilities	Restrooms at trailhead
Note	Bikes are allowed on roads, not trails, in Rocky Mountain National Park.

HIGHLIGHTS This exciting, short, high-altitude, tundra stroll features superb views and pretty wildflowers.

DIRECTIONS When you reach Estes Park on State Highway 34, continue to the third traffic light and you will see a sign for RMNP. Turn left at the sign and go up a hill, bear right at the stop sign, and then bear right at the intersection 0.5 mile after the next traffic light. You will see signs for the Beaver Meadows visitors center, which is worth a stop to see the overall map of the park, the fairly specific trail maps for areas such as Bear Lake, and a 3-D map graphically depicting the dramatic terrain you will be immersed in. You can also fill your water bottles there. From either entrance, take Trail Ridge Road (State Highway 34) up to the world of tundra at just under 12,000 feet. This is your third opportunity to stop once you crest the ridge and will be on the right (north) side of the road where you see a sign and restrooms.

Walk slowly uphill to avoid becoming light-headed if you aren't used to high altitudes. Enjoy hopping on the fun rocks along the way. The trail is bordered by rock formations on the right that are fun for scrambling if you feel okay. When you reach the end of the trail, you'll have a great view of the Mummy Range to the north; Chapin, Chiquita, and Ypsilon mountains are the closest summits.

TRIP 3 Mount Ida

Distance	11.5 miles, Out-and-back
Difficulty	Moderate
Elevation Gain	2110 feet (starting at 10,700 feet)
Agency	Rocky Mountain National Park
Map	Trails Illustrated *Rocky Mountain National Park*
Facilities	Restrooms at trailhead
Note	Bikes are allowed on roads, not trails, in Rocky Mountain National Park.

HIGHLIGHTS One of the most accessible high peaks in the park with a very high trailhead, this is a mountaineering experience and summit climb that can be accomplished with much less exertion than most. You will enjoy a spectacular 360-degree view from the top and the nonstop views along the way.

DIRECTIONS When you reach Estes Park on State Highway 34, continue to the third traffic light and you will see a sign for RMNP. Turn left at the sign on Moraine Street, and go up a hill, bear right at the stop sign, and then bear right at the intersection 0.5 mile after the next traffic light. You will see signs for the Beaver Meadows visitors center, which is worth a stop to see the overall map of the park, the fairly specific trail maps for areas such as Bear Lake, and a 3-D map graphically depicting the dramatic terrain you will be immersed in. You can also fill your water bottles there. Take Trail Ridge Road west, up and over Continental Divide, and past the Trail Ridge Road visitors center. Go to the Milner Pass parking lot that is about 4 miles west of the Trail Ridge Road Visitors Center.

Mt. Ida trailhead and Poudre River headwaters   *John Bartholow*

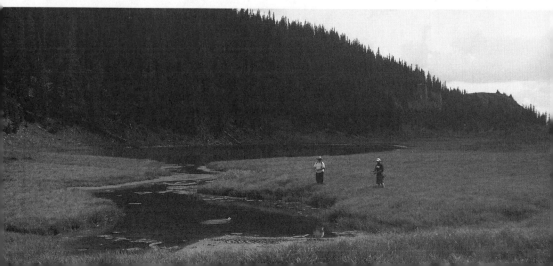

Mount Ida & Colorado River Trail

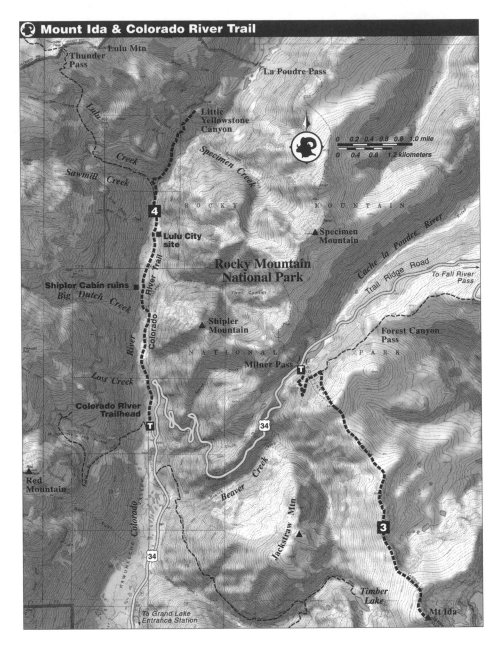

Don't be lulled by the easy accessibility of this peak climb as I once was; you should not undertake this trek unless you are well acclimated, fit, and well prepared for thunderstorms. Take the usual precautions by getting an early start and bringing waterproof cool weather gear.

The T-shirt, shorts, and poncho I wore when I hiked Ida the first time were inadequate.

The somewhat steep switchbacks start from the back of the parking and travel gradually to the east as they climb the steep slope toward treeline. As you climb toward the ridgetop, you have impressive views down-valley to the Never Summer Range. Once it tops out, the trail travels more gradually in a traversing fashion to the south and enters the world of tundra in another mile, approximately 2 miles from the trailhead. You are rolling next to the tundra with unnamed high spots nearby. The trail levels somewhat and then climbs gently. The trail climbs more steeply for the last 2 miles and becomes sketchier, but the route to the distant high spot is fairly obvious.

TRIP 4 Colorado River Trail to Little Yellowstone Canyon

Distance	7.4 miles to Lulu City, up to 10.0 miles to Little Yellowstone, Out-and-back
Difficulty	Easy to moderate, depending on distance
Elevation Gain	350 feet to Lulu City, 990 feet to Little Yellowstone (starting at 8950 feet)
Trail Use	Option for kids
Agency	Rocky Mountain National Park
Map	Trails Illustrated *Rocky Mountain National Park*
Facilities	Restrooms at trailhead
Note	Bikes are allowed on roads, not trails, in Rocky Mountain National Park.

HIGHLIGHTS This interesting, easy trail up a beautiful riparian valley goes through a mining ghost town that was home to 200 people and has many historic memories. Climbing up to see the appropriately named small canyon is a treat, not only for the canyon view, but because of the commanding, peaceful view of one the most idyllic looking river valleys on the continent.

DIRECTIONS You can reach Grand Lake from Denver by driving west on Interstate 70 to Berthoud Pass and then north on Highway 40, through Winter Park and Grandby. Follow signs to State Highway 34 and RMNP, Grand Lake entrance station. The Colorado River Trail parking lot is 10 miles east from the Grand Lake entrance station. It is the last lot before Trail Ridge Road goes steeply uphill. If you're approaching RMNP on State Highway 34, when you reach Estes Park continue to the third traffic light and you will see a sign for the park. Turn left at the sign on Moraine Street, and go up a hill, bear right at the stop sign, and then bear right at the intersection 0.5 mile after the next traffic light. You will see signs for the Beaver Meadows visitors center, which is worth a stop to see the overall map of the park, the fairly specific trail maps for areas such as Bear Lake, and a 3-D map graphically depicting the dramatic terrain you will be immersed in. You can also fill your water bottles there. Drive up and over Trail Ridge Road and look for the first trailhead on the right after reaching the bottom, or the last trailhead from the west.

The trail starts at the east end of the parking lot and goes straight uphill on a steep switchback before leveling off into a fairly gentle roll all the way to Lulu. It starts in unremarkable lodgepole pine for the first 0.25 mile but then gets interesting over the next 0.5 mile as the trail crosses the tributary streams (maybe even Squeak Creek) of the Colorado River three times. The trail is then riverside, and the small meadows and streambank make nice picnic spots for those with small children or ambitions. At the 0.5-mile mark continue straight when you reach an intersection with a trail to Thunder Pass (9.2 miles) and the Grand Ditch (2.8 miles). You will be 3.2 miles from Lulu, 4.0 miles from the lower part of Little Yellowstone Canyon, and 1.8 miles from the ruins of the Shipler Cabin. The meadows offer tantalizing peak views of Howard Mountain and Mount Cirrus to the north through the spruce trees and columbine flowers that grace the trail. At just over 1 mile, the trail climbs again, ascending about 70 feet, as it tracks away from the river.

At 1.5 miles it climbs again in earnest, ascending another 100 feet, and then

> **Great for Kids**
>
> The Shipler Cabin is a good turnaround point for families with small children or those hikers with modest goals. The cabin ruins are much more than you will see at Lulu City, where most traces of the town are long gone.

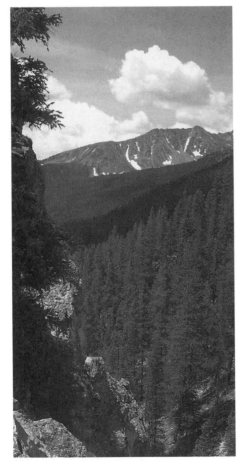

View from Little Yellowstone Canyon

drops through a meadow with cliffs soaring above. The trail edges next to the thousands of tons of rockslides that have thundered into the valley over time for the next 0.5 mile. You cross Crater Creek as Lead Mountain comes into view across the pretty meadow. You reach what is left of the Shipler Cabin at approximately 2.3 miles; there is a hikers' privy on the north side of the trail.

The trail steepens again and climbs around 200 feet over the next mile through thick trees; mosquitoes will keep you company if you feel lonely. Around the 3-mile mark you notice that the trees are draped with fungi commonly called Spanish moss. It is actually a parasite that can strangle a tree over time in its green gossamer web. When you reach another trail intersection, signs explain that you are 0.2 mile from Lulu, 2 miles from the Michigan Ditch, and 3.7 miles from Thunder Pass, 1 mile from Little Yellowstone, and 4.0 miles from Poudre Pass. Cross Sawmill/Specimen Creek, and the trees open up into mixed forest with aspen joining the Engelmann spruce and pine. Go downhill to the left (north) to the Lulu site if that is your goal. If you want to go all the way to Little Yellowstone Canyon, continue straight along an almost level path that travels along on a low ridge around 9500 feet that gives you a commanding view of the multicolored greens of riparian valley at your feet.

The trail then turns to the northeast as it climbs steeply into a wide, eroded drainage, showing nature in action carving a canyon. You come to another trail intersection, where you can go back 0.8 mile to Lulu or 1 mile to the Stage Road campsites. There is an impressive view back across the valley as you climb up and cross a bridge. Then you reenter trees and switchback uphill as the trail climbs quickly to 9800 feet. As you top the ridge, part of the Little Yellowstone opens up before you, and there is a nice two-person rock, good for a lunch or a snack. That is approximately the 4.5-mile mark projected as your destination. If you are willing to climb another 100 feet and hike another 0.5 mile you are in for a real treat—a much better view of the canyon, a spectacular view of the Kawuneeche (Native American for "coyote") Valley, a few peaks in the background, and a graceful waterfall. Cross two more drainages and climb to 9900 feet for your reward. If you didn't see Lulu on the way up, take one of the two available detours on the way back to see the town site; then merge into the main trail and head back to your starting point.

TRIP 5 Baker Gulch to Mount Nimbus & Mount Stratus

Distance	7.4 miles to Baker Gulch, 10.0 miles to Baker Pass, 12.0 miles to Mount Nimbus, 12.8 miles to Mount Stratus, Out-and-back
Difficulty	Moderate to challenging
Elevation Gain	2303 feet to Baker Pass, 3756 feet to Mount Nimbus, 3556 feet to Mount Stratus (starting at 8950 feet)
Agency	Rocky Mountain National Park, Arapaho National Forest
Map	Trails Illustrated *Rocky Mountain National Park*
Note	Bikes are allowed on roads, not trails, in Rocky Mountain National Park.

HIGHLIGHTS This is a hike across a river valley, through trees and vales, and into a gorgeous valley bordered by mountains with a riot of wildflowers in the spring and early summer, meadows that roll to the horizon, and the possibility of more challenging climbs to either Parika Lake or the top of Mount Nimbus.

DIRECTIONS You can reach Grand Lake from Denver by driving west on Interstate 70 to Berthoud Pass and then north on Highway 40, through Winter Park and Grandby. Follow signs to State Highway 34 and RMNP, Grand Lake entrance station. The Colorado River Trail parking lot is 6.5 miles east from the Grand Lake entrance station. It is the last lot before Trail Ridge Road goes steeply uphill. If you're approaching RMNP on State Highway 34, when you reach Estes Park continue to the third traffic light and you will see a sign for the park. Turn left at the sign on Moraine Street, and go up a hill, bear right at the stop sign, and then bear right at the intersection 0.5 mile after the next traffic light. You will see signs for the Beaver Meadows visitors center, which is worth a stop to see the overall map of the park, the fairly specific trail maps for areas such as Bear Lake, and a 3-D map graphically depicting the dramatic terrain you will be immersed in. You can also fill your water bottles there. Drive up and over Trail Ridge Road and look for the second trailhead on the right after reaching the bottom. Use the Baker and Bowen Trailhead, 6.5 miles from Grand Lake entrance station and visitors center.

From the trailhead you cross a long meadows area with beautiful views of the riparian valley and towering peaks. You then enter a lodgepole pine forest that might make you think this will be a dull hike. Your trek through the trees takes you out of RMNP and into Roosevelt National Forest. Once you hit Baker Gulch, the fun begins as you trek west and northwest. The lodgepoles give way to a beautiful mixed aspen forest, and then wildflowers begin to dot the landscape. The trail winds upward, opening up with a view of a very steep shoulder of Baker Mountain.

After 3.5 miles you reach the magnificent meadows of Baker Pass. If you go no farther, you will be very happy. If, however, you are mesmerized by the high mountain meadows and drawn by the blanket of wildflowers to go all the way up, north to the top of Baker Pass, continue on to the peaks. Around 5 miles from the trailhead, you see the tempting summit of Mount Nimbus with an unalluring scree and rock route to the top; scramble away. From the top of Mount Nimbus, you enjoy an unparalleled panorama. Thunderstorms permitting, you are but a short ridge walk away from Mount Stratus.

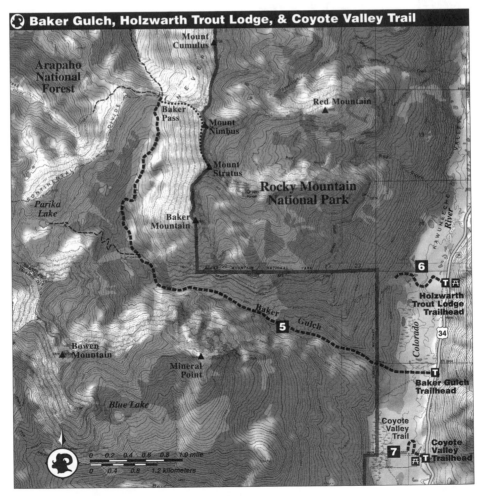

Baker Gulch, Holzwarth Trout Lodge, & Coyote Valley Trail

TRIP 6 Holzwarth Trout Lodge

Distance	1.0 mile, Out-and-back
Difficulty	Easy
Elevation Gain	Negligible (starting at 9000 feet)
Trail Use	Great for kids
Agency	Rocky Mountain National Park
Map	Trails Illustrated *Rocky Mountain National Park*
Facilities	Restrooms at trailhead
Note	Bikes are allowed on roads, not trails, in Rocky Mountain National Park.

HIGHLIGHTS This is the largest group of restored, historic structures in the park. This stroll through the middle of the Colorado River Valley includes a view of the Zirkel Range in the distance and gives you a sense of what life was like more than a century ago in what was once a remote piece of paradise. You may even see moose lurking about. During the summer months (June–September) a golf cart shuttle is available for the handicapped.

DIRECTIONS You can reach Grand Lake from Denver by driving west on Interstate 70 to Berthoud Pass and then north on Highway 40, through Winter Park and Grandby. Follow signs to State Highway 34 and RMNP, Grand Lake entrance station. The Colorado River Trail parking lot is 8 miles east from the Grand Lake entrance station. It is the last lot before Trail Ridge Road goes steeply uphill. If you're approaching RMNP on State Highway 34, when you reach Estes Park continue to the third traffic light and you will see a sign for RMNP. Turn left at the sign on Moraine Street, and go up a hill, bear right at the stop sign, and then bear right at the intersection 0.5 mile after the next traffic light. You will see signs for the Beaver Meadows visitors center, which is worth a stop to see the overall map of the park, the fairly specific trail maps for areas such as Bear Lake, and a 3-D map graphically depicting the dramatic terrain you will be immersed in. You can also fill your water bottles there. Drive up and over Trail Ridge Road and look for the first trailhead on the right after reaching the bottom. The lodge is 8 miles from the Grand Lake entrance station and visitors center.

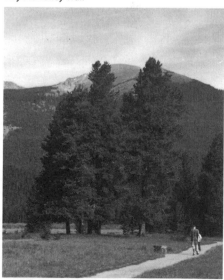

Coyote Valley Trail

One of the cabins is next to the parking lot while the others are a short, flat hop away on a two-track dirt road that is deal for family strolls. When you cross the Colorado River, look west and enjoy the view of the distant Zirkel range. Bear left when you reach the edge of the forest the road splits, and you will see the cabins slightly uphill. There is a golf cart shuttle for the handicapped. The walk up to the cabins is short and easy, and worth the trip back in time, to a different era.

TRIP 7 Coyote Valley Trail

see map on p. 170

Distance	1.0 mile, Out-and-back
Difficulty	Easy
Elevation Gain	Negligible (starting at 9000 feet)
Trail Use	Great for kids
Agency	Rocky Mountain National Park
Map	Trails Illustrated *Rocky Mountain National Park*
Facilities	Restrooms and picnic tables at trailhead
Note	Bikes are allowed on roads, not trails, in Rocky Mountain National Park.

HIGHLIGHTS Another terrific handicapped-accessible trail, this route is frequented by moose, elk, muskrats, otters, osprey, red-tailed hawks, voles, and shrews to mention a few of the critters highlighted in the nature stops. This pretty trail accompanies the river on a short loop with nice views of Baker Mountain.

DIRECTIONS You can reach Grand Lake from Denver by driving west on Interstate 70 to Berthoud Pass and then north on Highway 40, through Winter Park and Grandby. Follow signs to State Highway 34 and RMNP, Grand Lake entrance station. The Colorado River Trail parking lot is 6 miles east from the Grand Lake entrance station. It is the last lot before Trail Ridge Road goes steeply uphill. If you're approaching RMNP on State Highway 34, when you reach Estes Park continue to the third traffic light and you will see a sign for RMNP. Turn left at the sign on Moraine Street, and go up a hill, bear right at the stop sign, and then bear right at the intersection 0.5 mile after the next traffic light. You will see signs for the Beaver Meadows visitors center, which is worth a stop to see the overall map of the park, the fairly specific trail maps for areas such as Bear Lake, and a 3-D map graphically depicting the dramatic terrain you will be immersed in. You can also fill your water bottles there. Drive up and over Trail Ridge Road and look for the first trailhead on the right after reaching the bottom. The trailhead is 6 miles from the Grand Lake entrance station and visitors center.

The trail goes north from the parking lot and restrooms. After you cross the river, go left for a short picnic table loop or right for the guided nature tour along the river. There is a nice detour down to the river at the first stop. You pass some Engelmann spruce and lodgepole pine trees on the way, along with wildflow- ers, and, if you're lucky, some wildlife. You can enjoy Baker Mountain (12,397 feet) from anywhere along the trail. The farther you go on the trail, the more of the valley view you'll see. Plus you get to enjoy the Colorado River in its "infancy." Hawks often soar above the valley. Watch for moose and elk among the trees.

TRIP 8 East Inlet & Thunder Lake Trails

Distance	0.3 mile to 11.0 miles, Point-to-point
Difficulty	Easy to challenging
Elevation Gain	80 feet to Adams Falls, 3600 feet to Wild Basin Trailhead (starting at 8400 feet)
Agency	Rocky Mountain National Park
Map	Trails Illustrated *Rocky Mountain National Park*
Facilities	Restrooms at trailhead
Note	Bikes are allowed on roads, not trails, in Rocky Mountain National Park.

HIGHLIGHTS This stroll is ideal for photographers who don't want a major adventure but are looking for a real treat. The short trail offers several nice vantage points of the water-fall and the arroyo in which it resides. The lush meadows and wetlands just around the bend of the East Inlet Trail will tempt you to take a longer hike. You can take the trail for enjoyable hikes of almost any length, even an 11-mile trek to beautiful Lone Pine Lake or 17 miles one-way over the Continental Divide to Wild Basin if you like bushwhacking and route-finding, or take the all-day moderate hike to Lone Pine Lake.

DIRECTIONS You can reach Grand Lake from Denver by driving west on Interstate 70 to Ber-thoud Pass and then north on Highway 40, through Winter Park and Grandby. Follow signs to State Highway 34, RMNP, and the town of Grand Lake. Drive to the Grand Lake town entrance. Take an immediate left on the first paved road and follow it to the end 2.3 miles ahead. If you prefer, you can reach Grand Lake over Trail Ridge Road from Estes Park.

Go downhill immediately after leaving the parking lot and then uphill through aspen and lodgepole pine trees. When you reach the trail intersection, turn right and go downhill to Adams Falls. To complete the loop, go somewhat steeply uphill and intersect the main trail, where you turn left to return to the lot. I highly recommend going at least another 200 yards to the right to take in a little more of East Inlet Trail. After rounding the bend, enjoy a magnificent view of the expansive grassy meadows and distant rock outcrops carved by glaciers.

If you have time to explore farther, take the trail as it edges the lake before finally climbing gently after 0.75 mile. The farther you go, the higher you will go, letting you enjoy a more sweeping view of this gorgeous riparian scene. The trail rolls gently for 3 miles before

it climbs steeply out of the valley up to Lone Pine Lake, which is 5.5 miles from the trailhead. The trail to Lone Pine Lake is worth an adventure of any length. Just turn around when you become weary. The trail is a rolling route that steadily gains altitude to the lake with many nice viewpoints. If you have the time and energy and have set up a car shuttle at Wild Basin, you can continue over the Continental Divide and to the southern portion of RMNP in Wild Basin.

I have only hiked the route from east to west from Wild Basin via Thunder Lake and Grand Pass to Grand Lake. Either way you can enjoy the string of lakes—Verna, Spirit, and Fourth lakes, and more—that sit nestled in the thick evergreen forest. The trickiest and most challenging part of the hike is connecting from Grand Pass to the East Inlet Trail or

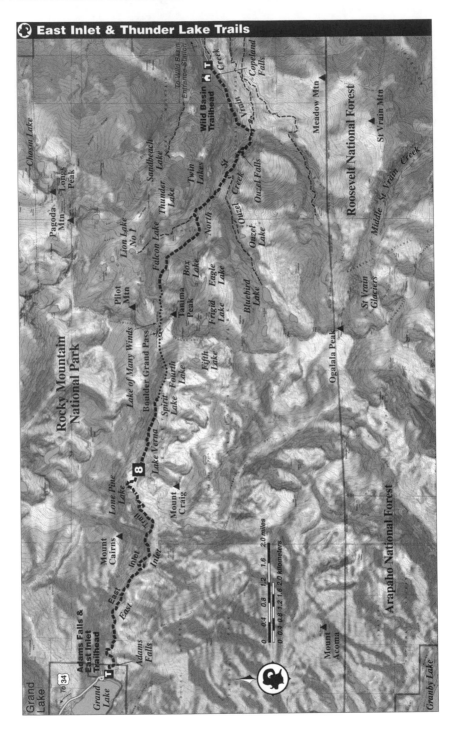

East Inlet & Thunder Lake Trails

vice versa. You must have good map and compass skills to traverse successfully and complete your trek in a single, very long day. Alternatively, you can turn it into a more relaxing backpack or an out-and-back to as many lakes as you want to see in a day.

TRIP 9 Monarch Lake to Brainard Lake

Distance	0.7 mile to end of Monarch Lake, 15.0 miles to Brainard Lake, Point-to-point
Difficulty	Easy to challenging, depending on distance hiked
Elevation Gain	4000 feet (starting at 8340 feet)
Trail Use	Camping, fishing, option for kids
Agency	Arapaho National Forest
Map	Trails Illustrated *Kremmling & Granby*
Facilities	Restroom and campground near trailhead
Note	Bikes are allowed on roads, not trails, in Rocky Mountain National Park.

HIGHLIGHTS Outside RMNP, this hike offers anything from an easy lakeside, wetlands, and meadow stroll to a challenging out-and-back trek to Pawnee Pass in the Indian Peaks on the east side of the Continental Divide or even a point-to-point adventure over the divide

The Continental Divide from Brainard Lake

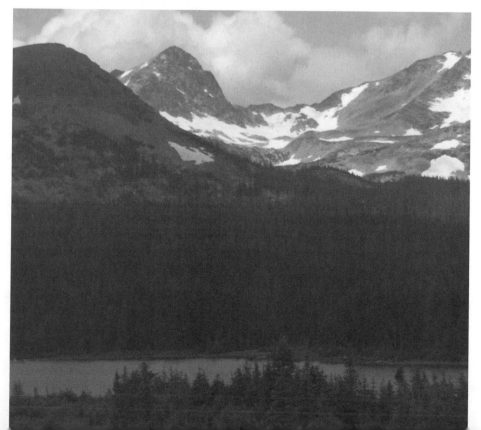

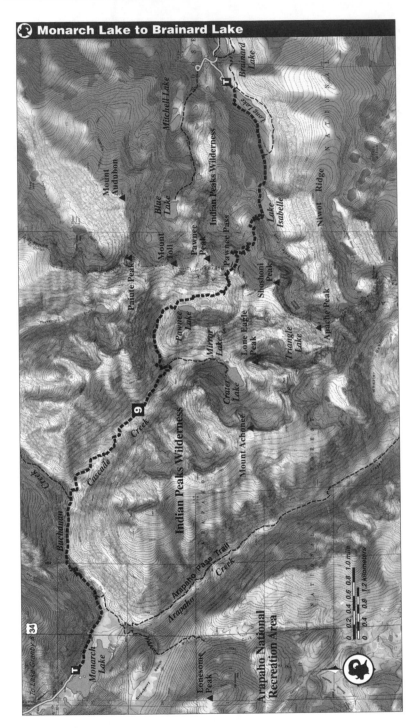

Monarch Lake to Brainard Lake

and to Brainard Lake. Along the way expect to hike next to a sparkling stream and to savor picturesque lakes. The trail is in Arapaho National Forest and is adjacent to RMNP.

DIRECTIONS The trailhead isn't easy to find, nor is it very difficult. You can reach Grand Lake from Denver by driving west on Interstate 70 to Berthoud Pass, and then north on Highway 40, through Winter Park and Grandby. Follow signs to State Highway 34 and RMNP, and the town of Grand Lake. Take State Highway 34 approximately 12 miles from Grand Lake to the south side of Granby Lake. Follow signs for Arapaho Bay left (east). The gravel road edges along Lake Granby and then Arapaho Bay, before winding its way back to the Monarch Lake Trailhead.

You can enjoy the beauty of Monarch Lake at the trailhead. The trail follows the cascading creek most of the way to the Buchanan and Pawnee Pass intersection and is a very nice round-trip of approximately 6 miles.

To go to Pawnee Pass, bear right (southeast). The intersection is near the Shelter Rock backcountry campsite, a good place for lunch or a snack unless you prefer to be streamside. The climbing begins in earnest after this intersection but is highlighted by tumbling, babbling Cascade Creek. It is a steep trek to Pawnee Lake, more than 6 miles from the trailhead, but the lake is a marvelous destination. It is another mile up steep switchbacks to the top of Pawnee Pass. From there you can either reverse course for a challenging 14-mile day or continue to Brainard Lake, around 3 miles below, and your car shuttle.

Great for Kids

The first 0.75 mile of trail is next to Monarch Lake and offers great scenery, wildlife, and photo opportunities. On hot days you might want to get your feet wet in the lake. You can take a nice family jaunt for a picnic hike and turn around when you have seen enough of pretty Buchanan Creek.

Chapter 8

Rocky Mountain National Park: South

One of the beautiful things about Rocky Mountain National Park is its size, making it an ecosystem onto itself, where the deer, elk, and bears can play, unscathed, unless they wander into the adjacent national forests. While bears are rare, the relatively tame elk, deer, and bighorn sheep are common, but striking sites throughout the park. This area is the geographically closest part of RMNP to Boulder and Denver because it is the farthest south, but is often overlooked because the town of Estes Park is associated as the east side entrance to the park. Wild Basin, a U-shaped glacier-carved valley, is a primary access point and a spectacular one at that with cascading streams, waterfalls, ridgetops, soaring peaks, and a magnificent forest. The highest mountain in northern Colorado and one of the highest in the state, Longs Peak is easily accessible just south of Estes Park and north of Allenspark, though it is also one of the most challenging 14ers.

To reach this section of the park, take State Highway 66 to Lyons and then State Highway 7 to State Highway 72. (Don't take State Highway 36 from Lyons to Estes Park because you will bypass Wild Basin and have to backtrack from Estes Park.) You can access Wild Basin and Longs Peak from State Highway 72, the highly scenic "Peak to Peak Highway," as you travel north toward Estes Park. If you live in Fort Collins, Loveland, or other points north, you can also, of course, drive to Estes Park and then south on State Highway 72.

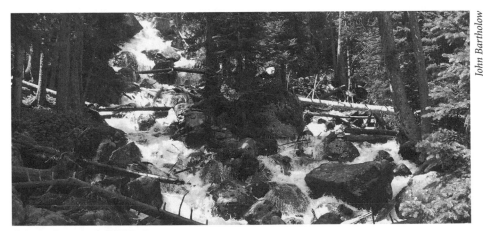

John Bartholow

Calypso Cascades in Wild Basin

Rocky Mountain National Park: South 179

Longs Peak Area

As Walter Borneman and Lyndon Lampert claim in *A Climbing Guide to Colorado's Fourteeners,* "Longs Peak is undisputedly the monarch of the northern Front Range, and one of the outstanding peaks of the entire North American continent." It was considered to be unclimbable from the time of its discovery by Stephen Long in 1820 until fearless, one-armed, Grand Canyon navigator John Wesley Powell did it in 1868 from the south side. His approach was especially remarkable because his party had to climb all the way up and over the Continental Divide and through uncharted terrain from Grand Lake before attempting the summit. It is, however, likely that Native Americans climbed the peak before he did.

It is one of those places, like many in Rocky Mountain National Park, that you never tire of no matter how many times you have visited, summited it, or attempted to summit it. It is a place that imparts a feeling of timeless immortality to us mere mortals. And the soaring and forbidding Diamond rock face never ceases to astonish climbers of all skill levels. Many an expert climber has spent an unplanned night bivouacked among its frigid granite cliffs praying for dawn.

The true beauty of Longs is the wide variety of trails that crisscross its massive expanse and make it possible for trekkers to partake of some piece of its high-altitude glory. In fact, during the frenzy of the summer months, thousands of poorly prepared hikers line up to be treated to the rigors of climbing almost 5000 feet in a little less than 7 miles and are rewarded with a down-climb of 5000 feet when their knees and feet are begging for an errant helicopter to whisk them away. Unfortunately the combination of geologic drama, death-defying heights, very fickle weather, and foolhardy trekkers has exacted a price of more than 35 fatalities since 1884. If you want to climb Longs, use any of the many excellent 14er guidebooks.

Wild Basin

This part of Rocky Mountain National Park offers its own kind of magic—sculpted by glaciers, sequestered by the stunning Mount Meeker massif to the south with Chief's Head in view, bordered on the west by the Continental Divide peaks (Ouzel, Tanima, and Mahana), and highlighted by Copeland Mountain. Few panoramas are its equal. You will also be inspired by the creativity of North Saint Vrain, Ouzel, and Coney Creeks as they tumble and fall through the valley, from serene lakes like Ouzel and Sand Beach. It is well south of Estes Park, making it a closer destination from the metro Denver and Boulder areas.

TRIP 1 Estes Cone

Distance	6.4 miles, Out-and-back
Difficulty	Moderate
Elevation Gain	1500 feet (starting at 9500 feet)
Agency	Rocky Mountain National Park
Map	Trails Illustrated *Rocky Mountain National Park*
Facilities	Restrooms, ranger station, and campground
Note	Bikes are allowed on roads, not trails, in Rocky Mountain National Park.

HIGHLIGHTS If you want a unique perspective and view of Longs Peak and Mount Meeker peaks as well as Twin Sisters, this hike is for you; it's an interesting ramble past an abandoned mining site with a minor rock scramble to reach the summit.

DIRECTIONS Take the Peak to Peak Highway (State Highway 7) south from Estes Park 7.5 miles to the turnoff on the west side of the road for the Longs Peak Trail and campground. Turn right (west) and go up the hill to the intersection and bear left into the parking lot. You can also reach the trailhead by driving north on State Highway 7 from either Lyons or Nederland. If you are driving north from the Denver area, the route through Lyons is the best alternative.

The Longs Peak Trail is the starting point for this hike, but you share the trail with the legions climbing that summit for only 0.5 mile of relatively steep climbing through lodgepole pine forest. The trail then veers to the northwest and levels off somewhat before climbing gradually to Eugenia Mine, where some aspen trees are mixed in with the pine. The area surrounding the abandoned mining site is a good place for a snack and water break.

After crossing the Inn Brook drainage, the trail travels northeast downhill into

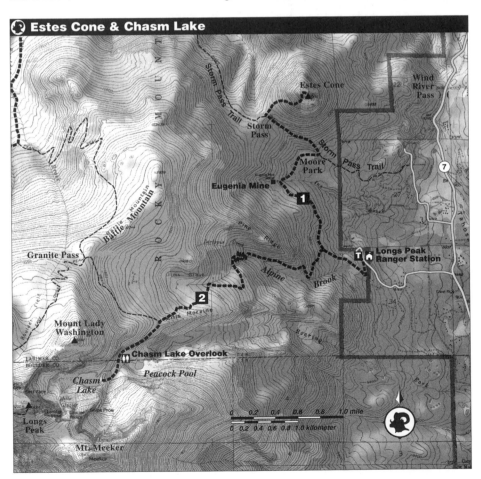

Estes Cone & Chasm Lake

Moore Park. It then joins the Storm Pass Trail and goes northwest (left) gradually uphill to Storm Pass, where the trees begin to thin out before turning northeast (right) and switchbacking more steeply uphill to the rock summit of Estes Cone. The most challenging section is the last, long switchback section because it climbs 1000 feet in approximately the last 0.5 mile, but this part of the trail rewards you with the best views of Longs Peak and Mount Meeker. Climb carefully on the sometimes slick, wet, and icy rock to reach the top of the summit rocks. The last climb to the summit is not recommended for young children. If you prefer not to climb the summit, you can go as far as Storm Pass and walk up enough of the switchbacks or to the summit rocks to enjoy a few photo opportunities and then turning around. Storm Pass can take you to Sprague Lake.

 Chasm Lake

Distance	8.4 miles, Out-and-back
Difficulty	Moderate
Elevation Gain	2300 feet (starting at 9500 feet)
Trail Use	Camping
Agency	Rocky Mountain National Park
Map	Trails Illustrated *Rocky Mountain National Park*
Facilities	Restrooms, campground, and ranger station
Note	Bikes are allowed on roads, not trails, in Rocky Mountain National Park.

HIGHLIGHTS Once you are above treeline you enjoy 360-degree views that include Longs Peak and Mount Meeker as well as Twin Sisters. The lake is in a magnificent setting with the heights of the Loft between Meeker and Longs soaring above. Hiking this early in the season before Longs Peak is accessible to climbers means far less crowding.

DIRECTIONS Take the Peak to Peak Highway (State Highway 7) south from Estes Park 7.5 miles to the turnoff on the west side of the road for the Longs Peak Trail and campground. Turn right (west) and go up the hill to the intersection and bear left into the parking lot. You can also reach the trailhead by driving north on State Highway 7 from either Lyons or Nederland. If you are driving north from the Denver area, the route through Lyons is the best alternative.

As with most of the trails described in this book, you can have a very satisfying, moderate, family adventure by planning a 2- to 3-hour round-trip adventure on the first 1.5 miles of the trail. Until you reach around 10,000 feet (around 1 hour into the hike) the trail is in a tree tunnel with tantalizing peeks, then you are afforded nice views of the summit of Longs Peak. At that point you could simply enjoy lunch or a snack and head back to the trailhead. The 500-foot climb is a good workout. This and the Longs Peak Trail are one and the same for most of the route, until you reach the junction on the ridge where the Longs Peak Trail goes straight (northwest) to Granite Pass while the Chasm Lake Trail takes Mills Moraine left (south and then west) to Chasm Lake Overlook.

Start at the Longs Peak Ranger Station, and walk 0.5 mile to the intersection where the Storm Pass Trail splits off to the north; you continue straight/left

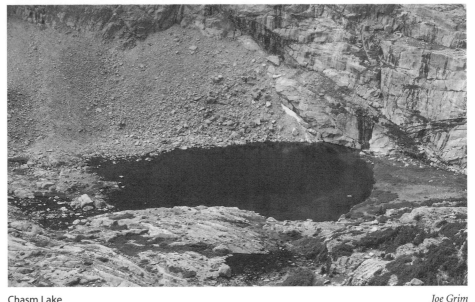

Chasm Lake   *Joe Grim*

(southwest) on a trail that steepens, climbing with occasional short switchbacks. When you aren't sufficiently warmed up to enjoy it, the trail is steep; it climbs up to 10,000 feet fairly quickly in thick tree cover over the next 0.5 mile. It then levels a little and more gradually climbs for the next 0.25 mile before steeply gaining another 500 feet. The trees thin out and allow you partial views of the summit of Longs, looking down from on high and daring you to climb it. On a clear day you enjoy an impressive view of the famous Diamond climbing route.

The trail climbs again, switchbacks, and turns more due south, edging its way up toward the stunted wind- and weather-gnarled trees of Goblin's Forest. Cross the small footbridge over Alpine Brook. Don't hesitate to turn around if conditions become challenging, particularly if early season snow or ice are present. Soon the krumholtz trees reveal a spectacular view of the slope all the way to the summit. Once you are above treeline at 11,000

feet you enjoy a panoramic view in all directions. Always keep an eye on the weather, and keep in mind that the trail down might not be as straightforward as you remember, allowing extra time for slower members of your party to make it back to the trailhead without the duress of a too rapid descent.

Once above treeline you gradually switchback your way to a ridge and steep slope that you have to traverse to the south to reach the final stretch up Mills Moraine to Chasm Lake Overlook where there is a privy. Here the trail splits again with the right branch going almost due north to Granite Pass while you veer to the south toward the lake. Follow the spectacular 11,600-foot-high ridge around the corner and be startled by the views of Longs Peak, Mount Meeker, and Chasm Lake itself. The final 200 feet to the lake from the privy can be a difficult and precarious ridge walk, depending on whether ice or snow lingers early in the season.

TRIP 3 Copeland Falls

see
map on
p. 184

Distance	2.6 miles, Out-and-back
Difficulty	Easy
Elevation Gain	195 feet (starting at 8320 feet)
Trail Use	Great for kids
Agency	Rocky Mountain National Park
Map	Trails Illustrated *Rocky Mountain National Park*
Facilities	Restrooms at trailhead
Note	Bikes are allowed on roads, not trails, in Rocky Mountain National Park.

HIGHLIGHTS This is a great family option because it is a short, easy hike to a spectacular, small waterfall in the magical Glacier Gorge, which also makes it a very popular destination, so arrive early or enjoy the national park camaraderie.

DIRECTIONS To reach Wild Basin from Estes Park, take State Highway 7 south approximately 12 miles. After you drive through Meeker, look for the sign on the right. Turn right (west) and proceed past the lodge and around the lake to the left. The road narrows to almost one lane. From Boulder or Denver, take State Highway 66 through Lyons to State Highway 7 past Allenspark. The close-in parking fills up early and that means an extra 1.5 miles of walking on the road or the trail next to it to reach the actual trailhead (the trail next to the road is more scenic).

The trail gains approximately 200 feet from distant secondary parking to Wild Basin Ranger Station (8500 feet). If the close-in parking is full or you have young children who prefer short hikes, Copeland Falls might be enough. You can always go farther though if you want to. The streamside stroll to the ranger station even features meadows along the way. When you reach the Wild Basin Ranger Station parking lot, bear left to see the falls off a well-marked side trail 0.25 mile from the ranger station. At that point you can rest and decide if you want to venture farther up the enchanted land of Wild Basin.

TRIP 4 Allenspark & Finch Lake Trails to Wild Basin

Distance	13.4 miles from Wild Basin to Finch Lake; 6 miles from Allenspark to over-look; 13.4 miles from Allenspark to Finch Lake
Difficulty	Easy to overlook, moderate to Finch Lake
Elevation Gain	952 feet (starting at 8960 feet)
Agency	Rocky Mountain National Park
Map	Trails Illustrated *Rocky Mountain National Park*
Facilities	Restrooms at Wild Basin Trailhead
Note	Bikes are allowed on roads, not trails, in Rocky Mountain National Park.

HIGHLIGHTS This trek offers two alternatives that go high above Wild Basin. You can hike to either the overlook at the trail intersection or Finch Lake. You can reach these destinations from either the Allenspark Trail or the Wild Basin Trailhead. The overlook offers spectacular views of this glacier-carved wonderland from above. You are also treated to

Wild Basin Area

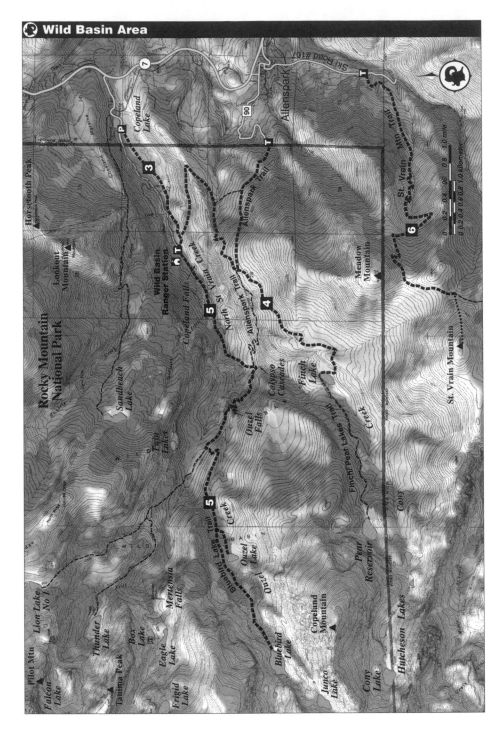

great views of Mount Meeker and Chief's Head to name just a couple. You can reach this overlook or Finch Lake by either taking a side trip or climbing up from the Wild Basin Valley or starting higher up on the Allenspark Trailhead.

DIRECTIONS You can access this trail from either the Allenspark Trailhead or Wild Basin. To reach Wild Basin from Estes Park, take State Highway 7 south approximately 12 miles. After you drive through Meeker, look for the sign on the right. Turn right (west) and proceed past the lodge and around the lake to the left. The road narrows to almost one lane. From Boulder or Denver, take State Highway 66 through Lyons to State Highway 7 past Allenspark. The close-in parking fills up early and that means an extra 1.5 miles of walking on the road or the trail next to it to reach the actual trailhead (the trail next to the road is more scenic).

To reach Allenspark Trailhead, take State Highway 7 approximately 10 miles south to Allenspark. Go to the post office and turn west on County Road 90. Drive a few miles until you see Meadow Mountain Drive, and turn right and look for the parking lot.

The trail gains approximately 200 feet from the distant secondary parking lot to the Wild Basin Ranger Station (8500 feet). Starting at Wild Basin requires climbing up from the valley floor. The Allenspark Trailhead is about 490 feet higher than the Wild Basin/Finch Lake Trailhead. The hiking distance on the main trails is about the same from either starting point.

Wild Basin Trailhead to Overlook

You will pass the Pear Lake/Finch Lake/Allenspark Trail on the left before you reach the ranger station. You don't have to hike to Finch Lake to enjoy a great view of Wild Basin. It is an interesting, short, out-and-back, side trip to climb to the ridge above Wild Basin, where you are rewarded with a terrific view of the glacier-carved valley and the peaks that surround it. It is about a 1.5-mile trek from the trailhead and a little less than 3 miles (one-way) to the viewpoint near the ridge top, with an 800-foot-plus climb on gradual switchbacks to reach it. When you arrive, great views of Mount Meeker, Longs Peak, Chief's Head, Pagoda Peak, and the entire Wild Basin stretch before you. At this point you can turn around and have a satisfying round-trip of less than 6 miles.

Allenspark Trail

The Allenspark Trail is more scenic than the trailhead on the valley floor. After approximately the first mile, you have breaks in the trees and start getting nice views of Chief's Head, Pagoda Mountain, and Meeker and Longs peaks. The last 0.5 mile to the overlook point provides even more nice views, with the grand finale being the overlook, where you get a 180-degree view of the peaks and the valley. It is a steady climb with variations all the way to the overlook. From the overlook you'll see the Finch/Pear Lakes Trail. Hike part of that trail for more great views.

Finch Lake

Once you reach the overlook and trail intersection, follow the Finch/Pear Lakes trail left (southwest). You reenter the trees and climb steadily toward the lake and pass through a small section of trail that was burned in the fire in 1978. After the first stream crossing, you dip into and out of the drainage. There is another stream crossing in about 0.5 mile; the trail then follows a small ridge down to the lake. Once there you have an impressive view of Copeland Mountain, a beautiful riparian area, and a dazzling lake.

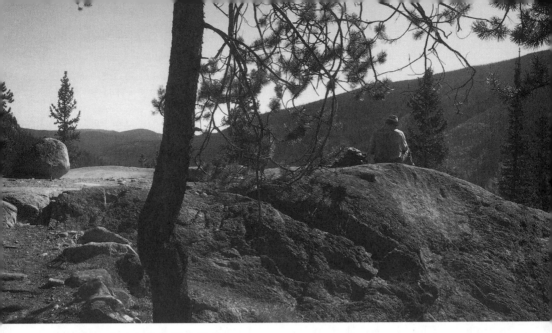

A snack break on the Ouzel Lake Trail

 **Calypso Cascades, Ouzel Falls,
& Ouzel Lake**

see map on p. 184

Distance	3.6 miles to the cascades, 5.4 miles to the falls, 10.0 miles to Ouzel Lake, 13 miles to Bluebird Lake, Out-and-back
Difficulty	Easy to cascades and falls, moderate to either of the lakes
Trail Use	Option for kids
Elevation Gain	880 feet to the cascades, 1130 feet to the falls, 1500 feet to Ouzel Lake, 2500 feet to Bluebird Lake (starting at 8320 feet)
Agency	Rocky Mountain National Park
Map	Trails Illustrated *Rocky Mountain National Park*
Facilities	Restrooms at trailhead
Note	Bikes are allowed on roads, not trails, in Rocky Mountain National Park.

HIGHLIGHTS Calypso Cascades and Ouzel Falls are very popular, easy, short hikes in Wild Basin that feature the beauty of a cascading stream and can be enjoyed by adventurers of all ages and abilities. It is most dramatic during spring runoff but fun year-round. Ouzel and Bluebird lakes are moderate almost all-day treks through almost every mountain climate zone. Ouzel is a pristine lake at the foot of Copeland Mountain, and higher Bluebird Lake affords a view of the Continental Divide.

DIRECTIONS To reach Wild Basin from Estes Park, take State Highway 7 south approximately 12 miles. After you drive through Meeker, look for the sign on the right. Turn right (west) and proceed past the lodge and around the lake to the left. The road will narrow to almost one lane. You can drive to the parking lot near the ranger station, but start early because it frequently fills up on weekends. The ranger station parking lot is approximately 1.5 miles from the highway. Take State Highway S66 and 7 west and north from Lyons, if you're coming from Denver/Boulder.

Proceed to the left through the parking lot to a route map and sign. Bear left and take the trail across the bridge. This trail offers a lot of variety as it winds, rolls, and steadily climbs through a pretty mixed forest of aspen and evergreens. The trail is next to the crystal-clear water and small waterfalls of North St. Vrain Creek, while at times you move some distance from it. Eventually you come to the bridge that crosses the creek about 0.4 mile below Calypso Cascades—a good spot for a snack break that usually offers nice photo opportunities of the stream. This bridge is approximately 1 mile beyond Copeland Falls; it is approximately another 0.25-mile climb to the intersection of North St. Vrain Creek and Coney Creek and the magical cascades that never look the same.

From the cascades it is another climb 0.7 mile to Ouzel Falls. At the cascades you see the Finch Lake/Allenspark Trail on the left, which has descended from the heights above to the floor of Wild Basin. Bear to the right and cross Coney Creek over two more bridges. At this point the trail levels for a bit and then steepens as it switchbacks straight uphill. Even if you don't plan to go all the way to Ouzel Falls, it is worth another 200 yards to enjoy the views of the west slopes of Longs Peak and Mount Meeker that open up. When you break out of the trees, you also see the dramatic scenery from the 1978 lightning-ignited fire that swept through this area and burned more than 1000 acres. Once you get beyond the steep switchbacks, cross Ouzel Creek and see Ouzel Falls. In another 100 yards you reach an overlook with spectacular views of Longs Peak, Mount Meeker to the northwest, Meadow Mountain to the southeast, and

> **Great for Kids**
>
> If you're hiking with young children, then you might take a snack break at the bridge that crosses the creek. Continue on to the intersection of North St. Vrain and Coney creeks to enjoy the cascades and turn around to retrace your steps to the trailhead.

Wild Basin and the North St. Vrain Creek below to the north.

At this point, you have a choice—continue up the trail steeply on switchbacks for the next 0.5 mile and then climb more gradually all the way to pristine Ouzel Lake or Bluebird Lake or to turn around and head for the parking lot. The hike to Ouzel Lake is one of my favorites in the park, but the later you start, the more heavily used it will be. You also have to consider getting caught in thunderstorms if you start late. If you see large clouds forming on the Continental Divide mountains to the west, it would be smart to turn around. If the sky is still clear and it is not yet midday, continue on the rolling, steadily climbing trail that offers a spectacular panorama of Wild Basin. In less than a mile you come to a fork in the trail with the right fork going to Thunder Lake and the left to Ouzel and Bluebird lakes, bear left. Thunder Lake is 1 mile farther one-way and offers access to a route over the Continental Divide.

When you are 0.5 mile from Ouzel Lake, you will reach another signed trail intersection. Go right for 1.5 miles, and climb steeply for another 1000 feet to reach the spectacular setting of Bluebird Lake. Go straight/left on a rolling but relatively flat trail for the more subtle beauty of Ouzel Lake's surroundings at the foot of Copeland Mountain.

TRIP 6 St. Vrain Mountain

see map on p. 184

Distance	6.6 miles, Out-and-back
Difficulty	Moderate
Elevation Gain	2423 feet (starting at 8970)
Trail Use	Horseback riding, camping
Agency	Rocky Mountain National Park
Map	Trails Illustrated *Rocky Mountain National Park*
Facilities	Restaurant and lodges in Allenspark
Note	Bikes are allowed on roads, not trails, in Rocky Mountain National Park or Indian Peaks Wilderness.

HIGHLIGHTS This is a great small peak climb into the Indian Peaks Wilderness near Allenspark that offers the spectacular scenery of RMNP without the crowds. The trail travels along the park border with superb views of the Meeker/Longs/Chief's Head massif and Wild Basin, as well as Twin Sisters and the plains sprawling to the east.

DIRECTIONS Take State Highway 7 to Allenspark and then go west on the right (north) side of the Allenspark Post Office. Turn left and follow gravel Ski Road (#107) south approximately 2 miles to the trailhead. Stay right when the road forks.

The trail goes gradually uphill through thick, mixed, beautiful aspen and lodgepole pines, making it a good fall color hike. It rolls uphill fairly gently through the trees for the first 0.75 mile, where it enters the Indian Peaks Wilderness. As the fir trees open up, the trail tracks into a broad drainage and steepens and then switchbacks. Early in the season, you'll see St. Vrain Creek below and hear the sounds of the small seasonal waterfall.

Go through a rocky section, and then the trail levels a little as it turns left (south) at around 1.9 miles, crosses a small stream, and then travels southwest steeply uphill, closing the distance to treeline while veering away from the drainage. Near treeline you are treated to wildflowers (early in the season) among the willows, and the start of the tundra, and there appears to be several ways up the broad slope to the summit. Late in the snow season after avalanche danger is over, this is a popular slope for telemark skiing and snowboarding.

The best route to the summit is on the right-hand ridge on the west side of the mountain unless you want to go directly up the very steep, facing slope and max out your heart rate. Look around and savor the mixed alpine flora and fauna and the 180-degree view. You can make the route a little less steep by making your own mini-switchbacks as you ascend the steep ridge. You see the boundary of Rocky Mountain National Park on the way up and great views of Mount Meeker and the other monarchs of Wild Basin. Near the summit you also see a trail going down into the park that eventually ends up near Wild Basin. The summit view is one of the best in the Front Range; enjoy the peaks of RMNP to the north and the Indian Peaks and Audubon and Paiute peaks to the south.

Chapter 9
Boulder Area:
Indian Peaks

Boulder is one of the most popular places to live in the U.S. because it is surrounded by wonderful places to escape urban living; the mountains west of the city, the Indian Peaks, a magnificent subset of the "Front Range," are among the best landscapes for escape and rejuvenation in North America. This rugged mountain range is lesser known to visitors but is extremely popular among locals for reasons that will become obvious should you have time to savor this awe-inspiring landscape. Ironically, they are virtually the only geographically significant natural or human-made wonders in the state that bear the names of the Native Americans that preceded Europeans by thousands of years. Take any of the following routes west from Boulder: Highway 119 through Boulder Canyon to State Highway 72 (the Peak to Peak Highway) or U.S. Highway 36 north to Lyons; west on State Highway 7 and then south on State Highway 72.

Indian Peaks Wilderness Boundary & Brainard Lake Road

This borderline of a wilderness area is one of the most popular places in the state for hiking, biking, and picnics. When you see the stunning setting you will know why. The Indian Peaks, including Navajo (13,409 feet), Apache (13,441 feet), Shoshone (12,699 feet),

Pawnee (12,943 feet), Mount Toll (12,979 feet), Pauite (13,088 feet), and Audubon (13,223 feet), form a formidable and thoroughly enticing backdrop that makes the crush of humanity bearable. This glacier-carved, Continental Divide, mountain "wall" was once considered as an addition to Rocky Mountain National Park to protect it, but many feared the designation would cause it to be overrun

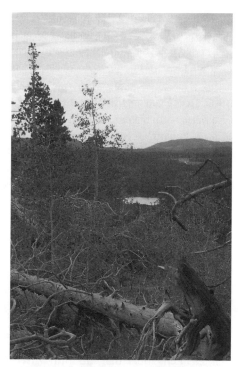

Beaver Reservoir from the Sourdough Trail

with people. Its beauty still makes it very popular. The 1970s wilderness designation for the area means that a permit system for camping and backpacking is now in place for summer—a regulation that was badly needed. I could see some point in the future when day use might require a permit too. I highly recommend that you visit during the week if you want to avoid your fellow *Homo sapiens*, though weekend visits are still enjoyable because of the sheer number of options. If you do plan to visit on the weekend, particularly in the more popular areas, arrive early to make sure you can secure a parking space. The Forest Service has made an effort to help users spread out and to maintain the wilderness appeal of the area; they ask that, if at all possible, you leave your pets at home. Some trails are designated as dog-free, but your furry friends are still allowed on many of the trails if you must bring them.

TRIP 1 Middle St. Vrain

Distance	Up to 9.0 miles, Out-and-back
Difficulty	Easy
Elevation Gain	1000 feet (starting at 8500 feet)
Trail Use	Mountain biking, camping, fishing, option for kids
Agency	Boulder Ranger District, Roosevelt National Forest
Map	Trails Illustrated *Indian Peaks & Gold Hill*
Facilities	Restrooms at campground, fee area

HIGHLIGHTS This area features multiple campgrounds, a beautiful mountain stream, access to Buchanan Pass, and some Indian Peak summits. It is an easy trek on a heavily used trail, starts on the road, and then parallels it from across Middle St. Vrain Creek, while passing through rolling, heavily forested terrain. It is wise to arrive early to avoid the large weekend crowds, or visit the area midweek.

DIRECTIONS Drive north from the Nederland and Ward area; the trailhead is approximately 6 miles north of Ward. You can also reach it by driving toward Allenspark from Lyons, and then turning left (south) on the Peak to Peak Highway (State Highway 72) toward Nederland and Peaceful Valley. Continue south when you see the turnoff for Peaceful Valley, which you're not taking. Do take the second turnoff on west (right) after Peaceful Valley. Look for signs that say FOREST ACCESS or CAMP DICK. Drive through the campground to the end of the road to reach the actual trailhead.

This trailhead also leads to the Sourdough Trail, which goes south toward Beaver Reservoir, Red Rocks Lake, and Rainbow Lakes Road in what is a major adventure. When you reach the trailhead parking lot, where the ORV trail begins, look for the Sourdough Trail on the left (south) side of the road. It is very well marked. Remember that the four-wheel-drive road is not the rolling, mellow trail.

The crossover trail is on the right (north), just beyond the Sourdough Trail. It is 200 yards from the parking lot and goes downhill to the stream on a wide, sturdy bridge. The trail is closed to motorized vehicles.

Some of the best views for photography are at the beginning of the trail and in the campground; if you want pictures of peaks, snap away before you reach the

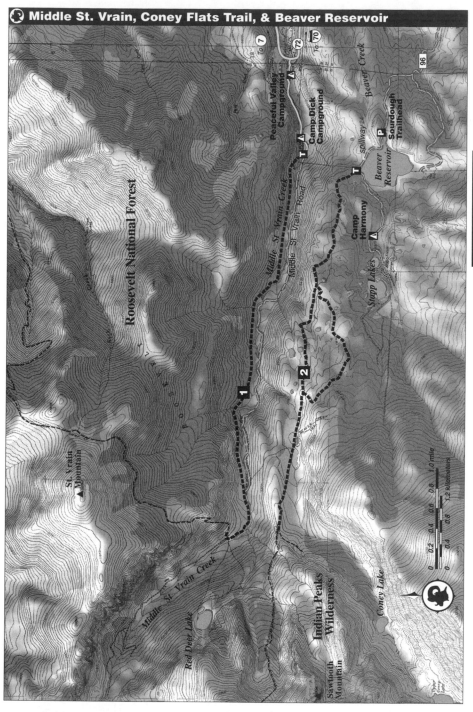

🜨 **Middle St. Vrain, Coney Flats Trail, & Beaver Reservoir**

Roosevelt National Forest

Peaceful Valley Campground

Camp Dick Campground

Beaver Creek

96

Spillway

Sourdough Trailhead

P

Beaver Reservoir

Camp Harmony

Middle St. Vrain Creek

Middle St. Vrain Road

To 7

72

To 70

Stupp Lakes

1

2

St. Vrain Mountain

Indian Peaks Wilderness

Middle St. Vrain Creek

Red Deer Lake

Coney Lake

Sawtooth Mountain

0   0.2   0.4   0.6   0.8   1.0 mile

0   0.4   0.8   1.2 kilometers

Great for Kids

Good for hikers of all ages and skill levels, this trail through a very wide valley climbs very gently to its high point, where it offers a variety of mountain scenery. It is a good place to go on windy or hot days because of the heavy tree cover that will shield you once you get beyond the campground. The trail parallels a beautiful mountain stream, and there are lots of informal spots where you can have a picnic when you have gone far enough to enjoy the riparian beauty. Drive to the end of the road for the closest access to the trailhead. Cross over to the trail from the four-wheel-drive road, and then stroll as far as you wish, until you find a nice picnic spot.

---

heavily forested trail. The trail scenery is varied, with riparian areas, open meadows, some aspens, and every species of evergreen: spruce and lodgepole, limber, and ponderosa pine. Go as far as you like before turning around. You have to start very early and move very fast if you want to make it to treeline and back. Buchanan Pass and the high mountain glacial cirques of the Indian Peaks await you if you make the complete trek. Buchanan Pass is an alternative for climbing up and over the Continental Divide, and trekking all the way to Monarch, Granby, and Grand Lakes. The farther you go, the rockier the trail gets, and the more stunning the high mountain scenery becomes.

TRIP 2 Coney Flats Trail & Beaver Reservoir

see map on p. 191

Distance	Up to 7.5 miles, Semiloop
Difficulty	Easy to moderate
Elevation Gain	600 feet (starting at 9200 feet)
Trail Use	Mountain biking
Agency	Boulder Ranger District, Roosevelt National Forest
Map	Trails Illustrated *Indian Peaks & Gold Hill*

HIGHLIGHTS This easy trek on a lesser known trail starts on the road and then parallels it while passing through rolling, heavily forested terrain. The trail rolls through the trees, offering some pretty vistas of the Indian Peaks along the way.

DIRECTIONS Drive south from Allenspark on the Peak to Peak Highway (State Highway 72) and take the turnoff south of Middle St. Vrain/Camp Dick Campground. The only sign says BOY SCOUT CAMP and Road 96 is on the west side of the highway. Drive approximately 5 miles north on the Peak to Peak Highway from Ward and look for the BOY SCOUT CAMP sign on the west side of the road. It's easy to miss, especially if you're driving too fast; if you reach Camp Dick, you've gone too far. Drive west past the entrance to the Boy Scout Camp until you reach the spillway of the reservoir and then look for the trail on the right (north) side of the road. You can turn around at a wide spot about 0.25 mile west, since the parking is tight when it fills up, and then park as close as you can get. You pass two access points for the Sourdough Trail on the left (south) side of the road on the way in; the first is near State Highway 72 and the second is near the reservoir. The second access is marked as the Beaver Reservoir Trailhead for the Sourdough Trail.

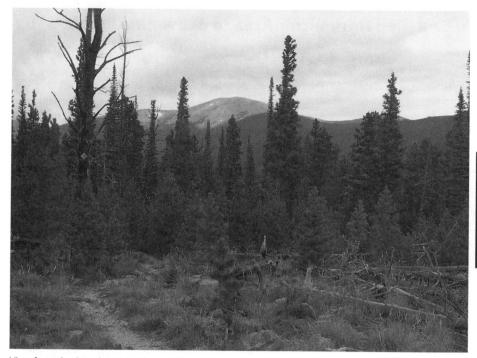

View from the Sourdough Trail near Coney Flats

There are some great views of the Indian Peaks, especially Sawtooth, from the reservoir. If the weather is iffy and you want peak pictures, take them before hiking the trail in case the weather socks it in. The trail starts a bit steeply, levels, and then rolls gently as you pass by several smaller lakes. You are in a lodgepole pine forest tree tunnel and then mixed aspen and pine for the first mile or so, and then the trees open up to some nice views of Sawtooth Mountain and Paiute Peak. When you reach a trail junction where the road leaves the trail and branches off to the south, you can use the gravel road for a short side trip but it isn't marked well and eventually becomes difficult to follow. Stay on the trail, or backtrack to it, unless you are experienced with a compass and topographic map or a GPS unit.

If you'd like a longer trip, take the Sourdough Trail from Beaver Reservoir south to the access at Brainard Lake Road. The northern route begins at the Coney Flats Trailhead, which you pass on the east side of the trail about 50 yards from the start. It goes downhill to the Middle St. Vrain and Camp Dick area described above and is a hilly, heavily forested route that can be a fun short car shuttle.

The southern route is about 0.25 mile short of the reservoir on the south side of the road and intersects with the Baptiste and Wapiti Ski Trails as it travels down- and then uphill until it finally joins the South St. Vrain Trail. From there you can go either to Red Rocks Lake Trailhead, or up to Brainard Lake. It is a long trek in any case.

More accessible, popular access points for the Sourdough Trail include the Brainard Lake Road and Red Rocks Trailhead; you could even go farther south to the Rainbow Lakes Road (County Road 116) Trailhead.

TRIP 3 Red Rock Picnic Area to Beaver Reservoir

Distance	Up to 15.0 miles, Out-and-back
Difficulty	Easy to moderate
Elevation Gain	860 feet (starting at 10,000 feet)
Trail Use	Mountain biking
Agency	Boulder Ranger District, Roosevelt National Forest
Map	Trails Illustrated *Indian Peaks & Gold Hill*

HIGHLIGHTS This is a less popular section of the Sourdough Trail for hiking but is more popular with intermediate mountain bikers, in spite of it being generally much rockier than going south. You break out of the thick tree cover from time to time for pleasing views but are sheltered from wind and sun most of the time.

DIRECTIONS The Brainard access is just east of the fee station for the recreation area and crosses the road at the Red Rock Trailhead parking area. From Boulder, take the Boulder Canyon Road to Nederland. At the intersection in Nederland, turn right or north on the Peak to Peak Highway (State Highway 72) for approximately 9 miles. Pass the funky town of Ward on the right (east) side of the road, and in 0.25 mile turn left (west) onto the Brainard Lake turnoff. From Boulder, you could also take U.S. Highway 36 toward Lyons and then turn left (west) on Left Hand Canyon Road to Ward. Bear right at all intersections along the way.

If you are coming from the north, you can take State Highway 66 west to Lyons and State Highway 7 west to Raymond. Then turn south on State Highway 72 toward Ward, and look for the area on the west side of the road. You can also access the trail near Beaver Reservoir on the north end (see directions for Beaver Reservoir in Trip 2).

Going north from the Red Rock Picnic Area, you have a slight climb over the first 0.25 mile and then a slowly descending stretch (a loss of about 200 feet) until just under a mile. Then the rocky trail descends another 200 feet to an intersection with the South St. Vrain Trail. This means, of course, that you'll have a bit of a climb on the way back. The next 0.5 mile is fairly level, and you come to another trail intersection where you should bear right to go toward Beaver Reservoir. You'll pass a small, seasonal pond and then roll over a 100-foot-high ridge, as the trail trends northwest and then turns sharply to the east and northeast over the next mile. The last mile includes climbs, descents, and switchbacks near the reservoir and then descends to the road. The last mile opens up with nice peak views.

Starting from the reservoir and going south has some immediate rewards for an out-and-back hike.

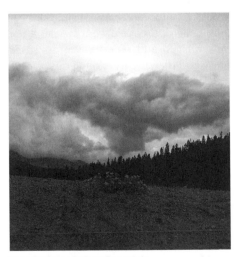

Clouds above Beaver Reservoir

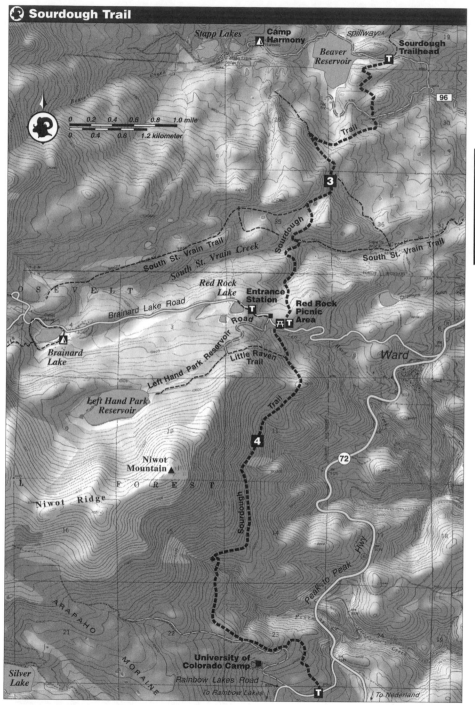

Sourdough Trail

Stapp Lakes

Camp
Harmony

spillway

Beaver
Reservoir

Sourdough
Trailhead

19

96

30

3

25

36

31

South St. Vrain Trail

South St. Vrain Creek

Sourdough

South St. Vrain Trail

Trail

35

R O S E V E L T

Red Rock
Lake

Entrance
Station

Red Rock
Picnic
Area

Brainard Lake Road

Road

Ward

Brainard
Lake

Little Raven
Trail

Left Hand Park Reservoir

Left Hand Park
Reservoir

Trail

9

10

4

11

72

Niwot
Mountain

F O R E S T

13

L

Niwot Ridge

Sourdough

14

16

15

18

A R A P A H O

M O R A I N E

21

22

23

24

16

Silver
Lake

University of
Colorado Camp

Rainbow Lakes Road

To Rainbow Lakes

To Nederland

Peak to Peak Hwy

0   0.2   0.4   0.6   0.8   1.0 mile
0   0.4   0.8   1.2 kilometer

TRIP 4 Red Rock Picnic Area to Rainbow Lakes

Distance	11.0 miles, Out-and-back
Difficulty	Moderate
Elevation Gain	900 feet (starting at 10,000 feet)
Trail Use	Mountain biking
Agency	Boulder Ranger District, Roosevelt National Forest
Map	Trails Illustrated *Indian Peaks & Gold Hill*

see map on p. 195

HIGHLIGHTS The Sourdough Trail, though popular, has much less traffic than trails in and around Brainard Lake. You won't get quite the stunning views of the Indian Peaks but you get beautiful views of the foothills, plains, and even snow-capped peaks in the distance. As you can see from the altitude information (gained and lost) on the map, both trail segments roller coaster, but the trail segment from Brainard to the south is more level overall, until you near Rainbow Lakes where the trail descends significantly.

DIRECTIONS The most accessible and popular access points for the Sourdough Trail are from the Brainard Lake Road or the Rainbow Lakes Road (County Road 116) parking area and trailhead. The Brainard access is just east of the fee station for the recreation area and crosses the road at the Red Rock Trailhead parking area.

From Boulder, take the Boulder Canyon Road to Nederland. At the intersection in Nederland turn right or north on the Peak to Peak Highway (State Highway 72) for approximately 9 miles. Pass the funky town of Ward on the right (east) side of the road, and in 0.25 mile turn left (west) onto the Brainard Lake turnoff.

From Boulder, you could also take Highway 36 toward Lyons and then turn left (west) on Left Hand Canyon Road to Ward. Bear right at all intersections along the way.

If you are coming from the north, you can also take Highway 66 west to Lyons and State Highway 7 west to Raymond. Then turn south on State Highway 72 toward Ward and look for the area on the west side of the road.

You can also access the trail near Beaver Reservoir on the north end (refer to the directions for Beaver Reservoir in Trip 2).

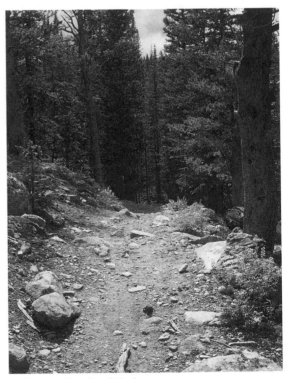

Rocky north Sourdough Trail

This most popular segment of the Sourdough Trail winds 7 miles south from the Red Rock Picnic Area to the parking lot at Rainbow Lakes Trailhead. A car shuttle is a good way to enjoy the trail though you can enjoy the trail with nice out-and-back romps. Much of the trail is sheltered by trees, a major bonus on the frequent windy days. The Sourdough Trail is a bit less scenic than the Brainard Lake area but is also much less heavily used and goes over, under, around, and through many pleasant hills and dales.

The route to the south is a bit easier overall than going north toward Beaver Reservoir. The trail does climb a bit initially and you pass the Little Raven Trail in a little less than 0.5 mile, coming in from the west. You can use this trail to hike up to Left Hand Park Reservoir, where it joins a road, or veer off to climb up Niwot Mountain. After climbing up to 10,200 feet in the first mile, the trail mellows and stays fairly level until you near Rainbow Lakes where it descends 1100 feet to the Rainbow Lakes Road. Needless to say, you will have a significant climb to start your hike if you travel north from the Rainbow Lakes parking lot.

TRIP 5 Red Rock Lake

see map on p. 198

Distance	100 yards, Out-and-back
Difficulty	Easy
Elevation Gain	Negligible
Trail Use	Great for kids
Agency	Boulder Ranger District, Roosevelt National Forest
Map	Trails Illustrated *Indian Peaks & Gold Hill*

HIGHLIGHTS This nice, short, easy side excursion on the left (south) side of Brainard Lake Road takes you 100 yards to the lake and gives you a spectacular view of the peaks, as well as a nice look at a beautiful small lake and riparian area. If you have young children, start with this very short, easy, and scenic round-trip to Red Lake. You can wander around the lake for an easy excursion of any length.

DIRECTIONS From Boulder, take the Boulder Canyon Road to Nederland. At the intersection in Nederland turn right or north on the Peak to Peak Highway (State Highway 72) for approximately 9 miles. Pass the funky town of Ward on the right (east) side of the road, and in 0.25 mile turn left (west) onto the Brainard Lake turnoff.

From Boulder, you could also take Highway 36 toward Lyons and then turn left (west) on Left Hand Canyon Road to Ward. Bear right at all intersections along the way.

If you are coming from the north, you can also take Highway 66 west to Lyons, Highway 7 west to Raymond, and then turn south on Highway 72 toward Ward, and look for the area on the west side of the road.

Pass the Red Lake Trail and side road on the left. Be careful not to confuse this with the Red Rock Trailhead that is the entry point for the superb but challenging Waldrop and St. Vrain Creek Trails. Out-and-back on the road is the easiest way to go, or if you feel a little more adventuresome and don't mind a small hill, take the right edge of the shoreline around the lake to the west where you are rewarded with additional views of the peaks and a nice view of the lake.

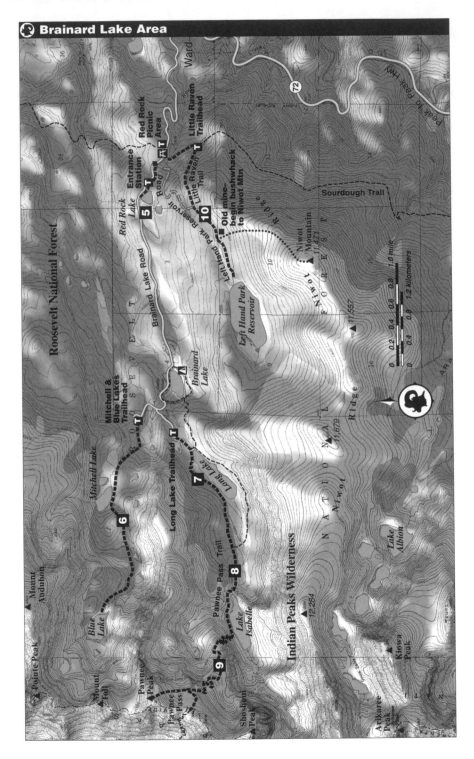

Brainard Lake Area

TRIP 6 Mitchell Lake & Blue Lake Trail

Distance	1.0 mile to Mitchell Lake, 4.8 miles to Blue Lake, Out-and-back
Difficulty	Easy to moderate
Elevation Gain	400 feet to Mitchell Lake, 1000 feet to Blue Lake (starting at 10,300 feet)
Trail Use	Option for kids
Agency	Boulder Ranger District, Roosevelt National Forest
Map	Trails Illustrated *Indian Peaks & Gold Hill*
Facilities	Restrooms at trailhead

HIGHLIGHTS High, pristine mountain lakes with the Indian Peaks as a backdrop are what you'll see for your efforts. The lakes are a very popular destination, so arrive early to find a parking spot. Mitchell Lake is an easy family stroll, while Blue Lake is a very pleasant hike.

DIRECTIONS From Boulder, take the Boulder Canyon Road to Nederland. At the intersection in Nederland turn right or north on the Peak to Peak Highway (State Highway 72) for approximately 9 miles. Pass the funky town of Ward on the right (east) side of the road, and in 0.25 mile turn left (west) onto the Brainard Lake turnoff.

From Boulder, you could also take U.S. Highway 36 toward Lyons and then turn left (west) on Left Hand Canyon Road to Ward. Bear right at all intersections along the way.

If you are coming from the north, you can also take State Highway 66 west to Lyons and State Highway 7 west to Raymond. Then turn south on State Highway 72 toward Ward, and look for the area on the west side of the road.

Follow the Brainard Lake Road 2.5 miles from the entrance station to reach the turnoff for Mitchell and Long Lakes on the right. Turn right at the fork in the road to get to the parking lot.

The trail climbs very gradually 1 mile up to the lake. The trail itself is a steady climb and somewhat steeper than the Long Lake Trail though not significantly so. (Long Lake is only 0.25 mile from the trailhead.) You are in trees most of the way but it opens up for several nice views of the glacial cirque and the pointed summit of Mount Toll at the lake. Climbing Mt. Toll is an adventure that requires very good mountaineering skills unlike Mount Audubon, which can be climbed easily with hiking skills.

The trail starts off by crossing Mitchell Creek on a footbridge and then goes north away from the creek for 0.1 mile before turning southwest toward the lake. It slowly climbs and winds through the pretty mixed forest before rejoining Mitchell Creek and getting steeper. You then climb in earnest and pass a small unnamed lake often mistaken for Mitchell Lake; another 100 to 200 yards is your first opportunity to drop off-trail to Mitchell Lake. After the first shoreline access to Mitchell Lake you continue to climb and pass several more opportunities to descend to the lakeshore. If you continue, you can hike another 2 miles up to Blue Lake, which is well above treeline. If you don't want to go all the way to Blue Lake but would like a nice view above the trees, climb the steep hill just beyond Mitchell Lake. It is worth the price of admission to see the view and won't add much to the return trip.

The trail from Mitchell Lake to Blue Lake is much steeper than the Mitchell

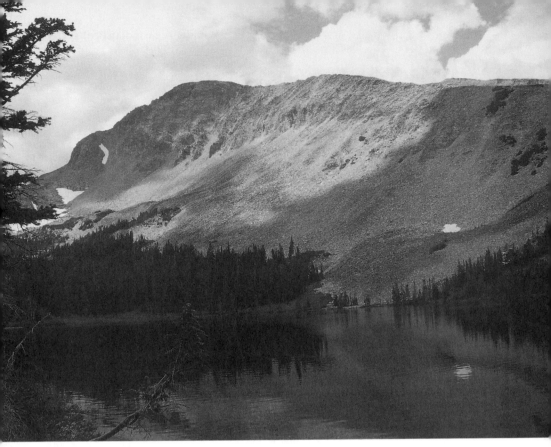

View from Mitchell Lake

Lake Trail throughout, although there are a few flat stretches. It is not a good early season trail, unless you don't mind lots of water and mud. It is much more enjoyable when it has dried out. You are out of the trees after the first steep hill beyond Mitchell Lake, and start enjoying spectacular ridgeline and peak views. On a clear day, the trail offers a steady diet of nice views all the way over the numerous waves of ridges rolling away under your feet, as you climb one false summit ridge after another. As with many of the trails in this book, even if you turn around short of Blue Lake, you will have had a very enjoyable, physically satisfying adventure. Just remember that the return trip will seem much longer and might actually take more time than your trip out because you will be tired.

Great for Kids

By definition and distance, the trek to Mitchell Lake is an easy, short, and highly scenic trip for families with small children or those not wanting an arduous outing. The trail goes up, over, and around rocks as it winds to the lake with a gradual climb and crosses a stream on a small footbridge. There are lots of intermediary sites and sounds to enjoy in the lodgepole pine and aspen forest. Take a picnic or snack for the lakeshore, and enjoy the sparkling water, cool breeze across the lake, and soaring cliffs before returning to your car. If you have additional time and energy, continue another 0.5 mile toward Blue Lake, and enjoy more spectacular views of Niwot Ridge and the high mountain scenery that surround you.

TRIP 7 Long Lake Trail

see map on p. 198

Distance	1.0 mile with side trips, Out-and-back
Difficulty	Easy
Elevation Gain	100 feet (starting at 10,500 feet)
Trail Use	Great for kids
Agency	Boulder Ranger District, Roosevelt National Forest
Map	Trails Illustrated *Indian Peaks & Gold Hill*

HIGHLIGHTS This nice family stroll for the uninitiated has nice views of Niwot Ridge along the way and a spectacular and unique view of the Indian Peaks when you reach the lake. The lakeshore is a delightful place for a lunch or snack break.

DIRECTIONS From Boulder, take the Boulder Canyon Road to Nederland. At the intersection in Nederland turn right or north on the Peak to Peak Highway (State Highway 72) for approximately 9 miles. Pass the funky town of Ward on the right (east) side of the road, and in 0.25 mile turn left (west) onto the Brainard Lake turnoff.

From Boulder, you could also take U.S. Highway 36 toward Lyons and then turn left (west) on Left Hand Canyon Road to Ward. Bear right at all intersections along the way. If you are coming from the north, you can also take State Highway 66 west to Lyons and State Highway 7 west to Raymond. Then turn south on State Highway 72 toward Ward, and look for the area on the west side of the road.

Follow the Brainard Lake Road 2.5 mile from the entrance station to reach the turnoff for Mitchell and Long Lakes on the right. Bear left at the intersection to the trailhead.

This high-altitude stroll leads to a beautiful mountain lake in a spectacular setting. Just follow the trail gradually uphill as it wends its way through the forest; up, over, and around rocks; and across one stream (on a footbridge) to the lake. Be sure to take a camera and a picnic or snack. If you keep going past the east end of the lake, you'll enjoy other nice views of the lake, and the high mountain ridgeline. The Jean Lunning Trail is a nice alternative for the return trip.

TRIP 8 Lake Isabelle

see map on p. 198

Distance	3.0 miles, Out-and-back
Difficulty	Easy
Elevation Gain	300 feet (starting at 10,500 feet)
Agency	Boulder Ranger District, Roosevelt National Forest
Map	Trails Illustrated *Indian Peaks & Gold Hill*
Facilities	Restrooms at trailhead

HIGHLIGHTS Lake Isabelle is another mile beyond Long Lake and is one of the more beautiful trails in the Front Range with spectacular Indian Peak views. It is a steady climb from Long Lake, but not particularly steep, until very near the lake.

DIRECTIONS From Boulder, take the Boulder Canyon Road to Nederland. At the intersection in Nederland turn right or north on the Peak to Peak Highway (State Highway 72) for approximately 9 miles. Pass the funky town of Ward on the right (east) side of the road, and in 0.25 mile turn left (west) onto the Brainard Lake turnoff.

From Boulder, you could also take U.S. Highway 36 toward Lyons and then turn left (west) on Left Hand Canyon Road to Ward. Bear right at all intersections along the way. If you are coming from the north, you can also take State Highway 66 west to Lyons and State Highway 7 west to Raymond. Then turn south on State Highway 72 toward Ward, and look for the area on the west side of the road.

Follow the Brainard Lake Road 2.5 miles from the entrance station to reach the turnoff for Mitchell and Long Lakes on the right.

You are rewarded with superb views almost all the way since most of the trail has openings through the trees to Niwot Ridge. At about 0.75 mile beyond Long Lake, you come to a very nice open meadow area that affords a terrific view of the ridge and some of the peaks beyond—a good place for a rest break because of its southern exposure and relative shelter from the wind. After this point the trail steepens considerably and switchbacks up through trees to the lake. The view from the lake of this section of the Indian Peaks is no less than stunning. From the lake you can continue higher up the Pawnee Pass Trail if you're looking for a longer trek or turn around and return to your starting point.

TRIP 9 Pawnee Pass & Peak

see map on p. 198

Distance	9.8 miles to the pass, 11.0 miles to the peak, Out-and-back
Difficulty	Moderate to challenging
Elevation Gain	2500 feet to pass, 2443 feet to peak (starting at 10,500 feet)
Agency	Boulder Ranger District, Roosevelt National Forest
Map	Trails Illustrated *Indian Peaks & Gold Hill*
Facilities	Restrooms at trailhead

HIGHLIGHTS The hike up to the top of Pawnee Pass is, along with climbing Mount Audubon, one of the most enjoyable moderate to challenging outings in the area. When you make the top of the pass, it is only a short scramble to the north to climb Pawnee Peak. From the top you have not only a great view of the Indian Peaks but also can see all the way over the Continental Divide and into the Monarch Lake and Winter Park area.

DIRECTIONS From Boulder, take the Boulder Canyon Road to Nederland. At the intersection in Nederland turn right (north) on the Peak to Peak Highway (State Highway 72) for approximately 9 miles. Pass the funky town of Ward on the right (east) side of the road, and in 0.25 mile turn left (west) onto the Brainard Lake turnoff.

From Boulder, you could also take U.S. Highway 36 toward Lyons and then turn left (west) on Left Hand Canyon Road to Ward. Bear right at all intersections along the way. If you are coming from the north, you can also take State Highway 66 west to Lyons and State Highway 7 west to Raymond. Then turn south on State Highway 72 toward Ward, and look for the area on the west side of the road.

Follow the Brainard Lake Road 2.5 miles from the entrance station to reach the turnoff for Mitchell and Long Lakes on the right.

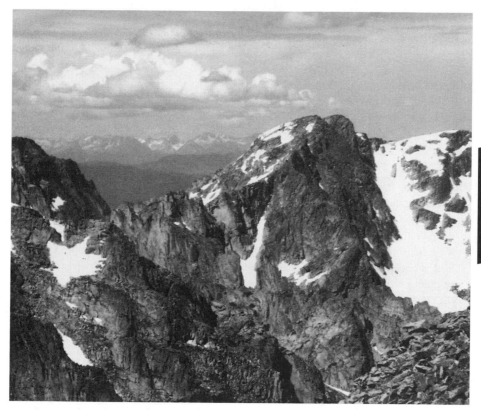

View from Pawnee Peak

You are rewarded with superb views almost all the way to Lake Isabelle because of openings through the trees to Niwot Ridge. At about 0.75 mile beyond Long Lake, you come to a very nice open meadow area that affords a terrific view of the ridge and some of the peaks beyond—a good place for a rest break because of its southern exposure and relative shelter from the wind. After this point the trail steepens considerably and switchbacks up through trees to the lake. The view from the lake of this section of the Indian Peaks is no less than stunning.

From Lake Isabelle continue up the Pawnee Pass Trail, so well marked and well-worn that it's almost impossible to lose. The trail switchbacks northeast from the lake and gradually gains elevation as it tracks mostly west, offering ever more spectacular views along the way. After the initial switchbacks, the trail goes directly and gradually west, narrowing and passing under and around some nice rock formations. It then travels on a broader but somewhat rocky trail for about 0.5 mile before hitting a stretch of short but very steep switchbacks—the crux of the climb to the pass. The peak is a short nontechnical scramble to the right (north) from the pass. Go up and over Pawnee Pass and then down into the Fraser/Grandby area, ending up at beautiful Monarch Lake. The trip to the lake makes a great car shuttle route because it is approximately 14 miles one-way.

TRIP 10 Niwot Mountain & Ridge

see map on p. 198

Distance	6.0 miles, Out-and-back
Difficulty	Moderate
Elevation Gain	1500 feet (starting at 10,000 feet)
Facilities	Restrooms at entrance station
Agency	Boulder Ranger District, Roosevelt National Forest
Map	Trails Illustrated *Indian Peaks & Gold Hill*
Notes	Bushwhacking, map and compass

HIGHLIGHTS Towering above Brainard Lake, this high ridge can be a fun adventure and offers a grand view of the majestic Indian Peaks and Longs Peak without having to travel the length of Brainard Lake to the other trailhead(s). This climb is best attempted on a calm, warm day since Niwot Ridge and Mountain are often windswept; bring extra layers if it is fall or spring. There are three approaches to Niwot Ridge (one of which isn't covered in this book): Left Hand Park Reservoir Road or Sourdough and Little Raven trails. Both originate at the entrance station near the Red Rock Trailhead parking lot.

DIRECTIONS From Boulder, take the Boulder Canyon Road to Nederland. At the intersection in Nederland turn right or north on the Peak to Peak Highway (State Highway 72) for approximately 9 miles. Pass the funky town of Ward on the right (east) side of the road, and in 0.25 mile turn left (west) onto the Brainard Lake turnoff.

From Boulder, you could also take U.S. Highway 36 toward Lyons and then turn left (west) on Left Hand Canyon Road to Ward. Bear right at all intersections along the way. If you are coming from the north, you can take State Highway 66 west to Lyons and State Highway 7 west to Raymond. Then turn south on State Highway 72 toward Ward, and look for the area on the west side of the road.

There is no marked trail to the top of Niwot Mountain, so this trip requires good route-finding and bushwhacking skills with a topographic map and compass. As mentioned, there are three routes to start this climb (one of which this book doesn't cover)—you can go up Left Hand Park Reservoir Road on the south side of the Brainard Lake Road about 200 yards from the Red Rock Trailhead parking area. Or, you can use the Sourdough and Little Raven Trails for the first mile and then travel the reservoir road to where the road and trail split. In both cases you are traveling to an old gravel pit or mine, approximately 1 mile up on the south side of Left Hand Park Reservoir Road. I recommend taking the trails on the way up and then the road on the way down.

To use the trails on the way up, take the Sourdough Trail south from the Red Rock parking area. The trailhead is across the road from the parking area and about 100 feet east. After leaving the road, take the Sourdough Trail approximately 0.5 mile south to the intersection with the Little Raven Trail. It rolls gently to the intersection where there should be a sign marking the Little Raven Trail. Turn right (west) onto Little Raven Trail while the Sourdough Trail to Rainbow Lakes continues straight (south). The Little Raven Trail alternates between steep and moderate climbing. As it nears Left Hand Park Reservoir Road, it levels out a little and climbs more slowly. You are on Little Raven Trail for approximately 0.6 mile to the intersection with the reservoir road. From there turn left (southwest) on the road and go approximately 0.5 mile uphill to the mined area. Leave the road for the ridge and when a sign indicates that Little Raven Trail is heading to Brainard Lake, get back on the road. When you reach the mined area, climb up the hill to the left (east) side of the mine. Then bear left or southeast when you enter the trees. You are climbing steeply and gaining about 200 feet in the first 0.25 mile through thick trees. After 0.25 mile you are on a more gradual ascent path at around 10,600 feet; pick the best route and angle to the southwest. After climbing another 0.3 mile and another 200 feet to 10,800 feet in elevation, you encounter stunted krumholtz pine trees. At this point you already have a great view of Longs Peak to

the north and Toll, Pawnee, and Audubon peaks to the west.

Turn around if the wind is howling, and you will have had a nice adventure. If it one of those rare beautiful, calm, summer days, note carefully where you emerge from the trees and pick your way west up the ridge. Look back frequently so you'll know where to reenter the trees on your return. From here you can decide how high and how far you want to go based on weather. If both are favorable, angle toward the rock shelter visible on the ridgetop. It offers a nice windbreak for a snack or photos. The Niwot Mountain/Bald Mountain summit is the high point at the east end of the ridge at 11,471 feet. If you are in a peak-bagging mood, check out the higher points along the ridge at 11,557 and 11,679 feet. Hike the ridge for as long and as far as you like and then turn around.

TRIP 11 Rainbow Lakes & Arapaho Glacier Overlook Trails

Distance	2.0 to 12.0 miles, Out-and-back
Difficulty	Easy to moderate
Elevation Gain	300 feet to Caribou Ridge, 1100 feet to Arapaho Trail (starting at 10,100 feet)
Trail Use	Fishing, camping, option for kids
Facilities	Campground and restrooms
Agency	Boulder Ranger District, Roosevelt National Forest
Map	Trails Illustrated *Indian Peaks & Gold Hill*

HIGHLIGHTS The four small Rainbow Lakes are in a spectacular high-mountain setting nestled next to the soaring tundra, glacier-carved Caribou ridgeline. The real treat is the view from the lakes, plus there's good fishing if the thunder isn't rolling. The Arapaho Glacier Overlook Trail is more challenging but an even more stunning spectacle. These trails and the campground are heavily used in the summer. The area melts out, and dries out, later in the summer (July/August) in an average snow year because of the elevation. Bring insect repellent.

DIRECTIONS From Boulder take Boulder Canyon 14 miles to Nederland. County Road 116 is between Nederland and Ward on the west side of the road. It is also the entry to the University of Colorado Research Station. There is a large parking lot for the southern

Rainbow Lakes & Arapaho Glacier Overlook Trails

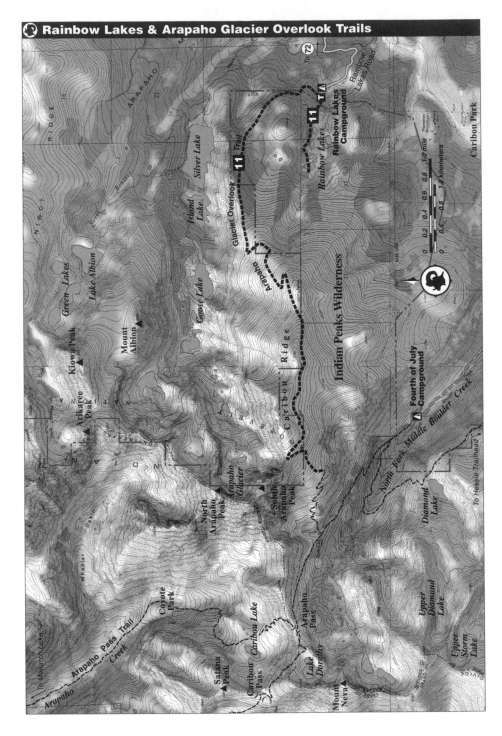

terminus of the Sourdough Trail and a rough but drivable road from that point 4.2 miles to the trailhead. Much of the rough road enjoys southern exposure and is relatively snow free much of the winter. Both trailheads are at the end of the road, and the western edge of the Rainbow Lakes Campground.

Rainbow Lakes Trail

This trailhead is at the very end of the road at the southwest end of the parking lot and is well signed. It rolls gently for 1 mile to the lakes, and you'll have some nice views along the way. The trail turns left (south) and then west at the watershed boundary sign. It gets steeper as you walk through the pretty mixed aspen and conifer forest. It widens and levels after climbing 150 feet and 0.5 mile to 10,250 feet. It is then only another 50 yards down to the first lake making this an easy jaunt for small children or the less ambitious. There is a slight climb to the second lake and overview. The first two lakes are essentially adjacent. The second lake offers a great peak view.

From there the trail gets very rocky, climbs up to 10,300 feet, passes wetlands, and then levels. In 0.25 mile you cross a stream that can be deep during spring runoff. Lakes 3 and 4 are like twin sisters and feature another nice peak view—a good lunch spot. If you go south and east around Lake 4 you will see a small pond with an informal campsite and illegal fire ring. I recommend going south and west between the lakes to the sheltered stream for quiet contemplation or a snack break. Pick your way around the rocks. It turns into a nice meadow stroll as the trail meanders in a southwest direction. Reverse course to the trailhead at your leisure.

Arapaho Glacier Overlook Trail

This trailhead is on the northwest end of the campground. The actual overlook is a distant 6 miles one-way from the trailhead, but you can make it to treeline and a stunning view in approximately 3 miles one-way. The trailhead is well marked, and the initial mile or so the trail is easy to track because it runs along the City of Boulder's watershed fence and then has a few blue ribbons once you leave the watershed boundary and enjoy a mixed conifer and aspen forest. Once the trail starts to climb and steepen, the switchbacks are difficult to see and are not well marked. You'll need a topographic map and good route-finding skills, but if you keep the lakes to your left (south) and the ridgeline to the right (north) you are generally traveling first north and then west on the south side of the ridge. There is much fallen timber everywhere except the trail, which is always a good clue as to its location.

Great for Kids

The trail to the four Rainbow Lakes is short and sweet with easy walking and nice views all around. This area is very popular for fishing and camping and hiking with families. It is a gently rolling, 1-mile trail to the lakes, so it is ideal for small children or casual excursions.

You have options for two Rainbow Lakes upon arrival: one to the right (west-northwest) and another to the left (southwest). The other two lakes are farther than 1 mile (approximately 0.5 mile beyond the first two). The trails around the lakes are quite narrow, but some lakeside spots are good for a snack or picnic stop between the lakes.

After following the winding trail to the treeline, walk over to the north side of the ridge to enjoy a superb view of the Boulder Watershed that includes the panorama of the Indian Peaks glacier-carved moraine. You have a great view of the rest of the Caribou Ridge route to North and South Arapaho Peaks as well as the glacier itself and Kiowa Peak and Niwot Ridge. The prevailing, west wind makes your visit above treeline an air-conditioned one even on hot days. The trail continues for another 3 miles one-way to the actual overlook of the small glacier.

TRIP 12 Woodland Lake Trail

Distance	10.0 miles, Out-and-back
Difficulty	Moderate
Elevation Gain	300 feet (starting at 10,000 feet)
Agency	Boulder Ranger District, Roosevelt National Forest
Map	Trails Illustrated *Indian Peaks & Gold Hill*
Facilities	Campground and restrooms

HIGHLIGHTS The Eldora town site and Hessie Trailhead are gateways to many excellent trails to serene high mountain lakes, and 13,000 foot North and South Arapaho peaks. This route to one of the closer lakes in this spectacular mountain park can be snowy or wet in late May or early June.

DIRECTIONS From Denver take State Highway 93 to Boulder and exit at Canyon Street. From Fort Collins go to downtown Boulder by your favorite route and take State Highway 119 west. From Boulder take Canyon St., which becomes State Highway 119 (also known as Boulder Canyon), west 18 miles to Nederland. Take the rotary around to the left (south) on State Highway 72/119. Turn right on Boulder County Road 130, where you'll see a sign for the Eldora Ski area. Continue straight past the second turnoff that goes up to the ski area; the Eldora town site and Hessie Road are straight ahead.

There is parking near the trailhead, but the road gets progressively rougher as you go. Do not go straight up toward 4th of July Campground. Hessie is left at the first major gravel road intersection, less than 0.5 mile from the Eldora town site. If you park near Eldora and walk down the road, bear left at the intersection, where there should be a sign for Hessie. Look for a short trail on the right side if the road to the trailhead is flooded with spring runoff. The final stretch, a walkable 0.5 mile, of road to the trailhead is a four-wheel-drive, high-clearance road.

After a large footbridge and stream crossing, you will travel on a rapidly ascending old mining road at the rate of 100 feet every 0.25 mile. The trail breaks out of the trees with a nice panorama of the high mountain valley at 9100 feet. The trail levels a little in another 0.25 mile around 9200 feet, or I should say that it is a little less steep before climbing another 200 feet over the next 0.25 mile to 9400 feet, reentering trees in the process. The next trail intersection signage gives the distances to some of the lakes—1.5 miles to Lost Lake, 4 miles to Woodland Lake, 5 miles to King Lake, 4 miles to Jasper, and 5 miles to Devil's Thumb.

Woodland Lake Trail

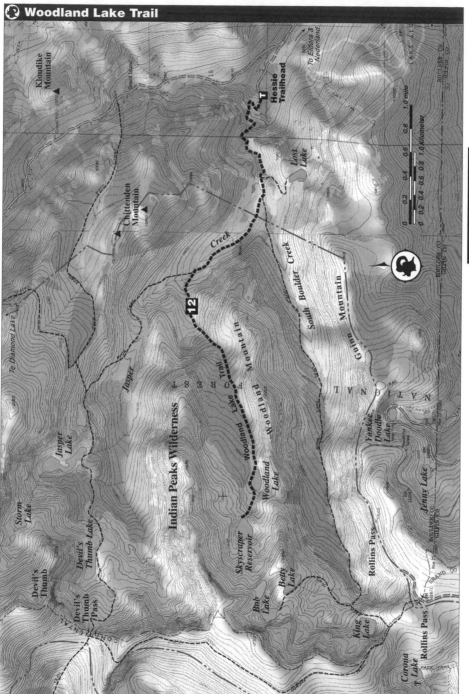

You have another footbridge stream crossing and reach another trail intersection at just under the 2-mile mark and around 9500 feet. Go right for Devil's Thumb Lake, left for your destination Woodland, and King's Lakes. You enjoy great views and a pretty cirque lake in the next 0.25-mile climb, a place where you could declare victory and turn around if your party has weary feet or lungs. The trail goes left back into the trees and then takes a sharp right northwest to another footbridge stream crossing. You'll enjoy a beautiful wildflower meadow and peak views (North and South Arapaho as well as the ridgelines) all around. When you reach the wilderness boundary in 0.25 mile, the trail levels and climbs more gradually, as it crosses more meadows with gorgeous wildflowers, while meandering next to the stream. (Yes, people can imitate nature and meander.) Look to the right to see a small waterfall just before you reach another trail intersection with signs telling you to bear left for Woodland Lake.

At 9600 feet the trail climbs more steeply at 100 feet per 0.1 mile. You have a great overview of the entire glacial moraine, or drainage, and several petite waterfalls at 9800 feet. At 9900 feet the trail levels again briefly and crosses a narrow footbridge to the south. It then turns west and back to the south sharply. You climb some steep switchbacks up to 10,000 feet, take a breath, and then climb in earnest up to 10,300 feet before leveling with a waterfall on the left. You enjoy lots of shade to keep you from overheating as you cross wetlands. The trail then turns south again and crosses open meadows with a ridgeline view at 10,600 feet. It actually descends a little before climbing to an even more spectacular view of the ridge at 10,800 feet and then levels as it reaches and skirts the lake.

Stay on the trail and climb up to a little less than 11,000 feet for an even better panorama of the lake. The trail continues in a stair-step fashion up to Skyscraper Reservoir. It isn't a pristine mountain lake like Woodland, but does have a great eagle's-eye view of the plains. The topmost ridge is surmountable from here, but because it would be a very steep scramble over scree and tundra I don't recommend it. Tiptoe across wetlands, meadows, or rocks. Look at the infinite variations of rock, sky, trees, flowers, grasses, and every angle of the universe at your feet. On the way down keep your eyes peeled for the gorgeous waterfall on the west side of the trail, near the second stream crossing if you missed it, as I did, on the way up!

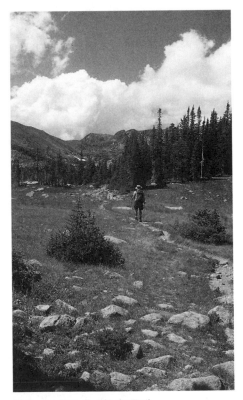

Author on Woodland Lake Trail

Chapter 10

Boulder Area:
Plains & Foothills

Few places on Earth offer as many recreational opportunities as the city and county of Boulder. Community leaders in the 1960s and 1970s very wisely passed tax initiatives to set aside a superb, almost endless variety of public open spaces. The city and county have done an excellent job of managing and protecting these special places from overuse and user conflicts. They can be used for hiking, biking, running, strolling, horseback riding, picnicking, or even just napping. Uses are often separated; making hikers, bikers, horseback riders, and dog lovers happy. You can enjoy foothills, prairies, canyons, arroyos, lakes, and riparian areas; urban and rural settings; rock outcrops for climbing and scrambling; or expansive ranches. A leash law for dogs

is strictly enforced, and dogs are prohibited on some trails and welcomed on others. (Please bring a plastic bag along for cleaning up after your pet.) There are hungry mountain lions in the hills, so keep a close eye on your children and keep your dog leashed to prevent them from becoming snack food.

Eldorado Canyon State Park

This world-class rock climbing mecca and delightful state park south of Boulder has more than death-defying rock climbing routes. It has an expansive picnic area, visitors center, and bookstore, a hot springs pool nearby, a wide variety of trails for children of all ages, and one of the most amazing settings along the Front Range only minutes from Boulder.

Sunrise over Boulder from Mount Sanitas

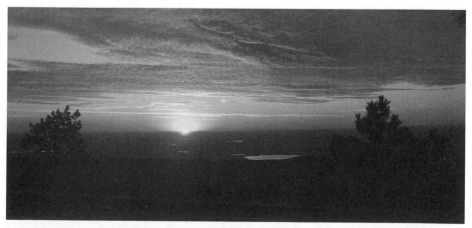

TRIP 1 Little Thompson Overlook Trail

Distance	3 miles, Out-and-back
Difficulty	Easy to moderate
Elevation Gain	500 feet (starting at 5490 feet)
Trail Use	Great for kids, leashed dogs OK
Agency	Boulder County
Maps	*Boulder County,* Trails Illustrated *Boulder & Golden*
Facilities	Restrooms and picnic tables at trailhead
Note	The nearby Indian Mesa Trail is a great mountain biking option.

HIGHLIGHTS This area was tropical lowland covered by rivers, swamps, and lagoons 140 million years ago. Dinosaurs and other reptiles wandered through the lush vegetation. In more recent history, Native Americans lived in this area for at least 5000 years. Eventually, battles were lost and treaties were signed and broken, and the Arapaho and Cheyenne were permanently removed from their lands by 1867; today their descendants live on reservations in Wyoming and Oklahoma.

Rabbit Mountain offers a variety of family-friendly trails that feature sweeping views of the plains, foothills, mountains, and hogback. There is some shade, but most of the ponderosa pine trees are scattered and not large; these trails are better on cool days, or in the spring and fall or even winter, unless you start early and avoid the midday heat. Rolling Little Thompson Trail has a nice perch for a hogback and foothills view. If you'd like a moderate day, combine this trail with the Eagle Wind Trail.

DIRECTIONS From Boulder, take U.S. Highway 36 north toward Lyons. At the intersection with State Highway 66 turn right. In 1 mile turn left on 53rd Street at the sign for Rabbit Mountain. Look for the parking lot in about 2 miles. From the parking lot, you have two options. If you are hiking, bear northeast and go up the hiking trail that switchbacks gently up the south-facing slope. If you're biking, hop on your bike, bear right, go due east on the road, and then turn left (north) in about 0.25 mile. After you turn left (north), you'll be going uphill on a trail that is more like a service or access road and is wide enough for cars.

If you are hiking, you immediately have changing hogback views to the northwest as you are going up. The steepest section is at the beginning, so don't be discouraged as the trail moderates after the first 0.25 mile. You can enjoy early season wildflowers, cactus, and trailside rocks that small people might like to perch on. After the switchbacks, the trail travels north-northeast, and you will see a biking route on the right (east) side of the trail. The trail climbs more gradually over the next 0.25 mile before reaching a level spot and a trail intersection. At this point you can bear left (northwest) to stay on the overlook trail, which is signed, or go downhill, cross the road, and take the Eagle Wind Trail loop (Trip 2). Though it is tempting to stop here, wait until you reach the overlook, so you can savor the view.

The Little Thompson Trail climbs a little more and then descends for approximately 0.25 mile, with pretty views of the dramatic rock formations to the north. You also have a nice view of the northeast slope of Rabbit Mountain as you traverse down and then up across the mountain-

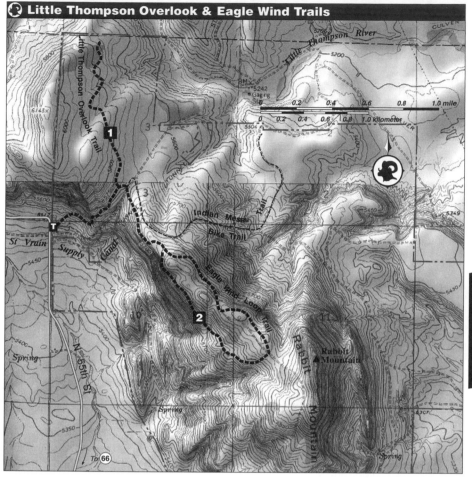

Little Thompson Overlook & Eagle Wind Trails

side. The trail gets somewhat steeper and is surrounded by a variety of shrubs that are taller as you reach the overlook. There is a bench for a snack break or other rock options if you want to rock scramble and escape your fellow travelers.

TRIP 2 Eagle Wind Trail

Distance	4.3 miles, Semiloop
Difficulty	Easy to moderate
Elevation Gain	380 feet (starting at 5490 feet)
Trail Use	Leashed dogs OK
Agency	Boulder County
Maps	*Boulder County*, Trails Illustrated *Boulder & Golden*
Facilities	Restrooms and picnic tables at trailhead
Note	The nearby Indian Mesa Trail is a great mountain biking option.

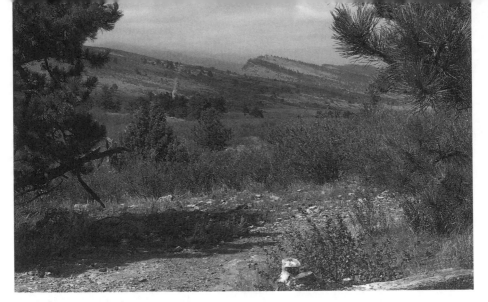

View from Rabbit Mountain, Eagle Wind Trail

HIGHLIGHTS The Rabbit Mountain area was tropical lowland covered by rivers, swamps, and lagoons 140 million years ago. Dinosaurs and other reptiles wandered through the lush vegetation. In more recent history, Native Americans lived in this area for at least 5000 years. Eventually, battles were lost and treaties were signed and broken, and the Arapaho and Cheyenne were permanently removed from their lands by 1867; today their descendants live on reservations in Wyoming and Oklahoma.

Rabbit Mountain offers a variety of family-friendly trails that feature sweeping views of the plains, foothills, mountains, and hogback. There is some shade but most of the ponderosa pine trees are scattered and not large; these trails are better on cool days or in the spring and fall unless you start early and avoid the midday heat. A pleasant, rolling jaunt with great views, the Eagle Wind Trail overlooks the plains and steep slopes of Rabbit Mountain from an easy loop. If you'd like a moderate day, combine this trail with the Eagle Wind Trail.

DIRECTIONS From Boulder, take Highway 36 north toward Lyons. At the intersection with Highway 66 turn right. In 1 mile turn left on 53rd Street at the sign for Rabbit Mountain. Look for the parking lot in about 2 miles. From the parking lot, you have two options. If you want to take the trail to the Eagle Wind loop, bear northeast and go up the trail that switchbacks gently up the south-facing slope. If you'd rather follow the dirt road, bear right, go due east on either the road, and then turn north in about 0.25 mile. After you turn north, you'll be going uphill on a trail that is more like a service or access road and is wide enough for two cars.

If you are hiking, you immediately have changing hogback views to the northwest as you are going up. The steepest section is at the beginning, so don't be discouraged as the trail moderates after the first 0.25 mile. You can enjoy early season wildflowers, cactus, and trailside rocks that small people might like to perch on. After the switchbacks, the trail travels north-northeast, and you see the biking route mentioned previously on the right (east) side of the trail. The trail climbs more gradually over the next 0.25 mile before reaching a level spot and a trail intersection. At this point you can bear left (northwest) to stay on the overlook trail, which is signed, or go downhill, cross the road, and take the Eagle Wind Trail loop.

If you've chosen the dirt road from the parking lot to reach the turnoff for the Eagle Wind Trail loop, look for the trail on the right (east) side of the road after you crest the hill. The loop begins in a saddle between the two humps that form Rabbit Mountain and traverses the easternmost broad ridge of Rabbit Mountain.

The loop starts uphill from the dirt road, and you have nice views of the distant Flatirons and foothills north of Boulder, to the south, through the occasional trees that border the trail. The first 0.25 mile from the road is uphill, then the trail climbs more gradually and levels as it reaches the top. You pass several social

(informal) trails on the right (south), but the actual trail is well marked—so stay on it to prevent erosion. Once you reach the actual loop trail intersection, if you go right/counterclockwise around the loop, you will emerge from the trees and shrubs to the aforementioned views to the south and the panorama of the Continental Divide that opens up to the west. The trail descends gradually with impressive arroyo views as it narrows and gets rockier. Sweeping views of the plains greet you as you roll around to the east side of the mountain. You have a slight climb on the way back either way because a section of the east end of the trail is lower than the west side, but not significantly so. The views and effort are equal regardless of the direction you choose and well worth the price of admission.

TRIP 3 Pella Crossing

Distance	Up to 3.0 miles total (1.9 miles on Braly Trails, 1.0 mile on Marlatt Trails, 0.5 mile on trail connecting them), Semiloop
Difficulty	Easy
Elevation Gain	Negligible (starting at approximately 5000 feet)
Trail Use	Mountain biking, running, horseback riding, fishing (catch and release bass, belly boat), leashed dogs OK, great for kids
Agency	Boulder County
Map	*Boulder County,* Trails Illustrated *Boulder & Golden*
Facilities	Restrooms, picnic tables, and a group shelter at trailhead

HIGHLIGHTS This delightful collection of peaceful, small lakes is circled by wide, flat, short trails ideal for easy-going strolls near Boulder. Circumnavigate Sunset and Webster Ponds, or Heron Lake on the Braly Trails on the eastern side of the park, or the smaller Poplar, Dragonfly, and Clearwater Ponds on the Marlatt Trails on the western side of the park—or perhaps connect the two for a longer outing. Both feature waterfowl, dragonflies, deer, foxes, and butterflies. Longs Peak peers over the top of the west side, while the distant foothills highlight the views of the east side ponds and even almost reflect in the still waters. Belly boat fishing is allowed.

DIRECTIONS From the informal village of Hygiene, which is north of Boulder, west of Longmont, and east of Lyons, turn south onto North 75th Street, or Hygiene Road. Pella Crossing is 0.5 mile south of town. The parking area is on the east side of road.

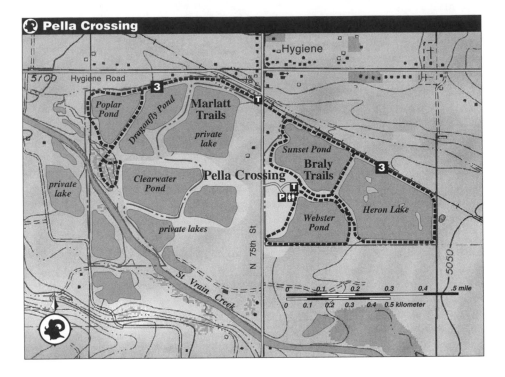

These lakes and ponds are reclaimed gravel pits that Boulder County purchased in 1995 and restored; the county did a beautiful job, making this a delightful natural area. The whole area is a great place for family strolls and mellow picnics. If you only have time to circle one lake, I suggest the largest one, Heron Lake. It has a few tiny islands that birds enjoy, as well as nice trees and views.

For the Braly Trails, go right (east) from the parking area between Sunset and Webster Ponds 0.25 mile to a trail intersection. Go left (north) between Sunset Pond and Heron Lake another 0.25 mile, then turn right (southeast) and enjoy the 0.5-mile jaunt along the northern edge of Heron Lake. Circle the lake back to Webster and Sunset Ponds, where you can circumnavigate either of them. Circle all three and you have completed a nice, almost 2-mile loop.

From the northwest edge of Sunset Pond, you can extend your excursion and walk 0.3 mile over to the Marlatt Trails on a connector trail. You get a nice farm-framed view of Longs Peak as your reward. You'll add another mile to your trek if you walk around this group of pretty ponds (Poplar, Dragonfly, and Clearwater).

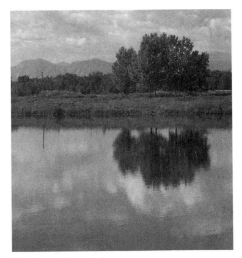

View from Heron Lake

TRIP 4 Lagerman Reservoir

Distance	1.6 miles, Loop
Difficulty	Easy
Elevation Gain	Negligible (starting at 5200 feet)
Trail Use	Mountain biking, fishing, great for kids, leashed dogs OK
Agency	Boulder County
Map	*Boulder County,* Trails Illustrated *Boulder & Golden*
Facilities	Restrooms, picnic table, and a group shelter at trailhead

HIGHLIGHTS This easy, flat loop trail is great for families with small children or anyone want-ing some quiet contemplation of the Flatirons/foothills views.

DIRECTIONS Take North 75th Street north from Longmont and turn left on Pike Road, which is called Clover Basin Road on the other side of 75th. Drive 0.5 mile west on Pike Road to the entrance on the left (south) side.

Circle the reservoir in a clockwise direc-tion to get the best foothills views. A thicket of beautiful sunflowers decorates the north shoreline in season. You will have a good, though distant, view of the Flatirons from the reservoir. This is a good place to bring small children for easy nature adventure. The trail is vir-tually flat, and you will likely see ducks and geese. The picnic area and restrooms make it easy for a picnic, too. Tie together routes with adjacent gravel roads for easy mountain biking.

Boulder Area:
Plains & Foothills

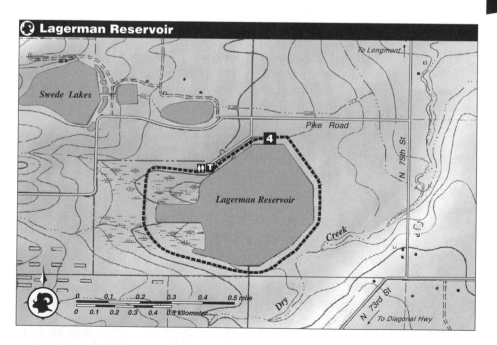

TRIP 5 Walden & Sawhill Ponds

Distance	2.6 miles, Semiloop
Difficulty	Easy
Elevation Gain	Negligible (starting at 5200 feet)
Trail Use	Fishing, leashed dogs OK, bird watching, mountain biking (bikes are prohibited on the boardwalk)
Facilities	Restrooms, picnic table, and a group shelter at trailhead
Agency	Boulder County
Map	*Boulder County*, Trails Illustrated *Boulder & Golden*

HIGHLIGHTS More than 19 small ponds and wetlands, once mined for gravel, are scattered on 113 acres of restored habitat. Some of it is rough around the edges since the restoration began only in 1975, but there is a great deal of natural beauty shining through; the Sawhill Ponds are the more attractive of the two areas. It is a nice setting for enjoying a variety of winged and feathered friends, including pelicans, great blue herons, belted kingfishers, gulls, and geese, to name just a few of the 20 species spotted regularly here.

DIRECTIONS From Boulder take Valmont Road to 75th Street. Turn left onto 75th Street and drive north. The preserve is 0.5 mile south of Jay Road on the west side of 75th Street.

Although you might not be impressed when you pull into the parking lot, persevere and take the Cottonwood Marsh Trail to the west. Keep an eye out for the bird watching boardwalk on the right (north) side of the trail and take a little detour to experience the marshland. Walk slowly and carefully and bring some binoculars to watch the waterfowl. Sink into the serenity of the place.

Walk on toward Duck Pond to the left (south) of the boardwalk. Walk south between the ponds and then turn right (west) and go between the Ricky Weiser Wetlands and Bass Pond. Take a left and walk south to Sawhill Ponds. Wander where your spirit takes you, weaving among the water, reeds, grasses, and birds—no goals permitted.

Family "on Walden Pond"

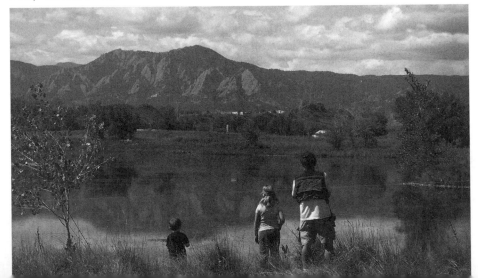

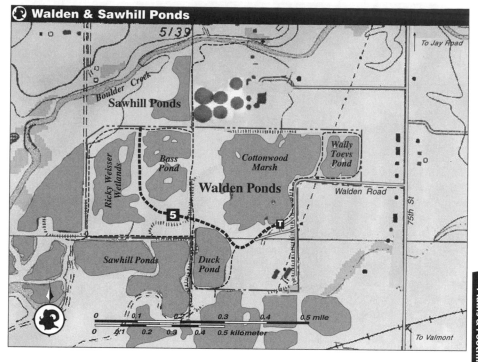

Walden & Sawhill Ponds

5/39

To Jay Road

Boulder Creek

Sawhill Ponds

Ricky Weiser Wetlands

Bass Pond

Cottonwood Marsh

Wally Toevs Pond

Walden Ponds

Walden Road

75th St

Sawhill Ponds

Duck Pond

0   0.1   0.2   0.3   0.4   0.5 mile
0   0.1   0.2   0.3   0.4   0.5 kilometer

To Valmont

TRIP 6 Hall Ranch

Distance	9.4 miles for the Nighthawk, Bitterbrush, and Antelope Loop; add 4.0 miles for the Button Rock extension; Loop
Difficulty	Moderate
Elevation Gain	1220 feet (starting at 5500 feet)
Trail Use	Mountain biking, running, option for kids, leashed dogs OK
Agency	Boulder County
Map	*Boulder County*, Trails Illustrated *Boulder & Golden*
Facilities	Restrooms at trailhead

HIGHLIGHTS This gem of the Boulder County Open Space Program features a beautiful loop trail popular with hikers, mountain bikers, and runners and a great view of Longs Peak at its highest point. It is also very busy on weekends, so an early start or a weekday visit is advisable. The trail is nestled in the foothills just west of the charming town of Lyons.

DIRECTIONS Lyons is north of Boulder, west of Longmont and south of the Loveland/Fort Collins area. From Lyons take State Highway 7 about 1 mile up the St. Vrain Canyon. Hall Ranch will be on the right (north) side of the road. From Denver take Interstate 25 to State Highway 66.

From the parking lot, start the loop hike on the Nighthawk Trail to the west and go clockwise if you are hiking.

Bicyclists are only allowed to start to the north and travel counterclockwise. If you are on foot and want to avoid bikes

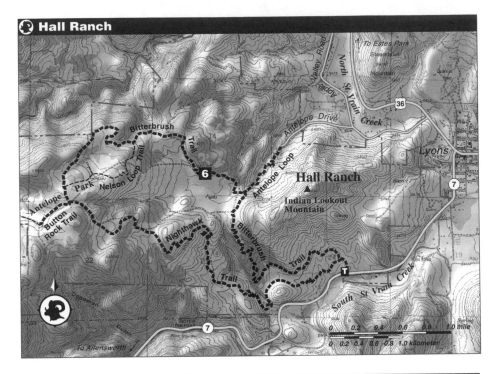

Hall Ranch

altogether, go west and then hike out and back rather than completing the entire loop. I describe this hike as a clockwise loop starting from the west side of the parking lot and joining the biking trail at the high point to return to the parking area.

From the parking lot go west as the trail rolls gently through tall yellow grass and crosses a service road. It goes uphill, steepening and getting rocky. The soaring cliffs offer some great sights behind you before you round the corner. The trail then travels north and west for 1 mile. When you come to the mile marker, you enjoy great foothills and vista views; that's what you will be climbing.

The trail turns south and gradually descends, losing almost 100 feet; a quarry and State Highway 7 are briefly visible from the trail. After you switchback down to the trickle of water, the trail turns right (north), regaining the lost altitude gradually as it climbs 100 feet up over the

> **Great for Kids**
>
> With its great views, the mile marker is a good turnaround for a 2-mile easy jaunt with small children. The 2.5-mile point is also a good place for families with small children to turn around for a 5-mile round-trip with superb scenery.

next 0.25 mile and away from the road and quarry noise. It then turns northwest through a beautiful meadow, where you see a fire marker and then the second mile marker at around 5900 feet. The trail climbs 200 feet in the next 0.5 mile as it offers nice views of a small canyon that it parallels. At around 6100 feet and 2.5 miles, the trail levels with superb 180-degree views.

The trail steepens for the next 0.5 mile and tracks to the southwest, becoming more narrow and rocky as it traverses the foothills terrain. It levels and morphs into long, easy, but uphill switchbacks

Hall Ranch panorama

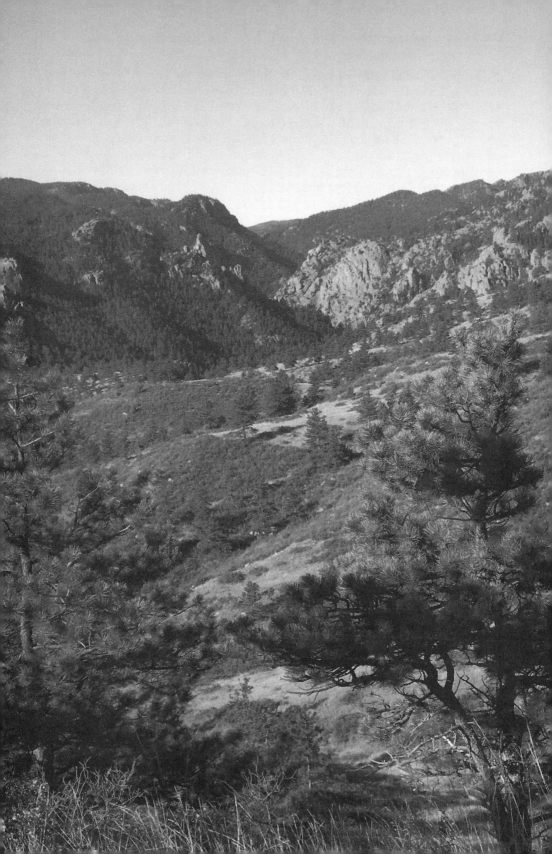

that top out at almost 6400 feet at around 3.2 miles. Enjoy the sunny flat spot or descend 50 feet into some nice trees and shade, as the trail tracks north, climbing across a pretty meadow, and then letting you enjoy a mountain view as it heads east. Another 0.25 mile brings you to around 6500 feet. The trail continues to climb, mostly in the open. You come to a trail intersection at around 4 miles, next to a lone shade tree; bear left. After crossing another nice meadow, the trail enters a stand of lodgepole pines and passes a stone retaining wall. The long, gentle climb of almost 0.5 mile brings you to the high point of 6700 feet, approximately 4.5 miles from the beginning of the trail—the highlight of the hike and a great place for lunch since you enjoy a spectacular view of Longs Peak and a superb panorama of the entire Rocky Mountain National Park massif. You also see signage that says you can add another 4.5 miles for the Button Rock Trail that travels west from this intersection. You also see a trail that goes right for the old ranch road; your route continues straight and takes you near a long-abandoned hotel complex.

Now the descent begins in earnest and you're sharing the trail with mountain bikers. In approximately 0.1 mile you intersect the Nelson Loop Trail, a pleasant detour that can add another 2.2 miles to your day if you circle the entire loop. If you continue to the left, you enjoy some better views as you trek 1.1

miles around the Nelson Loop Trail and eventually intersect the Bitterbrush Trail. From there you are approximately 4 miles from the trailhead. The trail descends rapidly across some classic mountain meadows with nice views of rocky cliffs, turning north to south at 6440 feet. It then crosses a drainage and stream, and you see a trail marker. You are enjoying nonstop views of the hogback, foothills, and St. Vrain Canyon while sharing the trail with frequent mountain bikers.

If you don't mind sharing the trail with bikers round-trip, this final segment of the Antelope Trail is also a nice, 8-mile counterclockwise out-and-back trip. The trail switchbacks in trees, crosses under a power line, and then levels for a wonderful panorama of meadows and foothills, and a prairie dog colony at 6200 feet. The trail descends to a drainage and then climbs gently to a bench that offers a nice view of the hogback and contemplation just off-trail from the legion of polite bikers. You are now 2.25 miles from the Antelope Trailhead, a side trail and alternate entrance to the area. The trail climbs briefly for 0.25 mile, before descending to the 8-mile mark and great views of Heil Ranch across the canyon. The next 2 miles are a steep, rocky 600-foot descent, and then it levels as you enjoy hogback-view heaven. The trail turns south, rolls over a drainage through pinyon pine trees, and provides an easy stroll to the trailhead with great views all around.

TRIP 7 Heil Valley Ranch

Distance	8.0-mile loop, plus a potential side loop, Semiloop
Difficulty	Easy to moderate
Elevation Gain	600 feet (starting at 6000 feet)
Trail Use	Mountain biking, leashed dogs OK, option for kids
Agency	Boulder County
Map	*Boulder County*, Trails Illustrated *Boulder & Golden*
Facilities	Restrooms and a tree-shaded picnic area

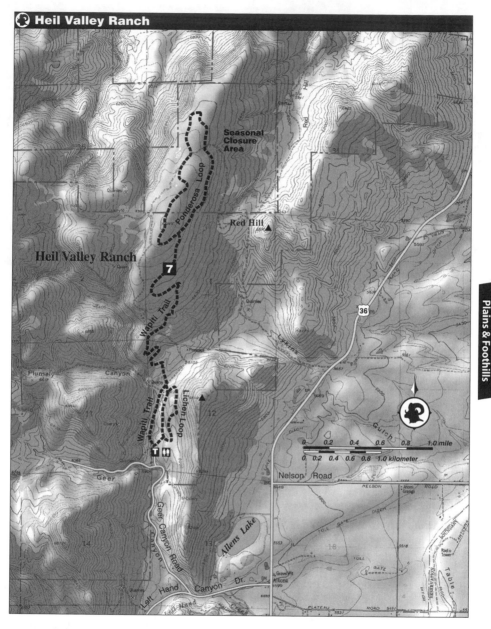

HIGHLIGHTS Another gem in the Boulder Space collection of precious jewels; it is just south of the Hall Ranch Trail. Although shorter and less challenging than the Hall Ranch loop, this trip offers a nice variety of scenery, including snow-capped peaks, wildlife, and the unique geology of fault and fracture foothills zone with the sedimentary rock of the hogback, and the lichen-covered boulders of the hills. You also enjoy views of Hall Ranch and St. Vrain Canyon on the northern corner of the loop.

DIRECTIONS The trail is approximately 1 mile west of U.S. Highway 36, between Boulder and Lyons. It is on the north side of Left Hand Canyon Drive.

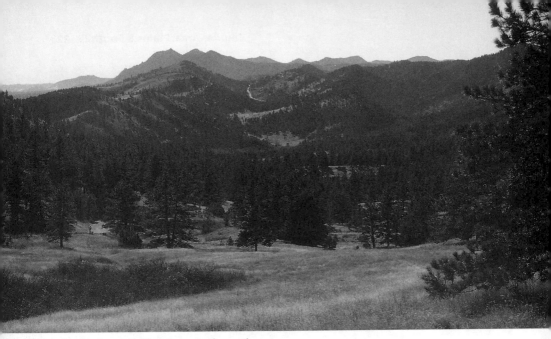

Heil Valley Ranch Trailhead, view to the south

Upon leaving the parking area, you immediately come to the Lichen Loop Trail on the right (east) side of the road. The main route, the Wapiti Trail, continues straight (north) 2.5 miles to the intersection with the Ponderosa Loop Trail, which is another 2.6 miles round-trip. Approximately 0.5 mile from the parking lot, you come to the second intersection with the Lichen Loop Trail. You could walk the portion just the other side of the fence out or back for variety. Continuing on the Wapiti Trail, when you encounter a closed segment turn left (west) on the Wapiti Trail as it goes more steeply uphill. As you cross over the meadow, you have a great view of the hogback to the south. The next mile becomes rockier under good tree cover, nice on hot or windy days. There's a trail marker at 1 mile, and then you pass an old, low wall at approximately the 2-mile mark. The trail then turns left (west), climbs, levels in 0.25 mile, and then climbs steeply through thick lodgepole pine trees to 6600 feet, 700 feet higher than the trailhead, at the 2.5-mile mark

> **Great for Kids**
>
> For an easy family with small children hike, take the 1-mile Lichen Loop Trail. It climbs around 120 feet to the top of a small hill with superb views of the geology of the foothills and hogback.

where you will reach the Ponderosa Loop Trail.

Your choice on the loop: Counterclockwise (left) means you'll have a steeper hike on the way out, while going right (clockwise) means your hike on the way out will be more gradual, but the return trip to the Wapiti Trail will be steep. Either way, you have to watch out for bikes; I would rather have bikes bombing down steep sections coming at me head-on so that I can see them instead of approaching me from behind. If, however, you don't want to hike the whole loop, and do want to see great views, then go right (northeast)—in another 1.5 miles you can enjoy the overlook and turn around.

Chief Niwot

The Arapaho Indians were the primary tribe in the 1800s when European settlers arrived in the area that would eventually become Boulder. Chief Niwot (*Niwot* is Arapaho for "left hand") was born in the 1820s and tried to live peacefully with whites in the Boulder Valley as an honorable, intelligent leader. Many Boulder County streets, towns, reservoirs, and canyons are named after him.

In the late 1850s settlers broke the Fort Laramie Treaty that the Niwot had negotiated in 1851, taking the Arapaho's land and decimating the buffalo herds they depended on for food. The tribe was devastated by disease and hunger and moved to the Great Plains to escape the white man's wrath. It was there, near Sand Creek, that Colonel John Chivington and 550 troops massacred 163 unarmed Arapahos, primarily women and old men. There is a new monument about this at the site.

Going counterclockwise (southwest and then west) the trail switchbacks broadly and then more narrowly as it climbs through the forest. It tops the hill at around 6750 feet, 150 feet higher than the beginning of the loop. It then levels and travels north. There is a nice view of snow-capped peaks off-trail on the left (west) side of the trail through lighter tree cover. The trail then descends through an open meadow with great views of Left Hand Reservoir and the plains to the east. The trail then enters nice ponderosa pines to confirm its name. In another 0.1 mile, you have good views of Longs Peak, the Indian Peaks, and Hall Ranch. The trail descends gently to 6500 feet to a nice overlook. (This previously mentioned overlook can be reached more quickly if you travel counterclockwise, right when you first reach the loop.) From the overlook the trail descends gradually to the beginning of the loop.

TRIP 8 Cobalt, Sage, & Eagle Loop

Distance	5.4 miles, Loop
Difficulty	Easy
Elevation Gain	100 feet (starting at 5200 feet)
Trail Use	Mountain biking, running, horseback riding, option for kids, leashed dogs OK
Agency	Boulder County
Map	*City of Boulder,* Trails Illustrated *Boulder & Golden*

HIGHLIGHTS The initial section of trail offers you a mellow option that travels downhill due east and then northeast from the parking lot. It rolls fairly gently in any direction you choose to take, except south, which is uphill. It is a wide, well-maintained trail popular with hikers, bikers, and people horsing around. You will enjoy superb views of the foothills, Boulder Reservoir, and even the Flatirons.

DIRECTIONS Take North Broadway to Highway 36/7, turn south 1 mile to Longhorn Road, turn right (east), and go approximately 0.75 mile to parking. You will see signs for the Boulder Ranch Open Space.

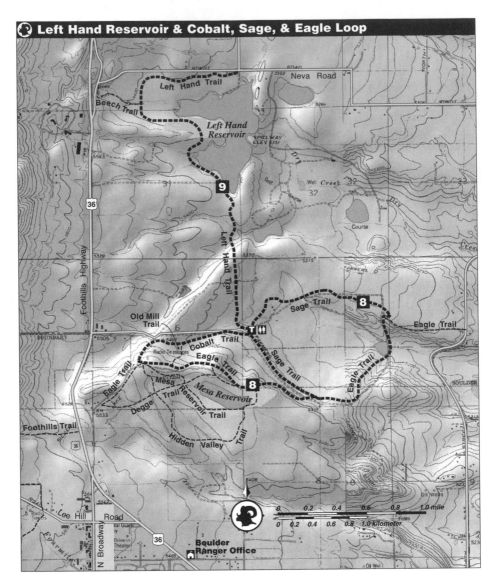

Left Hand Reservoir & Cobalt, Sage, & Eagle Loop

The trailhead at Longhorn road offers three options: the Sage-Eagle Loop Trail, the network of hilly trails to the south accessed from the uphill Cobalt Trail, or the Left Hand Reservoir/North Rim Loop Trail described in the next trip. The Sage-Eagle Loop Trail is the mellowest, goes straight east out of the parking lot (Cobalt goes uphill right, or south), and offers a gently rolling trail and nice scenery as it travels east and northeast before turning west and then southwest back to the parking area. The first section features Boulder Reservoir views and is downhill for 1.3 miles, bottoming out next to a pretty pond that reflects the foothills on still days. The next section is a gradual uphill and tops out at the trail intersection of the Eagle and Sage trails. Go right (east), and you will go around a mile to the Eagle Trailhead parking lot. Go left (north), and you will take the Sage

Great for Kids

The first 1.5 miles of the Sage-Eagle Trail is a very easy downhill and uphill return out-and-back. You will enjoy tall cottonwoods and end up at a pretty pond that reflects the foothills on calm days. This section is suitable as a short and easy mountain bike jaunt or a mellow hike.

Trail as it bends west and then south back to the Longhorn Road parking lot over gently rolling hills.

If you want a more challenging adventure, bear southeast and south out of the parking lot and choose either the Cobalt, Hidden Valley, or Mesa Reservoir trails to

climb up to the top of the ridge on the south side of the trail. It is a start that will get your blood pumping quickly, so make sure you warm up, and stretch sufficiently before charging uphill. This route is only for intermediate mountain bikers; take no chances on the steep downhill.

Once you mount the ridge, after an approximately 0.25-mile climb, you have a nice view of the reservoir in the distance to the east and the foothills to the west. The Hidden Valley and Mesa Reservoir trails go downhill after mounting the ridge and are nice roller-coaster loops that will take you back to the east edge of the Sage Trail.

TRIP 9 Left Hand Reservoir: North Rim Loop

Distance	6.0 to 11.4 miles, Out-and-back
Difficulty	Easy
Elevation Gain	200 feet (starting at 5200 feet)
Trail Use	Mountain biking, running, horseback riding, leashed dogs OK
Agency	Boulder County
Map	*Boulder County/City of Boulder*, Trails Illustrated *Boulder & Golden*
Facilities	Restrooms at trailhead

HIGHLIGHTS This nice rolling trek to Left Hand Reservoir is somewhat more suitable for mountain biking or running than it is for hiking. It has nice foothills views, open fields, and a small sparkling reservoir.

DIRECTIONS Take North Broadway to Highway 36/7, turn south 1 mile to Longhorn Road, turn right (east), and go approximately 0.75 mile to parking. You will see signs for the Boulder Ranch Open Space.

This trail starts north across the gravel road from the parking lot. Pass through the gate, and take a sharp left (west) turn to start. The trail goes up an easy uphill and then is a real roller coaster for the 2.9 miles to the parking area on Neva Road. There is one very steep downhill, about 1 mile north of the trailhead, that isn't advisable for kids or beginner mountain bikers. There is a covered picnic area with restrooms at the north end

of the trail in the Beech Open Space area. When you reach the north parking lots for Beech Open Space and private Left Hand Reservoir, your best bet is to simply turn around for an out-and-back trek. Trying to complete the loop by going east on Neva Rd. and then through the Lake Valley golf community is not worth the trouble.

If you start at the Eagle/Cobalt Trailhead, you can add an additional 5.8 miles onto your venture with the Eagle/Cobalt round-trip. Take this route to the west side of the reservoir and then return by the same route for 6.0 miles total. Completing the Sage-Eagle loop will bring your total miles to 11.4.

TRIP 10 Foothills Trail: Hogback Ridge Loop

Distance	2.3 miles, Semiloop
Difficulty	Moderate
Elevation Gain	300 feet (starting at 5900 feet)
Trail Use	Leashed dogs OK, mountain biking (technical)
Agency	Boulder County
Map	*Boulder County/City of Boulder*, Trails Illustrated *Boulder & Golden*

HIGHLIGHTS This steep trail includes great views and is a close-to-town alternative for a short hill workout. Most of the trail is subject to traffic noise, but the top of the rocky ridge is tree covered, fairly serene, and opens onto a beautiful meadow that attracts deer.

DIRECTIONS In Boulder, go to the intersection of North Broadway and Highway 36, travel 0.1 mile north, and immediately turn right (east) onto a gravel road. Follow it north to the parking area 0.25 mile on the left (west). The other access point is from a parking lot on Lee Hill Road. Take Lee Hill Road west from North Broadway to a parking lot 0.25 mile on the south side of the road. If you prefer to access the trail from Lee Hill Road, cross the road to the north, the trail edges a subdivision before turning west and then north 0.6 mile to the loop.

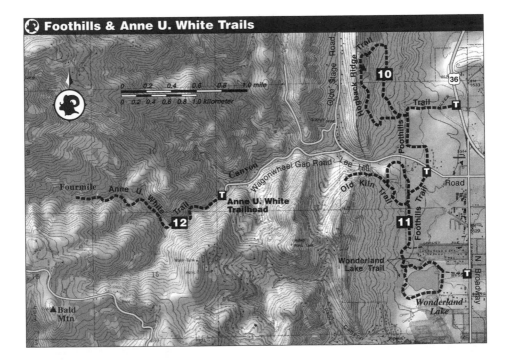

Foothills & Anne U. White Trails

This trail goes west under Highway 36 and gradually uphill for the first 0.5 mile. As it begins to climb, you will see a Foothills Trail sign pointing uphill to the south. There is an unmarked trail that travels uphill to the north. It is bike-free but travels within earshot of the highway so, unless you are up early, ignore the traffic. A better option is to turn left (south) on the actual Foothills Trail and take it 50 yards to a second intersection on the right side of the trail with the Hogback Loop. If you prefer to access the trail from Lee Hill Road, cross the road to the north; the trail edges a subdivision before turning west and then north 0.6 mile to the loop.

When you reach the loop intersection, either go west and steeply uphill over widely spaced steps or turn north and go uphill more gradually—your choice depends on how you like to encounter steep sections, on the outbound uphill or on the return downhill. If you want to get your heart in gear as soon as possible go left, or clockwise, to head straight uphill and see the meadow sooner. If you prefer a mellower warm up, go north and gradually switchback up to the ridge. The view from the top is somewhat better going counterclockwise. Either way, you experience a fair amount of traffic noise unless you are hiking very early.

TRIP 11 Foothills Trail: Wonderland Lake Loop

Distance	Up to 6.6 miles (add 1.3 miles for Old Kiln Loop), Semiloop
Difficulty	Easy
Elevation Gain	Negligible (starting at 5200 feet)
Trail Use	Mountain biking, running, leashed dogs OK
Agency	Boulder County
Map	*City of Boulder*, Trails Illustrated *Boulder & Golden*

HIGHLIGHTS This delightful close-in trail, part of which is paved, can be used for hiking and running. You benefit from the beauty of the Boulder foothills and have the option of circumnavigating Wonderland Lake.

DIRECTIONS There are many entry points along North Broadway and neighborhood streets and parks. The primary parking lot can be accessed by turning west from North Broadway onto Lee Hill Road. Drive and driving 0.25 mile; the lot is on the south side of the road for the Four Mile Creek Trailhead.

The trail goes south out of the parking lot. The trail rolls gently to Wonderland Lake with lots of side trail options. If you want a flat route, go straight south. The first option you reach after 0.4 mile on the west side is the fairly steep Old Kiln loop that goes up into the foothills. It is a nice 1.3-mile option that climbs quickly with nice views, as the trail tracks north and then west, paralleling Lee Hill

Road, before going south and reaching a gate and sign that says private road. You then reach a 0.4 mile out and back that climbs and rolls to moderately challenge your heart, lungs, and joints. Another windy, hilly 0.3 mile takes you back to the Foothills Trail.

Traveling south on the Foothills Trail is straightforward. In 0.5 mile you can take the paved Wonderland Lake loop.

You can continue south on the main trail with nice foothills views for as long as you wish before turning around. It is a gently rolling trail, making it ideal for easy jogging or walking. It can become icy in the winter after snowfalls and thaw/freeze cycles. The foothills shade the trail in late afternoon, so it does occasionally stay frozen in midwinter. Be sure to use appropriate footwear.

TRIP 12 Anne U. White Trail

see map on p. 228

Distance	3.0 miles, Out-and-back
Difficulty	Easy
Elevation Gain	200 feet (starting at 5500 feet)
Trail Use	Great for kids, leashed dogs OK
Agency	Boulder County
Map	*Boulder County/City of Boulder,* Trails Illustrated *Boulder & Golden*
Notes	Bikes are prohibited. Parking is very limited.

HIGHLIGHTS Proximity to Boulder and a very pleasant arroyo environment make this a Boulder favorite for casual hikers and dog lovers. It features a delightful riparian area and rock gardens.

DIRECTIONS Take Lee Hill Road west from North Broadway. Bear left just before Lee Hill Rd. turns sharply north onto Wagonwheel Gap Road. Turn left on Pinto Road to the very small parking area.

After the first 0.3 mile the trail jogs across a stream bed and travels north while going uphill. It passes a nice small meadow and then climbs some rock steps where you see a nice bench for snack or water breaks. It then rolls as it meanders through the creekbed and opens up onto a nice rock garden at 0.5 mile. You'll pass another small meadow at 0.7 mile. The trail steepens around the 1-mile mark as it climbs into a pretty tree canopy.

Turn sharply left when you reach a steep rocky section; you'll see two tree stumps on the left as markers. The trail rolls more steeply uphill, levels out, and abruptly ends at private property, blocking access to the Bureau of Land Management property ahead.

TRIP 13 Red Rocks Trail & Mount Sanitas

Distance	1.5 miles to Red Rocks, Semiloop; 3.3 miles to Mount Sanitas, Loop
Difficulty	Easy (Red Rock), moderate (Mount Sanitas)
Elevation Gain/Loss	200 feet (starting at 5430 feet) for Red Rock; 1343 feet (starting at 5520 feet) for Mount Sanitas
Trail Use	Mountain biking, great for kids (Red Rocks), leashed dogs OK
Agency	Boulder County
Map	*City of Boulder,* Trails Illustrated *Boulder & Golden*

HIGHLIGHTS Enjoy a little touch of Utah in this red rock garden. These are actually separate trails and can be experienced separately. Combining them gives you a longer, more satisfying workout, but hiking them individually can also be great fun.

DIRECTIONS The Red Rocks Trailhead and parking lot is at the west end of Pearl Street in Boulder, where it ends and merges into Canyon Boulevard. Mount Sanitas has its own trailhead off the west end of Mapleton Avenue. This description assumes a starting point of Red Rocks Trailhead and hiking north. If you start there and loop Mount Sanitas, you will walk about 4 miles. If you take one of the side loops, you can hike a total of 6 miles.

Red Rocks

If you just want a short family outing, exploring this area is a treat. When you leave the parking lot, you'll see the bike route to Pearl Street or west to Eben Fine Park. If you walk the bike trail, watch out for high-speed bikers. The next trail is the short out-and-back Settler's Quarry. As you travel straight up the dirt path, you see the Red Rocks Loop Trail. The whole loop is approximately 1.2 miles. Left takes you up into the drainage next to the first set of pretty sandstone sculptures. Right takes you up the switchbacks and a sweeping view of Boulder. Go straight to mount the small ridge, where you'll have nice views to the west and can scramble onto the rocks for photos or relaxation.

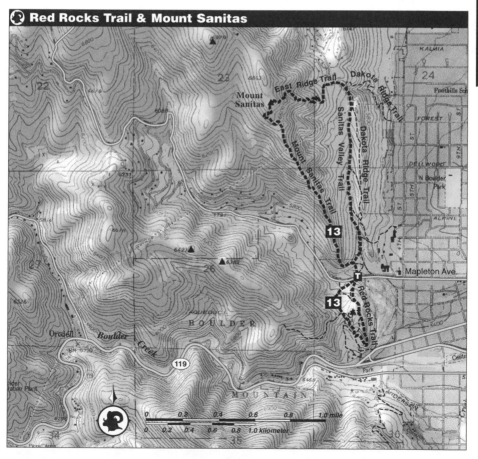

Red Rocks Trail & Mount Sanitas

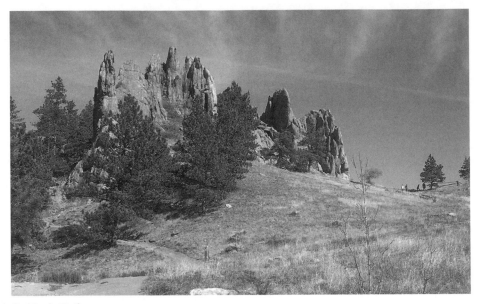

Red Rocks Trail

The more dramatic rocks are yet to come. Go through a short shady section that opens up to even more pleasing views of the next coxcomb set of red rocks. The right-hand trail intersects with the rest of the loop as you travel uphill to the saddle and finish the first 0.3 mile; you have a great view of Mount Sanitas and the wide trail that will take you there, as well as nice photo opportunities of the impressive rock monument. You can clamber on to the rocks for quiet contemplation before returning or continue down the trail to the north another 0.3 mile, through the trees to cross Mapleton/Sunshine Canyon Road, and discover the Mount Sanitas Trailhead.

Mount Sanitas

This wide, well-groomed trail can be used for moderate hikes, though the top requires some minor rocky trail scrambling. If you don't want to combine this trail with Red Rocks, start at the trailhead on Mapleton and go up the easier Sanitas Valley Trail on the right (east) side of the valley. It is a more moderate grade in the beginning and gives you time to warm up for the steeper trails near the top. The downside of going counterclockwise is that you will have some steep downhills on the return. If you prefer to start steep and finish mellow, then go clockwise up the steeper Mount Sanitas Trail that travels straight uphill 1.4 miles to the summit, gaining more than 1300 feet in the process. Take your time and enjoy the interesting rock formations and ponderosa pines along the way.

At around the 0.7-mile mark you are on a spectacular ridge with great views to the west. You then descend via the steep East Ridge Trail for 0.9 mile to the mellow Sanitas Valley Trail. If you go up Valley Trail, you climb up the steep, breathtaking East Ridge Trail as you push for the summit of Mount Sanitas. From the top you'll have a nice canyon view to the west, and the twinkling lights of Boulder spreading out into the plains below, if you visit at twilight (or sunrise).

TRIP 14 Switzerland Trail

Distance	3 to 5 miles, Out-and-back
Difficulty	Easy
Elevation Loss	300 feet (starting at 5900 feet)
Trail Use	Mountain biking, motorized recreation, leashed dogs OK
Agency	Boulder County
Map	*Boulder County,* Trails Illustrated *Boulder & Golden*

HIGHLIGHTS This beautiful trail near Gold Hill is used primarily for mountain biking but can also be a fun hike. It starts high and then is a gradual descent on a wide double-track, four-wheel-drive road that is almost passable for regular cars. There are great views of the ridgelines, valleys, and some distant peaks. Unfortunately there is some motorized use, especially on the weekends, but it is worth dodging the infrequent usage.

DIRECTIONS From Boulder take Mapleton Avenue to Sunshine Canyon and then on to Gold Hill. The trail is 3 miles west of Gold Hill at a four-way intersection with a large brown sign labeled LITTLE SWITZERLAND.

From the above intersection, you can go left to reach the Mount Alto Picnic Area in 1 mile and the Sunset town site in 4 miles. I recommend going right on a more scenic part of the trail that starts on a gradual downhill. In 0.25 mile you come to a short secondary trail on the right (north) side of the road that is closed to motorized vehicles. If you want a nice quiet meadow for a picnic, this is a good spot. There are lots of aspen and ponderosa pines. It is a better trail for hiking than biking because of how short it is. The first 0.1 mile switchbacks downhill from Little Switzerland and then levels into the expansive meadow, bordered by private property, cabins, and a ridgeline palace. Lots of wildflowers and

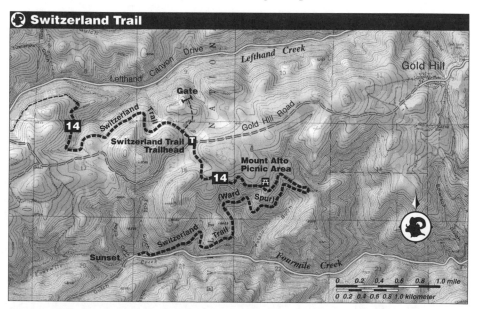

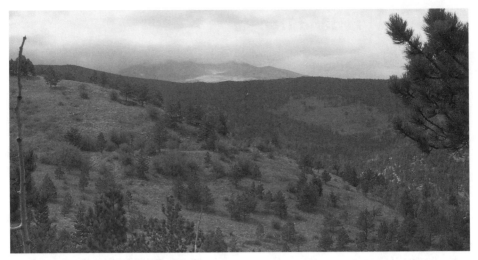

Mountain view from the Switzerland Trail

the soft trail make it an inviting side trip. Unfortunately the trail ends at a locked gate in only 0.5 mile.

Back on the trail continue downhill as the constantly changing scenery opens up with mountains, valleys, rock formations, and sweeping ridgelines of trees. The trail levels after around 0.5 mile and then turns north in a wide arc. You can go up, over, or around a hillock. Avoid the trail you see going straight up a hillside unless your name is Lance or you want your heart to pound. The trail continues fairly level and enters tree cover for another mile before plunging downhill in earnest for the valley below. Turn around at any point for an experience of your choice. Extend your ride on other gravel roads.

TRIP 15 Mesa Trail: Northern Segment

see map on p. 236

Distance	Any distance up to 14.0 miles , Out-and-back
Difficulty	Moderate
Elevation Gain	800 to 1000 feet, depending on route taken (starting at 5700 feet)
Trail Use	Running, leashed dogs OK
Agency	Boulder County
Map	*City of Boulder,* Trails Illustrated *Boulder & Golden*
Facilities	Ranger station, visitors center, and restrooms

HIGHLIGHTS Hiking nirvana in Boulder cannot be attained without a jaunt on the well-known and venerable Mesa Trail—one of the original foothills trails networks and open space parks that inspired the creation of so many other pieces of paradise in Boulder County. This rolling trail climbs high onto the side of Green Mountain and travels below the landmark Flatiron rock formations all the way south to Eldorado Springs Road. It features great vistas to the west and east as it roller coasters ever southward. You can also access the trail from several places along the way; consult a map. Aside from Chautauqua, one of my favorite starting points is at the south end off of the Eldorado Springs Rd. The trail climbs up to spectacular views of the Flatirons in about 1 mile. A variety of loop trail options make for delightful outings of varying difficulty.

DIRECTIONS   A good starting point, but challenging place for parking (I recommend that you carpool or take the bus), is Chautauqua Mountain Park. It is straight uphill from the famous Hill district near the university and on the way up Flagstaff Mountain. Take 9th Street south from downtown until it dead-ends into Baseline Road, or take Baseline Rd. west from Broadway. You will see the Flatirons and the park on the left (south) side of the road, just past 9th Street off of Baseline. Arrive early if you want a parking place in the park. If you arrive late on a weekend, you will have to park down the hill in the neighborhood and walk up.

The trails begin west of the circular park drive, past the visitors center, through the gate to the fire road. It goes uphill either to the south, or more directly west, to the foot of the Flatirons. It is at the east edge of the beautiful meadow that sprawls across the hillside at the foreground of the Flatirons graced with wildflowers in the spring. I recommend that you bear left to travel south and then west, unless you plan to climb one of the Flatirons or want to take the loop trails that circle the Flatirons. You can clamber around on the Flatirons without ropes for grins, but don't go very high without technical climbing gear.

Since the southern route is a roller coaster, you will have some uphill sections on the way back; they are moderate if you do an out-and-back trip. As the trail travels south, you find it goes up, down, and sideways in almost every direction. For a nice out-and-back route of approximately 3 miles, go to the area behind the National Center for Atmospheric Research (NCAR) and then turn around. You pass lots of options for picnics or snack and water breaks along the way. It is a generally a good winter trail option unless there has been a recent Front Range snowstorm.

Going south from Chautauqua, bear right (west) and go uphill at the first intersection at the end of the buildings,

at around 0.4 mile. The trail traverses at first gradually and then more steeply uphill for approximately 0.5 mile. When it enters the trees, it levels temporarily. You can go either uphill to the right (north) or roller coaster up and downhill along and in the enchanting foothills ecosystem to the south. I recommend the southerly route, unless you want a shorter challenging uphill workout on the loops to the north. So go left (south) at the next trail intersection, and travel more gradually uphill for 0.5 mile to a loop trail. Bear left (straight) unless you want to explore the steeper 0.5-mile loop that offers some nice views to the west and is worth the detour. You can see the other end of the loop trail in a little more than 0.25 mile if you skip it. The trail then zigzags and offers the option of traveling east 1.5 miles downhill to Table Mesa Drive, just north of NCAR. The trail then travels downhill for more than 0.5 mile, goes uphill briefly, and then meets an intersecting trail that heads east, switchbacking downhill to a point just north of NCAR.

The trail splits at the next intersection in 0.25 mile, offering either a steep uphill or downhill section. This is a good turnaround point unless you want to take a major plunge through Bear Canyon. You can cross the canyon and make this a major adventure by climbing Bear Peak.

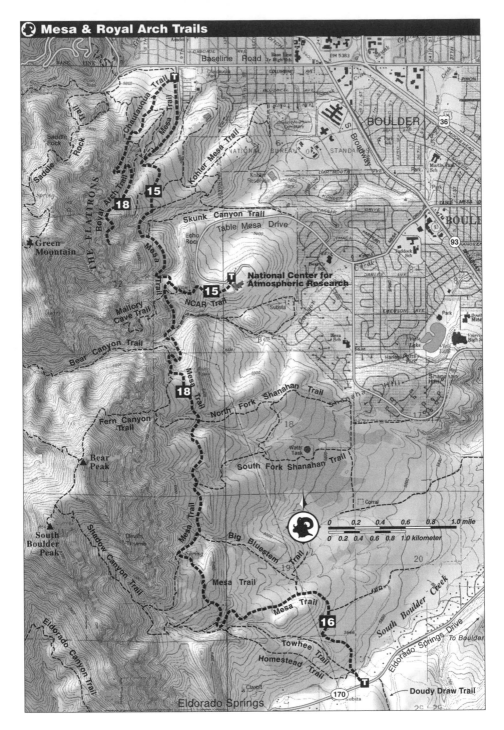

Mesa & Royal Arch Trails

TRIP 16 Mesa Trail: Southern Segment

Distance	Up to 13.5 miles, Out-and-back
Difficulty	Moderate
Elevation Gain	900 feet (starting at 5700 feet)
Trail Use	Leashed dogs OK
Agency	Boulder County
Map	*City of Boulder,* Trails Illustrated *Boulder & Golden*
Facilities	Restrooms at trailhead

HIGHLIGHTS You can access the Mesa Trail from the south and travel north to enjoy another beautiful stretch. Walking north on this section of trail offers one of the most spectacular views of the Flatirons rock formations. It is a winding, somewhat steep trail initially but then mellows and rolls along.

DIRECTIONS Take Broadway south toward Golden, turn right on Eldorado Springs Road, and look for the trailhead on the north side of the road, across from Doudy Draw.

From the parking lot, cross the creek, pick one of the intersecting loop trails (Towhee or Homestead), and then bear west and north, going straight uphill. All of the trails merge as you climb and then you are on the Mesa Trail, which is well signed. Go as far as you wish and then reverse course, or set up a car shuttle.

The Mesa Trail connects to the Towhee Trail, Homestead Trail, and Big Bluestem Trail. A very scenic round-trip can be had by going to the National Center for Atmospheric Research (NCAR) from the south and back. It is 13.5 miles round-trip to Chatauqua Park.

TRIP 17 Doudy Draw Trail

see map on p. 238

Distance	Up to 6.2 miles, Out-and-back
Difficulty	Easy
Elevation Gain	300 feet (starting at 5700 feet)
Trail Use	Leashed dogs OK
Agency	Boulder County
Map	*City of Boulder,* Trails Illustrated *Boulder & Golden*
Facilities	Restrooms at trailhead

HIGHLIGHTS This short, very scenic, and easy trail is wheelchair accessible to a picnic area. It features spectacular views once you climb out of the draw.

DIRECTIONS Take Broadway south toward Golden, turn right on Eldorado Springs Drive, and look for the trailhead on the south side of the road, across from the South Mesa Trailhead.

The trail starts out flat, for the first 0.5 mile and then climbs gradually to a picnic area, where the paved trail ends. You will see the Community Ditch Trail on the left, continue straight south, crossing a creek on a footbridge. The gravel trail climbs more steeply toward the top of a small mesa area that tops out at

South Boulder Creek & Doudy Draw Trails

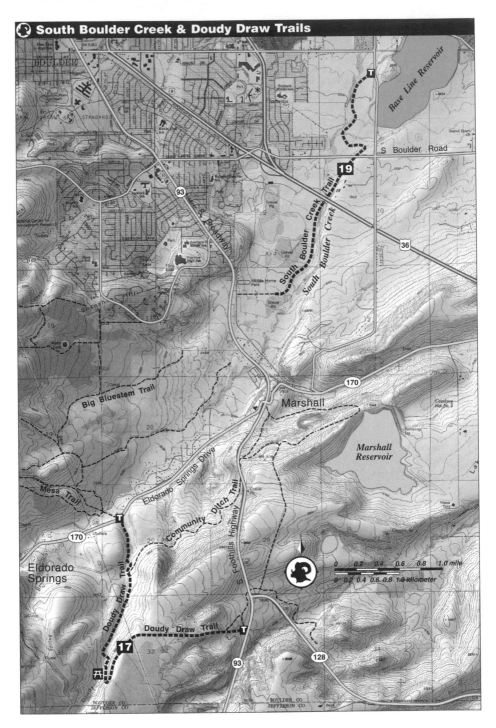

around 6100 feet. The views are enhanced with every step, especially to the north, as the dramatic Flatiron formations come into view.

Once on the mesa you will be in a pretty ponderosa pine forest and will have nice views to the west of Eldorado Canyon and the soaring foothills. You can even see some snow-capped peaks if you're lucky. The trail continues north for 1 mile from the picnic area and then descends from the ridge, turning first north and then east as it goes the final 1.6 miles to the parking area on State Highway 93. It rolls and then descends a little more steeply to the parking lot.

TRIP 18 Royal Arch Trail

see map on p. 236

Distance	3.3 miles, Out-and-back
Difficulty	Moderate
Trail Use	Leashed dogs OK
Elevation Gain	800 feet (starting at 5710 feet)
Agency	Boulder County
Map	*City of Boulder*, Trails Illustrated *Boulder & Golden*
Facilities	Ranger station, visitors center, and restrooms at trailhead and near Bluebell Shelter

HIGHLIGHTS One of the somewhat challenging options along the Mesa Trail is an interesting trail in its own right because you end up at a small arch with striking views, especially to the north, and you have unique glimpses of the Flatirons along the way. It has the feel of a high mountain hike even though it is close to town. The challenging part is the fairly steep, rock garden trail that makes you feel like you're on a short Himalayan trek with all of the twists, turns, and ups and downs, without the altitude or length. If you go at a slow pace, the challenge becomes a fun, moderate clamber rather than a heart-thumping workout.

DIRECTIONS A good starting point, but challenging place for parking (I recommend that you carpool or take the bus), is Chautauqua Mountain Park. It is straight uphill from the famous Hill district near the university and on the way up Flagstaff Mountain. Take 9th Street south from downtown until it dead-ends into Baseline Road, or take Baseline Rd. west from Broadway. You will see the Flatirons and then park on the left (south) side of the road, just past 9th Street off of Baseline. Arrive early if you want a parking place in the park. If you arrive late on a weekend, you will have to park down the hill in the neighborhood and walk up.

You have two options at the trailhead: Take the gravel road uphill due south from the ranger station and travel next to Chautauqua if you want fast access. If you want a much more scenic but less direct approach, go uphill toward the Flatirons and angle southwest and then watch for the intersection of the Bluebell Shelter trail on the left (east) side of the trail. Backtrack downhill past the shelter to the Royal Arch Trail. The former option is fast and less scenic, while the latter is a hiking trail that requires an extra 0.1 mile. If you're on the road, bear right at the first intersection and continue uphill to near the Bluebell Shelter, where you will bear left (south) onto the actual Royal Arch Trail. There are restrooms trailside near the shelter. The trail travels uphill, narrows, and passes a group of picnic tables in the trees. You can picnic either at Bluebell Shelter or under the trees.

Past the shelter the trail crosses two streams on footbridges and gets steeper as you climb through a major rock slide. To the west you see the interesting Flatirons mountainside that make you feel like you're in a national forest miles from nowhere. The trail then rolls a little but generally climbs steeply uphill, often on stone steps, as it winds through the thick tree cover that is a bonus on hot days. After 1.25 miles you encounter steep switchbacks that take you to the top of a small ridge. You then get to travel steeply downhill for 0.1 mile, climbing over rocks, and, yes, you climb uphill on the way back. You have another 0.1 mile push uphill to get to the arch, but the view is well worth the finale.

TRIP 19 South Boulder Creek Trail

see map on p. 238

Distance	Up to 8.0 miles, Out-and-back
Difficulty	Easy
Trail Use	Running, mountain biking, leashed dogs OK
Agency	Boulder County
Map	*City of Boulder*, Trails Illustrated *Boulder & Golden*
Note	Dogs are not allowed beyond the gate.

HIGHLIGHTS This gently rolling trail has great views of the foothills and Flatirons and meanders through a pretty riparian area that is close to Boulder. It features woods, wetlands, and more than 30 varieties of wildflowers.

DIRECTIONS Take Baseline Road east of the Foothills Parkway to Cherryvale Road. Take Cherryvale south less than 0.5 mile to the turnoff for the parking area on the right (west) side of the road.

Foothills view from the South Boulder Creek Trail

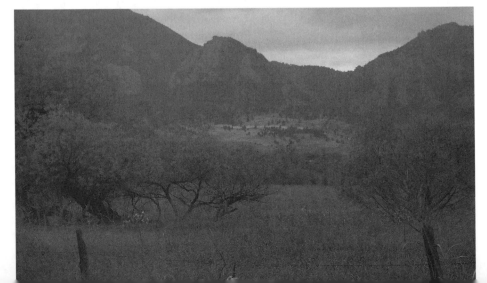

Since it's crowded on weekends, try to visit during the week when possible. The bikers are offered a paved path, while hikers and runners have a soft path option closer to the creek. The trails intertwine at times along the way, but it isn't possible for a biker and runner to stay together. You enjoy a short grass prairie and creekside trees at the outset, the latter offering some shade late in the day. The trail loops east and then south before crossing under South Boulder Road via a tunnel. After you emerge from the tunnel, either go west, parallel to the road, for another 0.3 mile to a dead end or go through the gate on the south side of the road. This is a dog-free (as in no dogs allowed) extension that continues on for another 1.8 miles to State Highway 36 and then a dead end at the State Highway 93 intersection.

Once you pass South Boulder Road, you enjoy a very peaceful section of the trail, as it meanders as much as the creek and plays tag with some lofty, old cottonwoods. You also have nonstop foothills and Flatirons views.

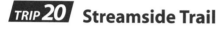

TRIP 20 Streamside Trail

see map on p.242

Distance	0.6 miles, Out-and-back
Difficulty	Easy
Elevation Gain	Negligible (starting at 5900 feet)
Trail Use	Great for kids, leashed dogs OK
Agency	Eldorado Canyon State Park
Map	*Eldorado Canyon State Park,* Trails Illustrated *Boulder & Golden*
Facilities	Restrooms at trailhead

HIGHLIGHTS Ideal for mellow family strolls and contemplation if you arrive early, this short and easy stroll along South Boulder Creek accesses the climbing routes. You will likely see the rock jocks up close and get a breathtaking view of them on the Bastille rock south across the creek and road. If the climbers look glassy eyed, it is because they have once again defied the mortal grasp of gravity.

DIRECTIONS From Boulder, take State Highway 93 south from Boulder. Turn right on State Highway 170 and continue to the park entrance west of Eldorado Springs, about 8 miles southwest of Boulder. From Denver, take Interstate 25 north to State Highway 36 (west toward Boulder). Exit at Louisville-Superior and turn left (south) at the light. Take the first right (west) onto State Highway 170 and follow it 7.4 miles to Eldorado Canyon State Park. Park immediately after you pass the entrance station.

Walk on the trail on the right (north) side of the road, and cross the footbridge that is 50 yards from the stylish restrooms and changing rooms. Cross the stream and go another 0.3 mile before the trail dead-ends into rocks and trees. You can continue by climbing up, over, and around but that isn't recommended for children. You'll see several small side slot canyons that are used for climbing access. Bring your climbing gear—harness, hard hat, rope, and so forth—if you really want to explore them. If not, contemplate the ageless rock and babbling brook.

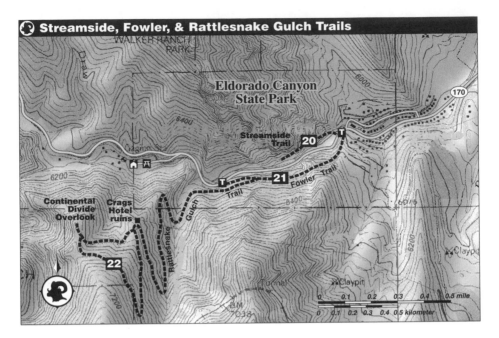

Streamside, Fowler, & Rattlesnake Gulch Trails

TRIP 21 Fowler Trail

Distance	1.4 to 4.0 miles, Out-and-back
Difficulty	Easy
Elevation Gain	100 feet (starting at 6000 feet)
Trail Use	Wheelchair-accessible, leashed dogs OK
Agency	Eldorado Canyon State Park
Map	*Eldorado Canyon State Park*, Trails Illustrated *Boulder & Golden*

HIGHLIGHTS This short, easy uphill climb's chief advantage is that it allows hikers to savor the soaring cliffs and rock climbers perched on them or dancing their way to the top across the valley. The trail provides views of the magnificent rock garden made of grayish quartzite rock that started off as eroded sand 1.6 billion years ago. The reddish Fountain Formation rocks were compacted into sandstone 300 million years ago and are the same formation and from the same era as Boulder's Flatirons and the Red Rocks amphitheater. The Lyons Formation sandstone rocks are the youngsters of the canyon at 240 million years old. These silent monuments give you a new perspective on the precious, brief span of a human's life and the necessity of savoring every moment. Combining this hike with the longer Rattlesnake Gulch Trail is a very doable adventure.

DIRECTIONS From Boulder take State Highway 93 south from Boulder, and turn right on State Highway 170 and continue to the park entrance west of Eldorado Springs, about 8 miles southwest of Boulder. From Denver take Interstate 25 north to State Highway 36, and turn west towards Boulder. Exit at "Louisville-Superior" and turn south (left) at the light. Take the first right (west) onto State Highway 170 and follow it 7.4 miles to Eldorado Canyon.

The trailhead for the Fowler and Rattlesnake Gulch Trails are one and the same and are 0.5 mile uphill from the entrance station. There is limited parking so you might have to walk up the road from the entrance, or back from the visitors center. The latter is the better, shorter option for walking on the road.

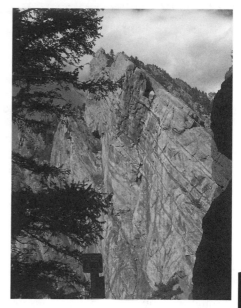

View from Fowler Trail at Eldorado Canyon State Park

Once you find the trailhead simply walk up the gradual incline to the east and follow the nature guide stations. Gaze across the canyon to see a wonderful rock climbing exhibition as climbers test their skills. There is even a free telescope if you want an up close and personal view of these limber and fearless rock aficionados. You see the magnificent panorama of rock ridges, from west to east: Quartzite Ridge, Nest Ridge, Redgarden Wall, Hawk Eagle Ridge, and Rotwand Wall. They are topped off by Rincon Wall and 7240-foot Shirt Tail Peak. The trail continues gradually uphill until you are above the out-of-view, famous Bastille rock wall, which is on the same side of the canyon as the trail.

Beyond the state park boundary, the trail travels slightly downhill until it intersects a dirt road. There is no access to the entrance station, and it mean-ders with the curving low ridgeline for another 1.3 miles until it dead-ends at private property. Although this trip has some great views, more interesting scenery can be found in nearby Rattlesnake Gulch (Trip 22).

TRIP 22 Rattlesnake Gulch Trail

Distance	2.8 miles, Semiloop
Difficulty	Moderate
Elevation Gain	800 feet to Crags Hotel ruins, 1200 for loop (starting at 6000 feet)
Trail Use	Leashed dogs OK
Agency	Eldorado Canyon State Park
Map	*Eldorado Canyon State Park,* Trails Illustrated *Boulder & Golden*
Facilities	Restrooms at visitors center, none at trailhead

HIGHLIGHTS This trail features excellent views of the main canyon, an interesting side canyon, Crags Hotel ruins, the Continental Divide, and the Burlington Northern-Sante-Fe/Amtrak rail line. The switchbacks are almost as ambitious as the Eldorado Trail if you complete the entire loop. You gain 800 feet in a little more than 0.6 mile on the widely sweeping, fairly gradual switchbacks to reach the ruins of the Crags Hotel, which burned down in 1912, only four years after it was built. There is a historic marker about the hotel at the site and a limited view of the Indian Peaks. If you also want to see the Continental Divide, it is a short, easy stroll uphill from the ruins. If you'd like, it's quite possible to combine this hike with the short Fowler Trail.

DIRECTIONS From Boulder take State Highway 93 south from Boulder, and turn right on State Highway 170 and continue to the park entrance west of Eldorado Springs, about 8 miles southwest of Boulder. From Denver take Interstate 25 north to State Highway 36, and turn west towards Boulder. Exit at "Louisville-Superior" and turn south (left) at the light. Take the first right (west) onto State Highway 170 and follow it 7.4 miles to Eldorado Canyon.

The trailhead for the Fowler and Rattlesnake Gulch trails are one and the same and are 0.5 mile uphill from the entrance station. There is limited parking so you might have to walk up the road from the entrance, or back from the visitors center. The latter is the better, shorter option for walking on the road.

Go up the Fowler Trail for 100 yards and access the Rattlesnake Gulch Trail approximately 100 yards up on the right. The trail starts sharply uphill through trees and is rocky but opens up fairly quickly and widens. Since it is a former road, it is often wide enough for two. It has very good sun exposure, so snow and ice can melt much of the year, making it accessible to hikers well into the late fall. The first 0.3 mile is a little steep, but then the trail mellows and even goes downhill. After the S turn you see some minor ruins, but the trail to them is blocked off so they are best ignored. The next 0.3 mile is uphill, and the Burlington Northern-Sante-Fe/Amtrak train line comes into view. The rail line is also the route of the ski train to Winter Park Resort and the bright red hematite and iron ore hillsides are precipitous and striking high above.

You next come upon the Crags Hotel ruins with a superb 180-degree view back to the east of the soaring cliffs and a snow-capped Indian Peak or two to the northwest. An old wall or fireplace still stands from a century ago. This is a good place for a water and rest break and there is a bench. The overlook is closer than it

appears to be on the state park map. It is a fairly easy 0.1-mile jaunt up an easy hill to the overlook. The overlook has limited space, so use the ruins area if you want more breathing space for your snack or lunch break. The overlook has another bench and features an even better view of the Continental Divide.

You see the loop option as you leave the overlook; it is well worth the extra effort and extends what might otherwise be a short hike. The 0.8 mile loop is best taken counterclockwise from the overlook since it is less steep and rocky in that direction. You can save the steep and rocky sections for the downhill trip. The trail goes steeply uphill on the right (west) side of the trail. As it climbs you realize that you are climbing toward the railroad tracks. The loop levels after the 0.25-mile mark and then climbs more gradually until you are almost next to the stretch of train track framed by two tunnels. If you're lucky and are there either first thing in the morning or in early evening, you'll see an Amtrak train go by. The trail goes steeply and then more gradually downhill through the trees back to the main trail. Once you reach the main trail, retrace your steps to the trailhead.

TRIP 23 Eldorado Canyon Trail

see map on p.246

Distance	Any distance up to 9.0 miles, Out-and-back
Difficulty	Moderate to challenging
Elevation Gain	1000 feet (starting at 6000 feet)
Trail Use	Leashed dogs OK
Agency	Eldorado Canyon State Park
Map	*Eldorado Canyon State Park,* Trails Illustrated *Boulder & Golden*
Facilities	Restrooms, visitors center with bookstore, and a hot springs pool

HIGHLIGHTS See the panorama of 1.7 billion years of geologic history that has become some of the most renowned rock climbing terrain in North America, with countless climbers dangling from vertical cliffs on hundreds of challenging routes—all in the first mile you travel through the park on the trail. The state park is a fee area but is worth the price of admission. One of the best Front Range trails for scenery in one of the most accessible areas takes hikers along the top of a spectacular canyon with views of the Indian Peaks and the occasional Amtrak or coal train chugging along on the Moffat Road high above. Soak in the Eldorado Springs pool after your adventure. A hike of any length is rewarding. Allow most of a day for the 9-mile round-trip.

DIRECTIONS From Boulder take State Highway 93 south from Boulder, and turn right on State Highway 170 and continue to the park entrance west of Eldorado Springs, about 8 miles southwest of Boulder. From Denver take Interstate 25 north to State Highway 36, and turn west toward Boulder. Exit at "Louisville-Superior" and turn south (left) at the light. Take the first right (west) onto State Highway 170 and follow it 7.4 miles to Eldorado Canyon. Continue 1 mile through the canyon to the visitors center.

Parking is limited and challenging on weekends so carpool and arrive early. The visitors center is surrounded by a large picnic area with a lot of tables. The trail begins east of the visitors center, crosses the road to the north, and then stair steps quickly uphill. You experience steep switchbacks that climb around 300 feet in the first 0.5 mile and offer good photo opportunities. Enjoy the cluster of trees; most of the trail is open to the sun and can become warm if you get an early start. Around 0.75 mile the trail mellows with spectacular 180-degree views, including often snow-capped Indian Peaks in the distance.

The trail temporarily descends and turns northwest, heading around a rock-

> **Great for Kids**
>
> The 0.75-mile mark is a fine turnaround point for small children or the altitude challenged. Its great views make for a satisfying, brief trip.

fall area and downed tree at around the 1-mile mark. It then climbs through a steep switchback to around 6700 feet with even better peak views. At 1.5 miles it mellows into a ridge walk with sweeping views. It then descends gradually through ferns and poison ivy before roller coastering a bit.

After hiking for about 1½ hours, you reach the point where the trail makes a short climb to the next ridge before

Walker Ranch Loop & Eldorado Canyon Trail

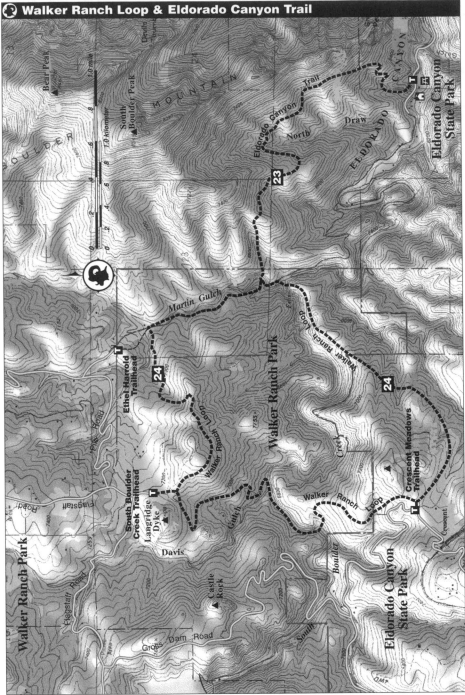

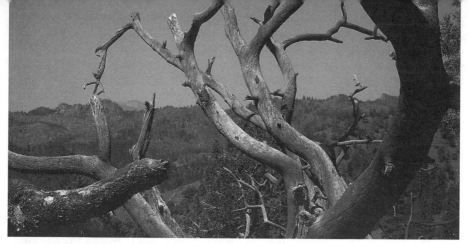
View from Eldorado Canyon Trail

plunging 500 feet down to the creek. It is a rewarding round-trip but pushes the hike into the more difficult range for most people since you'll have to climb back out and then descend what you just climbed.

TRIP 24 Walker Ranch

Distance	Up to 7.6 miles, Loop
Difficulty	Moderate (hiking), challenging (mountain biking)
Elevation Gain	1500 feet (starting at 7300 feet)
Trail Use	Mountain biking, leashed dogs OK
Agency	Boulder County
Map	Trails Illustrated *Boulder & Golden*
Facilities	Restrooms at trailheads

HIGHLIGHTS This beautiful, rugged foothills area features high ridges and a beautiful canyon with sparkling Boulder Creek running through it. The ranch is almost 3778 acres—more than 1000 acres were scorched in the Eldorado fire, but the vegetation was generally reinvigorated by it. It features the mountain version of sparkling Boulder Creek, old ranch homestead buildings, and a dazzling display of wildflowers, ponderosa pines, and wildlife. The ranch is a premiere mountain biking area and a superb hiking environment. If you're a hiker who wants to avoid bikers, visit during the week or be prepared to dodge lots of biking enthusiasts. If you're a biker, be prepared for some challenging, technical terrain.

Experiencing the entire loop is a delightful challenge at a fast pace on foot. You can enjoy very nice out-and-back hikes down to the creekside canyon from either the South Boulder Creek (or nearby Ethel Harrold Trailhead) or Crescent Meadows Trailhead. Or you can hike all the way over from Eldorado Canyon State Park and use a car shuttle or enjoy a nice bike-free out-and-back adventure.

DIRECTIONS The most popular trailhead is South Boulder Creek, accessed from Boulder by taking Baseline Road west to Flagstaff Mountain Road and going up and over Flagstaff Mountain. If the parking lot is full, you can just as easily use the nearby Ethel Harrold Trailhead and Picnic Area. Getting down to the creek is less scenic but 1.75 miles shorter than the South Boulder Creek Trailhead.

The Crescent Meadows Trailhead is closer to Denver and Golden and is 8 miles from Highway 93. Take Highway 72 west and watch for signs for Gross Dam Road, which takes you near the trailhead.

Crescent Meadows Access

You can, of course, use this access point to hike or bike the entire 7.6-mile loop. Or you have two choices for shorter out-and-back hikes to get down to Boulder Creek Canyon. If you go north-northwest (left), it takes only 1.5 miles to reach the pretty canyon but the trail parallels the road a short time. You also have views of the often snow-capped peaks of the Continental Divide. It is a steep, short plunge to the creek.

If you want a longer trek (2.5 miles to the canyon), then go right (northeast) across the beautiful meadow that gives the trailhead its name. It is a more gradual descent with long sweeping switchbacks and almost constant views of the rock formations that top Eldorado Canyon and the plains to the east. The last 0.25 mile to the creek is very steep steps with nice views of the arroyo on the way down.

South Boulder Creek Trailhead

From this trailhead I recommend starting off to the right (southwest) toward the South Boulder Creek Picnic Area. This is the shorter trek down to the creek. If you decide that all you want to do is hike to the creek, this is definitely the way to go. If you want to hike or bike the entire loop, this is also the less steep, wider trail to start on for the descent into the canyon. You will have an uphill on the way back regardless of the way you go. This description goes counterclockwise (southwest or right) on the loop and starts toward South Boulder Creek Picnic Area 1.6 miles ahead—a good goal for families.

The trail immediately goes downhill with a view of two large, striking rock formations. In 0.25 mile there is an overlook of the dramatic valley that uplift and the creek have created. The wide, very well-maintained trail descends gradually through the burn area and the thinned forest, where there is already much new growth. You lose about 600 feet in a little less than 1 mile. The soothing sounds of the stream are loud and clear and at the 1-mile mark as the trail climbs gently before its final descent to the shaded picnic tables at around 6500 feet. There is a sculpted wall of rock on the other side of the jostling water. Since the riparian area was untouched by the fire, the trees are stately. Once you are streamside, the wonderful arroyo opens up as you hike or bike next to the cascading water. You pass small waterfalls and then cross the stream on a footbridge.

The trail turns sharply northeast as it passes a bench. It is time to regain elevation as you climb 200 feet in the first 0.25 mile on the more narrow and rocky trail. Disregard a side trail to an unremarkable overlook unless you want a snack break. At the 2-mile mark you are back up to 7150 feet and have an impressive view across the canyon from whence you came of the entire trail and the distant parking lot high above.

The trail levels and then turns left (north-northeast) toward the Crescent Meadows Trailhead. You are climbing 100 feet every 0.25 mile in this steep trail section, back up to 7200 feet quickly. You then parallel the Gross Mountain Reservoir Road for 0.25 mile and see the dam face. At the Crescent Meadows Trailhead take a sharp left (northeast) and cross the gorgeous meadow as the trail descends 150 feet to the 3-mile marker. You enjoy sweeping views all the way to the top of Eldorado Canyon and the plains beyond. When I scouted this trail, I reached the 4-mile marker at 6800 feet in about 2 hours from the start of the hike.

The trail switchbacks down more steeply to an option for a less technical mountain biking route that's also easier for hikers. At around 4.5 miles, you begin to hear the sounds of the stream again as you negotiate very steep steps that wind around 0.25 mile to the creek. Enjoy the panorama of the rock garden arroyo on the way down to the cool waters.

When you reach the water, you have to look carefully ahead to see the trail going northwest uphill. You can hear the small waterfalls producing a good roar. Watch for water ouzels as you cross the bridge and prepare to climb 900 feet back up to the parking lot. The trail roller coasters through the valley and then screams straight uphill past an old mill site. Watch

---

Great for Kids

If you started at Crescent Meadows and have family along, the waterfall is a good turnaround point. It is 3 miles (round-trip) for an outing to streamside. The return trip is uphill, so be sure to maintain a leisurely pace to keep it fun for small people. A long, restful picnic next to the stream is highly recommended.

---

for the sharp left turn to stay on the South Boulder Creek Trail in 0.5 mile. If you don't turn, you will end up at the Ethel Harrold Trailhead. At 6800 feet, after gaining 300 feet from the creek, you roll through Columbine Gulch drainage until it tops out on a ridgeline. From there you have a commanding view as you make the final climb to the ridgetop at 7282 feet, where you're looking again at the scorched earth as you enjoy the panoramic ridge walk (with one short uphill section) back to the parking lot.

Chapter 11

Denver Area:
Plains & Foothills

Denver's urban renewal has made it one of the better U.S. cities to live in. What many nonresidents don't know is how rich and varied the nearby natural resources and wonders are. Because of space constraints, I am covering only a tiny slice of the many trails, parks, and opens spaces that abound in the Denver metropolitan area. You don't have to suffer the traffic on Interstate 70 to enjoy spectacular scenery or escape from urbanity on your bike or with your hiking boots. The following natural wonders are short and easy commutes you can enjoy without a deadline. The hiking, biking, and horseback riding is exceptional and ranges from easy strolls to heart-pumping challenges but always with time to stop, listen, relax, breathe deeply, and recreate.

White Ranch Open Space

This inspirational place is a former ranch draped on the side of foothills mountains that are 8000 feet high and offers pretty meadows, a pristine canyon, rock formations, and buttes. These mountains are the equal of many stretches of mountain ranges like the Appalachian Mountains but are mere foothills to the Rockies. The open space is almost 4400 acres and was the home of nomadic Ute and Arapaho Indians until settler James Bond set up a ranch on the property in 1865. The Whites purchased it in 1913 and maintained a ranch on it until 1969, when it was purchased as open space.

There are 18 miles of trails to hike, bike, or horse around on. Either start all of your hikes uphill from the northeast access point at 6300 feet, or drive 10 miles up to the west access at 7700 feet and begin your hikes going downhill and finishing uphill. The open space includes two camping options: Sawmill Hikers Camp and Sourdough Springs Equestrian Camp.

Golden Gate Canyon State Park

Although for many years this state park was not well developed for recreation, it has finally been expanded into a hidden treasure that is easily accessible from the Denver, Boulder, and Golden areas. The park offers mellow trails for hiking and biking, abundant wildflowers, spectacular vistas of the Front Range, and almost every type of tree seen in the mountains of Colorado.

Roxborough State Park

A geological spectacle, Roxborough State Park is one of the Front Range's most dramatic displays of monumental rocks and is part of the same 300-million-year-old Fountain Formation visible in Boulder's Flatirons and the Garden of the Gods in Colorado Springs. Roxborough has a wide variety of earth's geologic history displayed within its relatively small confines, including 280-million-year-old, light-colored Lyons sandstone; 260-million-year-old Morrison rocks colored by ancient blue-green algae; and 1-billion-year-old granite on Carpenter Peak. The Dakota hogback sandstone, deposited a mere 100 million years ago, when Colorado was covered by a sea that stretched from the Arctic to the Gulf of Mexico is also a highlight. It is a patch of serenity near a growing swell of suburban development and foothills subdivisions. Trails range from easy to moderate, and an informative visitors center is open year-round. Bikes and horses are not allowed

on the trails inside the park. (Also check out nearby Douglas County and Pike National Forest trails that connect with the park.)

Indian Creek Trailhead & Campground: Pike National Forest

South of Roxborough State Park, this little-known and little-used area has lots of recreational trail assets. This trailhead offers two major options for hiking, biking, or horseback riding: the Indian Creek Trail north to the Elk Valley Trail and the Ringtail Trail north to the Swallowtail and Sharptail trails.

TRIP 1 White Ranch: Belcher Hill Trail

Distance	8 miles, Semiloop
Difficulty	Moderate (hiking), challenging (mountain biking)
Elevation Gain	1700 feet (starting at 6300 feet)
Trail Use	Mountain biking, horseback riding, leashed dogs OK
Agency	Jefferson County Parks
Map	*Jefferson County*, Trails Illustrated *Boulder & Golden*
Facilities	Restrooms, backcountry camping

HIGHLIGHTS This most challenging and rocky of the ranch trails offers a great workout and excellent views of the buttes, mountains, plains, and canyon. It starts in a suburban setting that is distracting for the first couple of miles but then opens up to the magic panorama of these high foothills. You can access easier trails along the way (Whippletree, Longhorn, Maverick, and Sawmill) and make the trek much easier and shorter if you wish. It is popular with very fit mountain bikers and is as wide as the former ranch road it once was.

DIRECTIONS This trailhead is 1.7 miles north of Golden on Highway 93. Turn west on 56th Avenue and then Pine Ridge Road for 1 mile. Look for the parking lot on the right (north) side of the road. This is a much closer access point to drive to for the open space, but you'll get to view several estates on the way.

You travel north from the parking lot and go downhill, passing through two gates. The trail then goes uphill gradually through lots of rocks on a sandy creek bottom. It climbs onto the hillside, crosses the stream on a bridge, and

continues uphill more steeply. The trail then begins to switchback, and when you reach the 1-mile mark you see the easier Whippletree Trail on the right (north) side. The Whippletree Trail climbs up through a major drainage of mixed forest

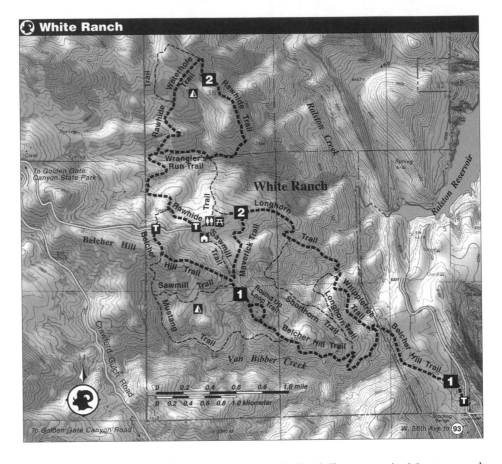

with nice butte views and becomes the Longhorn Trail, traveling through meadows as it climbs. That trail combination doesn't climb as high or as steeply as the Belcher Hill Trail, and you won't get away from views of suburbia as quickly. It merges with the Belcher Trail, where you can continue to climb or descend to the trailhead on the Belcher Trail if you prefer a short loop instead of a long out-and-back trip.

The Belcher Trail switchbacks up the mountainside and travels southwest toward the canyon. At 6700 feet you see Golden's characteristic table top mountains and downtown Denver in the distance. Around the 2-mile mark, at 6900 feet, you get sweeping views of high foothills that are reminiscent of foothills

in similar hill country in Montana and California. The Longhorn Trail branches right at around 7200 feet, and you have an extensive canyon view with striking rock formations on your left. The trail has fewer steep sections as it climbs up to 7400 feet and levels out as the Mustang Trail takes off downhill to the southwest into canyon country. You can of course explore the canyon views on the Mustang Trail and then return to the Belcher Hill Trail, avoiding another 600 feet of climbing. There is a bench available for a rest or snack break.

In 100 yards you see the short Round Up Loop Trail that travels about 0.1 mile out for a northerly view rejoining the Belcher Trail in short order. Another 100 yards take you to the Maverick Trail, another easier but scenic option that goes downhill to the broad meadows of the Longhorn Trail. In around 50 yards or so you reach an intersection with the Sawmill Trail and the route back to the Sawmill Hiker campsites (left). Take Sawmill right (north) for a short, easy trek downhill to the westside parking area.

The Belcher Hill Trail gets much steeper again as it climbs quickly up to 7800 feet, levels temporarily, and then climbs to around 8000 feet. The final panorama of views is well worth the effort with 8000- to 9000-foot foothills all around and even distant 14,000-foot Pikes Peak to the southeast.

TRIP 2 White Ranch: West Access Trails

Distance	Up to 10.0 miles, Out-and-back
Difficulty	Moderate
Elevation Gain	1500 feet (starting at 7700 feet)
Trail Use	Mountain biking, horseback riding, leashed dogs OK
Agency	Jefferson County Parks
Map	*Jefferson County,* Trails Illustrated *Boulder & Golden*
Facilities	Restrooms, backcountry camping for hikers or equestrians

HIGHLIGHTS The western access to White Ranch is peaceful and bucolic. Soft, rounded hills, stately foothills, and the buttes in the distance make this a rural rather than suburban entry point. There are two picnic tables 100 yards from the parking lot, and many of the trail options are mellow. This trailhead is 1400 feet higher than the east access, so you can more easily limit your level of exertion versus scenic density if you so desire.

DIRECTIONS Take Colorado Highway 93 north from Golden approximately 1 mile to Golden Gate Canyon Road. Travel west approximately 4.1 miles to Crawford Gulch Road (Highway 57). Turn right onto Crawford Gulch Road and follow the signs to White Ranch Park.

View north from the top of the White Ranch western access trails

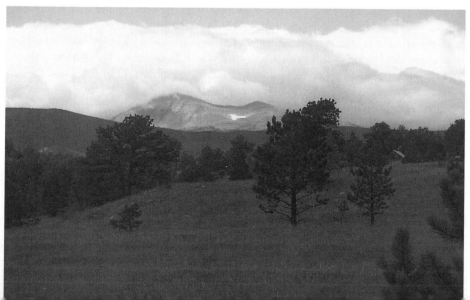

Longhorn Trail

This trail gently descends for the first 0.5 mile and then gradually steepens for 3 miles with meadow and butte views. Descend as far as you like and climb back up or take the Whippletree or Belcher all the way down if you set up a car shuttle.

Maverick Trail

For superb views of the canyon, take this roller-coaster, 2.2-mile trail down from the west access and then climb back up (up to 530 feet of gain/loss), or access the Maverick Trail off of the Belcher Hill Trail on your way up.

Sawmill Trail

This relatively mellow 1.6-mile trail with up to 700 feet of gain/loss is the primary route to the campground, or the Belcher Hill Trail from the west side. You can just walk the first 0.5 mile up and back to the Belcher Hill Trail if you want a short and easy adventure.

Rawhide Trail

The most interesting and challenging of the west side trails, the Rawhide Trail lunges and climbs and rolls over hill and gorgeous dale and meadow (up to 1400 feet of gain/loss).

TRIP 3 Coyote, Mule Deer, & Elk Trails Loop

Distance	8 miles, Loop
Difficulty	Easy
Elevation Gain	600 feet (starting at 8860 feet)
Trail Use	Fishing, mountain biking, leashed dogs OK
Agency	Golden Gate Canyon State Park
Map	*Golden Gate Canyon State Park*, Trails Illustrated *Boulder & Golden*
Facilities	Campgrounds, picnic areas, and restrooms at trailhead and along trail

HIGHLIGHTS Although for many years this state park was not well developed for recreation, it has finally been expanded into a hidden treasure easily accessible from the Denver, Boulder, and Golden areas. The park offers mellow trails for hiking and biking, abundant wildflowers in spring, spectacular vistas of the Front Range, and a broad range of almost every type of tree seen in the mountains of Colorado. The rampant aspen make it a superb place to visit in the fall. This route in particular is an excellent spring wildflower loop.

DIRECTIONS From central or north Boulder take State Highway 119 up Boulder Canyon and then south toward Rollinsville. After passing Rollinsville, cross the railroad tracks and continue past Highway 72. In a few more miles, look for the park on the left (east) side of the highway.

Or take State Highway 93 south from South Boulder or north from Golden, and then turn west on State Highway 72 (Coal Creek Canyon). When you come to a little village, turn left on Twin Spruce Road, and watch for a brown state park sign. Enter the park between Rifleman Group and Aspen Meadow campgrounds. Another campground you'll notice on the map, Renegade Ridge, includes yurts and cabins, too. Go right (north) toward Aspen Meadows. The Panorama Point overlook, 1.5 miles from the campground, is worth a stop. Look for the Bootleg Bottom Trailhead, where you park.

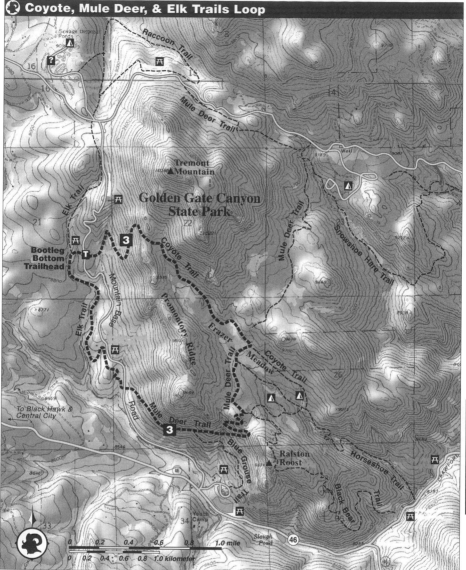

Coyote, Mule Deer, & Elk Trails Loop

Downhill from the parking area there is a restroom; it will be a very long time before you see another. The Coyote Trail goes gradually downhill from the parking area between the picnic tables, traversing the side of a small, heavily forested hill that would be a mountain in many other states with expansive views of slanting meadows and lofty foothills rolling off into the horizon. The downhill lasts approximately 0.1 mile and, in the spring, you immediately see geraniums, white bedstraw, and sulfur flowers among the aspen and ponderosa pine trees. The trail turns very sharply left and crosses a meadow with great views, before it climbs gradually and then more steeply uphill. If your timing is right, you will see wild roses, cow parsnip, black-eyed Susans, and blanket flowers. The trail then travels uphill steeply for 0.25 mile, where you see remains of a bootleggers' cabin from the 1920s, or Prohibition, when alcohol was illegal in the U.S.

The trail turns right and then switchbacks broadly uphill. Look for cinquefoil flowers and enjoy the subalpine zone Douglas fir trees. As you walk you also see lodgepole and limber pine and Engelmann and blue spruce trees. The views open up as you reach some rock outcrops that are a good spot for a snack or water break. You can see part of the Front Range, with James Peak (13,296 feet) in the distance, as well as Grey and Torrey peaks and even Mount Evans. Far to the right side are Arapaho and Audubon Peaks. Look carefully and you might see chiming bluebells, shooting stars, cow parsnip, and wallflowers, as well as lots of aspens.

The trail climbs to the west from the rocks, descends steeply, and then mellows into gorgeous meadows. The Frazer backcountry campground and a covered shelter for picnics are on your left. Turn around to see the striking rock outcrop of Promontory Ridge (9442 feet) behind you. This can be used as a turnaround point if you want a shorter out-and-back hike. Ahead are signs for more backcountry campsites (Rim and Greenfield Meadow) and the intersection with Mule Deer Trail. Turn right onto Mule Deer (southwest and south) and continue the loop. Where you see signs for the Frase, Black Bear, and Blue Grouse trails, turn sharply to the right. Mule Deer eventually morphs into Homestead, which becomes the Elk Trail. The trail

then goes uphill for 0.25 mile as it turns west. After some short, steep switchbacks, it rolls for another 0.25 mile, veering from west to north.

On the way, you see an intersection for the Blue Grouse Trail that goes left downhill to Kriley Pond. If you want to detour for fishing or soaking your feet, a car shuttle would make your trip easier. You will see Mountain Base Road below, as the trail turns north, opens up, goes gradually down a very long hill, and then crosses the road. You then have a steady uphill on the Elk Trail and can enjoy a different view of Promontory Ridge as you pass restrooms and picnic areas along the way. Watch for the sign for the Coyote Trailhead on the right to go back to the starting point at Bootleg Bottom.

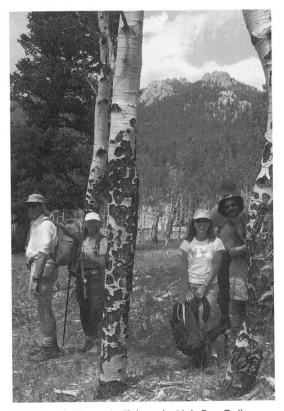

The Colorado Mountain Club on the Mule Deer Trail

TRIP 4 South Valley Park: Coyote Song Trail

w/ Jim + Deb
8/7/2010

Distance	Up to 3.2 miles, Semiloop
Difficulty	Easy
Elevation Gain	300 feet (starting at 5800 feet)
Trail Use	Mountain biking, leashed dogs OK
Agency	Jefferson County
Map	*Jefferson County Parks*
Facilities	Restrooms and picnic area at South Valley Road entrance

HIGHLIGHTS A pretty foothills area that includes the hogback and the usual striking rock formations, South Valley Park is great for hiking or biking. Part of the trail system is for hikers only, while the rest is open to bikers too. Coyote Song Trail is a great, perhaps the best, option in the park. Farthest from the road, it weaves through the beautiful rock formations and low foothills. The trail has more of an uphill start from the parking lot at the south entrance off of Deer Creek Canyon Road, more downhill from the north.

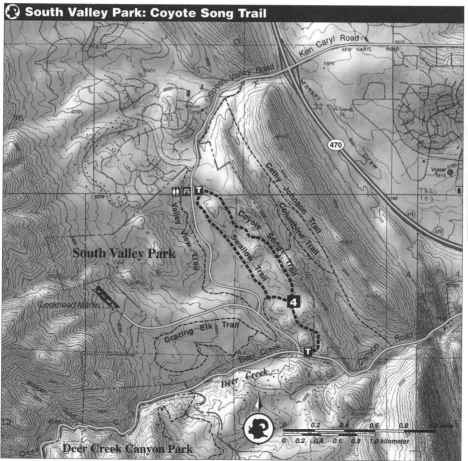

South Valley Park: Coyote Song Trail

DIRECTIONS Take State Highway 470 south to the Ken Caryl exit and turn west. Turn left on to South Valley Road to the park's north parking area. Or from the South Wadsworth and State Highway 470 intersection take Deer Creek Canyon Road west to the south parking area.

If you want a mellower start, go to the north lot, although the hill you immediately encounter at the south entrance isn't terribly steep. From the south entrance you climb the short hill through a very pretty, small canyon with inspiring rock walls. You crest the primary part of the hill after a little more than 0.25 mile, where a small rock formation on the west side of the trail can be used for a rest break.

At the 0.4-mile mark you come to an intersection with the Swallow Trail. If you are on foot, you can go downhill to the left (west) and take the Swallow Trail as your outbound loop, which is closed to bikes. The Swallow Trail is closer to relatively quiet South Valley Road. If you want to stay farther from the road, go straight and stay on the Coyote Song Trail. You go very gradually uphill and into the more intimate surroundings of the rock and foothills. It is 0.9 mile to the restrooms, picnic area, and water (summer only). The trails continue up to the north parking area where they rejoin.

TRIP 5 Fountain Valley Trail

Distance	2.2 miles, Semiloop
Difficulty	Easy
Elevation Gain	200 feet (starting at 6200 feet)
Trail Use	Leashed dogs OK
Agency	Roxborough State Park
Map	*Roxborough State Park*
Facilities	Restrooms at visitors center

HIGHLIGHTS Roxborough State Park is a red rock wonder that shouldn't be missed. This trail gets the award for highest scenic density and beauty for the smallest amount of physical effort.

DIRECTIONS Take State Highway 470 to Wadsworth Boulevard (State Highway 121) and go south to Waterton Road. Turn left (east) on Waterton Road 1.5 miles to Rampart Range Road. Turn right (south) and drive 2.5 miles to where the road narrows at the Golf Club. Turn left onto the Roxborough Park Road and then take an immediate right onto the park road. It is approximately 1.4 miles to the visitors center. This loop trail originates at the visitors center.

The trail goes uphill north from the visitors center, with a short detour for the Lyon Overlook on the west side. Although a nice overlook with two benches, it is marred by a subdivision to the west. The views to the north and south, up valley, are still worth the side trip. Descend down the gradually sloping trail to the loop intersection. I suggest going clockwise to the left (west) on the trail for the best views of the dazzling leaning towers; an out-and-back

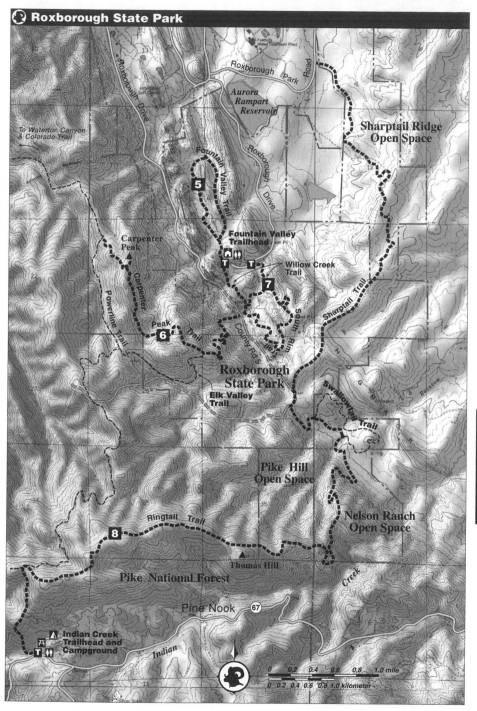

Roxborough State Park

Foothills Water Treatment Plant

Roxborough Park Road

Roxborough Drive

Christine Gulch Open

Aurora Rampart Reservoir

To Waterton Canyon & Colorado Trail

Sharptail Ridge Open Space

5

Fountain Valley Trail

Roxborough Drive

Carpenter Peak

Fountain Valley Trailhead

Willow Creek Trail

Carpenter Trail

7

Powerline Trail

Peak

South Rim Trail

Sharptail Trail

6

County Rd 5

Roxborough State Park

Elk Valley Trail

Swallowtail Trail

Pike Hill Open Space

Ringtail   Trail

Nelson Ranch Open Space

8

Pike National Forest

Thomas Hill

Creek

Pine Nook (67)

Indian

Indian Creek Trailhead and Campground

Silver State

0   0.2   0.4   0.6   0.8   1.0 mile

0 0.2 0.4 0.6 0.8 1.0 kilometer

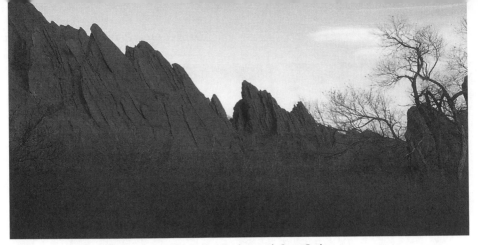

Rock formations on the Fountain Valley Trail at Roxborough State Park

venture on only the west side of the loop was more enjoyable to me than the less scenic east side. As you round the turn, you get a 180-degree view of the rock garden with soaring fingers, parapets, and fins. The trail wanders through scrub oak and comes to a magnificent view of the rock formations, with willows in the foreground and a bench for meditating on the last 300 million years and humankind's recent appearance.

At 0.6 mile the trail flattens, the wet meadow widens, and the giant flakes of sandstone stand as sentinels. You can round the end of the loop and follow the trail as it turns northeast into a pretty arroyo. Here I suggest turning around and retracing your steps on the west side of the loop, rather than completing the loop, so you can enjoy the inspirational rocks from a different perspective.

TRIP 6 Carpenter Peak

see map on p. 259

Distance	2.2 to 6.4 miles, Out-and-back
Difficulty	Easy to moderate
Elevation Gain	900 feet (starting at 6200 feet)
Trail Use	Option for kids, leashed dogs OK
Agency	Roxborough State Park
Map	*Roxborough State Park*
Facilities	Restrooms at visitors center

HIGHLIGHTS Roxborough State Park is a red rock wonder that shouldn't be missed. You can enjoy a short and easy route by hiking the Carpenter Peak Trail over to County Road 5. The road route isn't mentioned in park literature but it is one of the most scenic and easy (2.2 miles) out-and-back treks. You can savor intimate views of the dark red "sculptures" while strolling along the road. You have to cross the road to access the Carpenter Peak Trail. If you're ambitious, continue on to the summit of Carpenter Peak.

You don't have to go all the way to enjoy golden eagle views of the park from the Carpenter Peak Trail. The views of the park on your return from the Carpenter Peak summit are better than the outbound views, which are somewhat marred by an intrusive subdivision. The main visual benefit of summiting is seeing Waterton Canyon and the distant snow-capped peaks near the Continental Divide.

DIRECTIONS Take State Highway 470 to Wadsworth Boulevard (State Highway 121) and go south to Waterton Road. Turn left (east) on Waterton Road 1.5 miles to Rampart Range Road. Turn right (south) and drive 2.5 miles to where the road narrows at the Golf Club. Turn left onto the Roxborough Park Road and then take an immediate right onto the park road. It is approximately 1.4 miles to the visitors center. This trail originates at the visitors center, across from the roundabout.

The first 0.5 mile of the trail is a flat meander to the south-southwest with views of the green-hued Lykin/Morrison Formation rocks that frame the Willow Creek Loop Trail. It's easy to picture them as part of the landscape in the sea that once blanketed the area. At the 0.5-mile mark the Willow Creek Trail splits off to the left (southeast). Bear right or straight for County Road 5, the South Rim, and Carpenter Peak trails. In another 0.1 mile bear right when you see the South Rim Trail on the left. Go uphill past the pretty meadow to see the colorful rocks towering next to County Road 5 and some scattered cabins. If you want to savor the rocks, go left (south) along the road for 1.1 miles to the gate.

If you want to enjoy them from an eagle's height, continue straight ahead on the Carpenter Peak Trail, which then bends to the right and into switchbacks. You'll see a sign that says you have 2.6 miles to go for the summit, which means that the road is the 0.8-mile mark. You still have about 900 feet of gain for the peak. The switchback sweeps steeply up to the southwest; you reach a bench in about 0.1 mile that is a nice place for a water break or stretch. The bench has a commanding view at around 6400 feet that is worth the effort.

After climbing to almost 6600 feet over the next 0.25 mile, you finally have more shade and another bench. The trail levels for a bit and then climbs under tree cover to an intersection with the Elk Valley Trail, which climbs and then goes

> **Great for Kids**
>
> If you have small children or breathless friends, combining a trip to the first bench with County Road 5 could be a nice, easy round-trip.

down to the Indian Creek Trailhead and Campground at 6800 feet. The next 0.5 mile is a very gradual uphill with cooling shade, nice on a warm day. You emerge out of the trees onto a nice ridge walk with some peaks peeking through in the distance to the north. The trail tops out on a ridge with another bench at around 7100 feet, about the same elevation as Carpenter Peak.

Unless you are a peak bagger and want the workout or want to see the Continental Divide peaks, you can just as easily turn around after reaching this ridge top bench and be satisfied. After a snack and water break at the bench, follow the trail downhill into a gulch, dropping about 100 feet. You enjoy a relatively mellow trail with lots of shade for the next 0.3 mile where you reach the intersection of Waterton Canyon and the possible connection to the eastern end of the Colorado Trail 4.4 miles away; you are 3 miles from the Waterton Canyon Trail.

The summit is another 0.25 mile; from there at 7140 feet, where you can see distant snow-capped peaks and the canyon. The best part of this hike is the return, where you get a view of the ancient Rox rocks that will soothe your soul.

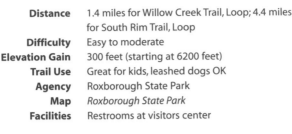

TRIP 7 Willow Creek & South Rim Trails

see map on p. 259

Distance	1.4 miles for Willow Creek Trail, Loop; 4.4 miles for South Rim Trail, Loop
Difficulty	Easy to moderate
Elevation Gain	300 feet (starting at 6200 feet)
Trail Use	Great for kids, leashed dogs OK
Agency	Roxborough State Park
Map	*Roxborough State Park*
Facilities	Restrooms at visitors center

HIGHLIGHTS Roxborough State Park is a great red rock display. The Willow Creek Trail is essentially a connector trail to the South Rim Trail but can be used as a pleasant almost flat loop alone if you prefer. It provides good views of some of the rock formations. More ambitious and interesting, the South Rim Trail features a sweeping switchback that climbs 300 feet to an overlook with a bench. You'll experience the 260-million-year-old Morrison Era rocks with their characteristic blue-green algae tinge more intimately.

DIRECTIONS Take State Highway 470 to Wadsworth Boulevard (State Highway 121) and go south to Waterton Road. Turn left (east) on Waterton Road 1.5 miles to Rampart Range Road. Turn right (south) and drive 2.5 miles to where the road narrows at the Golf Club. Turn left onto the Roxborough Park Road and then take an immediate right onto the park road. It is approximately 1.4 miles to the visitors center. This loop trail originates at the visitors center.

Both trails originate across from the visitors center. Walk west and then south and watch for the signs on the left that take you southeast. You then cross a meadow and see the trail continuing to the top of the rock outcrop to the southeast. The view from the top is worth the gently climbing switchbacks. There are great views all the way with a bench at the top for the weary. From there you get a 360-degree view of the park and especially the plains to the east, but some of the rock formations are obscured by the ridge to the west.

Rock arch window at Roxborough State Park

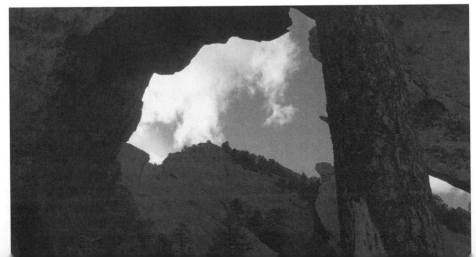

TRIP 8 **Ringtail Trail**

see
map on
p. 259

Distance	12.2 to 16.0 miles, Out-and-back
Difficulty	Moderate to challenging, depending on distance
Elevation Gain/Loss	1500 feet (starting at 7000 feet)
Trail Use	Mountain biking, horseback riding, leashed dogs OK
Agency	Pikes Peak Ranger District, Pike National Forest
Maps	*Pikes Peak Ranger District, Pike National Forest, Douglas County*
Facilities	Restrooms and campground

HIGHLIGHTS Adjacent to Roxborough State Park and well worth a visit, this rolling trail is better for biking than hiking and offers everything from sagebrush to foothills views.

DIRECTIONS This trailhead and campground is 10 miles west of Sedalia on County Highway 67. To reach Sedalia, drive south from State Highway 470 on State Highway 85 or take Interstate 25 about 30 miles south of Denver to Castle Rock and then County Highway 67 to Sedalia.

This trail climbs up and over Thomas Hill and then travels down into a major drainage and back up the other side to the Swallowtail Trail. You'll experience forest, plains, and rock formations and get a significant workout.

Bikes are not allowed in Roxborough State Park, so this is a way to enjoy the area with a bike. You cannot do a car shuttle without two cars. The conflicting reports on the actual length of this adventure range from 12.2 to 16.0 miles round-trip. Head off for an out-and-back trek of your chosen length, and turn around in time to beat the sunset.

Other Trails to Explore

Great for hiking or horseback riding, the Sharptail Trail adjacent to Roxborough State Park in Douglas County is 4.4 miles of rolling prairie that travels to the southern boundary of the park and County Road 5, which exits the park there. It rolls over hill and through dale climbing 700 feet gradually over the ridgeline that continues beyond the park. From there the trail intersects with the Swallowtail and Ringtail trails that travel south through the Nelson Ranch Open Space 6 more miles to the Indian Creek Trailhead and Campground.

Approximately 7 miles one-way, Indian Creek Trail connects to Elk Valley Trail in Roxborough State Park. The trail itself has rugged, rolling terrain and is great for mountain biking (although bikes are prohibited in Roxborough) and horseback riding.

**Denver Area:
Plains & Foothills**

Chapter 12
Denver Area: Mountains

The mountains west of Denver are the magic kingdoms that attract sojourners from around the world, but if you're a resident, they're at your feet. All you have to do is avoid the weekend snarls to truly enjoy the experiences. Though many of the treks are daytrips, I encourage you to spend the night in tents or lodges whenever possible so that you can spend more time on the trails and less time in your car. Quite a few of these trips aren't easily doable in a day, but they are too incredible to leave out of the book. From South Park and Como to Steamboats Springs and points in between like Vail and Summit County, there is enough to explore for a lifetime. So clear your schedule, travel at off-peak times, carpool, and savor this amazing panorama of experiences.

Georgetown & Guanella Pass Area

This popular area south of Georgetown offers many recreational options that are close to Denver and don't require a trip through the Eisenhower Tunnel. Turn-of-the-century mining village Georgetown is a bonus with restored Victorian architecture and a wide variety of great dining options. Allow for a snack or meal break in Georgetown to add to your appreciation of this once bustling mining region.

Summit County: Loveland Pass

The top of the pass is one of the best places in the state for panoramic views. The 12,000- to 13,000-foot ridgelines are stairways to mountain heaven and are often above the clouds. You can see 14,000-foot Grey and Torrey Peaks, as well as 13,000-foot Grizzly Peak and Sniktau Mountain, 12,500-foot Baker Mountain, and the Loveland, A-Basin, and Keystone ski areas. You will also see the Continental Divide and the more distant Gore and Tenmile mountain ranges. Take short strolls to enhance the view or climb the aforementioned 13ers, with a major head start by launching your expedition from 12,000 feet. If you want to summit a 13,000-foot peak and take in the bracing views from the top of Colorado's world with a lot less effort, this is one of the best opportunities. It is wise to have foul weather gear and warm, back up clothes, as the weather in the mountains can change suddenly without warning. Heavy hail storms and sudden, summer snowstorms are not uncommon; and a stiff, cool breeze is the norm.

Vail/Minturn

This lovely area has lots of options. I have included my favorite near the Holy Cross Wilderness Area, a super wildflower hike to Lake Constantine. Vail is known for very steep hikes into the Gore

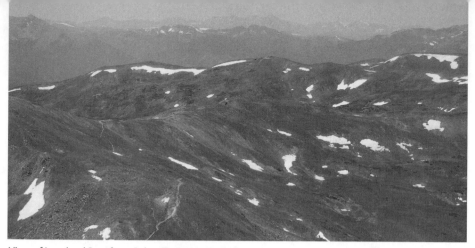
View of Loveland Pass from Baker Mountain Trail (Trip 5)

Range. This hike is an exception—a gently rolling trail near a popular wilderness area. The ambiance of Minturn is a bonus for some.

Steamboat Springs

It is impossible not to mention one of the true all-season wonderlands of the Rockies—Steamboat Springs. Although Aspen is well named for its abundance of trees of the same name, Steamboat also has some of the most impressive aspen forests in the state. They quake in soft mountain breezes, are surrounded by wildflowers during the summer, and are covered in shimmering golden leaves against an iridescent blue sky in the fall. Entire mountainsides covered by wildflowers in the spring and early summer are reason enough to visit.

Buffalo Pass Area

The Buffalo Pass area, just northeast of Steamboat, is one of the richest recreational areas in the state. It offers superb hiking and biking trails in summer and hard-to-match cross-country skiing and snowshoeing trails in winter.

Rabbit Ears Pass

Rabbit Ears is a popular year-round recreation destination simply because it is simply spectacular. The trails are easily accessible and varied, offering high ridge walks, riparian rambles, and beautiful aspen and conifer trees. The east end of the pass is dominated by motorized recreation while the west side is for hiking, biking, skiing, and snowshoeing.

Dunckley Pass

Nestled in the Dunckley Flattops, these lightly used trails offer a subtle beauty away from the hustle of Steamboat Springs and Rabbit Ears Pass. Imagine countless groves of aspen and wildflowers, butterflies, and sparkling mountain lakes. This area is especially stunning in the fall and spring.

Approximately 40 miles south of the Steamboat Area are the Flattop and Dunckley Flattop Mountains. This lesser known area is a little farther from Denver and less convenient than Rabbit Ears Pass but well worth the price of admission. It doesn't draw the crowds in spite of great scenery. Gravel Dunckley Pass Road is much lower and slower than Rabbit Ears and is only open before the snow flies.

Leadville Area

Leadville is rarely thought of as a recreation mecca, losing out to more fashionable locales such as Aspen and Vail. Lest we forget, it is the highest-elevation incorporated city in the U.S. and is a charming town surrounded by some of the most stunning scenery and mining devastation in the state. Colorado's highest mountain, Elbert, is southwest and the views of it and its neighbor, Mount Massive, would be the envy of any town in the Alps. It is the gateway for these two 14,000-foot mountains. Half Moon Campground, southwest of the city, is the jumping-off point for climbing these peaks or enjoying the part of the Colorado Trail that travels past them.

The infamous open pit mine at Climax is also nearby with its massive tailings pond—what happens when reclamation is not enforced—surrounded by the scars of the gold and silver mines that dotted the area during the mining boom that started in 1878 and peaked by 1890 with 24,000 people. The town is now undergoing a renaissance fueled by recreation. It is well worth a visit because the historic downtown has been rebuilt and refurbished and offers a variety of dining options. Though little of the surrounding terrain has not been mined, it still enjoys some spectacular and unique outdoor opportunities. The trails aren't crowded because of the mixed reputation created by the mining.

Kenosha Pass & Colorado Trail

Kenosha Pass is in a splendid location for gazing down upon the unique high country plains of South Park and the soaring mountains that surround and majestically frame it. Accessible from Kenosha Pass, the Colorado Trail begins at 10,000 feet. Superb views of South Park and the 14,000-foot peaks of the Mosquito Range are just off-trail.

Como

A good base camp and little-known recreational area, Como features a magnificent backdrop and is the gateway to Boreas Pass and the Gold Dust Trail, both of which are delightful ways to enjoy the scenic backdrop of the Tarryall Mountains and the Tenmile and Mosquito Ranges. Don't expect any support services in Como, but Fairplay is nearby and offers a variety of lodging and food options.

TRIP 1 St. Mary's Glacier & James Peak

Distance	2.0 miles to the top of the glacier, 8.0 miles to James Peak summit, Out-and-back
Difficulty	Moderate to the glacier, challenging to James Peak
Elevation Gain	270 feet to top of the glacier, 3250 feet to James Peak (starting at 10,000 feet)
Trail Use	Leashed dogs OK
Agency	Clear Creek Ranger District, Arapaho National Forest
Map	Trails Illustrated *Winter Park, Central City, & Rollins Pass*
Note	Avalanche danger is generally low in winter and summer, but check with the U.S. Forest Service office in Idaho Springs before frolicking in the snow.

HIGHLIGHTS This very climbable permanent snowfield, or glacier, with a spectacular setting is an easy drive from Denver. When it shrinks in the summer, trails go around it. If you have an ice axe and know how to use it for self-arrest, you can have fun glissading on the snowfield. Don't attempt it otherwise because it is easy to careen out of control onto the rocks and remove valuable brain cells or body parts.

DIRECTIONS Take Interstate 70 west from Denver, past Idaho Springs, to the Fall River Road/ St. Mary's Glacier exit onto County Road 275. Follow the signs approximately 8 miles to the glacier parking area. (It is essentially a dead end road so you can't miss it.) On a clear day you can see the glacier from the road.

You have a lot of recreational options when visiting St. Mary's Glacier. Many people enjoy the climb from the lake to the top of the glacier, and you can enjoy the nonstop round-trip views of the Front Range and call it a day.

When you reach the area near the summit of the glacier, you enjoy an impressive panorama of James Peak and its Front Range neighbor, Bancroft Peak. Some hikers find this sight an irresistible invitation and decide on an extended adventure to the summit of James Peak. The distance to the summit of James is 4 miles one-way.

From the parking lot follow the drainage toward the lake, approximately a 1-mile trek. Once you reach the lake, circle it to the right (east). When you reach the edge of the lake, continue to the east side

and climb up-slope to the saddle. By the end of June the east edge of the snowfield shrinks and the snow-free corridor widens, making snowshoe and crampon-free travel possible. The climb to the saddle is a moderate, fairly steep challenge that requires catching your breath more than once. Take your time and switchback as much as possible, enjoying the ever-expanding view as you climb. From the saddle either finish your hike to the top of the glacier to the west or bear east toward James Peak.

Continuing northeast toward James Peak is a nice, easy climb in clement weather. The route to the peak is very obvious because it is well traveled. If you cannot see James Peak because of weather, reconsider unless you are an experienced mountaineer. The route is a

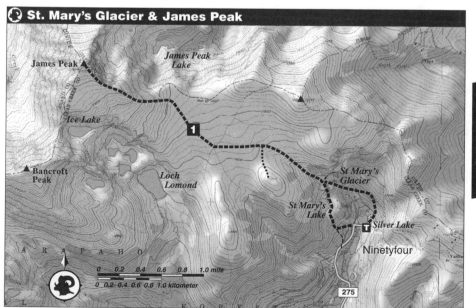

St. Mary's Glacier & James Peak

gradual uphill until you reach the foot of the peak; then it climbs steeply, and you'll have to employ some route-finding skills. The best route follows the right or northeast slope. Stay just below the top of the ridge, and you can angle your way to the summit. Don't track too far to the northeast, or you will climb a false summit and end up on cliffs. Enjoy the views!

TRIP 2 Jones Pass

Distance	Up to 7.0 miles, Out-and-back
Difficulty	Easy to challenging
Elevation Gain	2600 feet (starting at 10,000 feet)
Trail Use	Mountain biking, leashed dogs OK
Agency	Clear Creek Ranger District, Arapaho National Forest
Map	Trails Illustrated *Winter Park, Central City, & Rollins Pass*

HIGHLIGHTS This beautiful mountain valley is close to Denver and doesn't require a drive over Berthoud Pass. There are several trails you can explore at this popular location near the Henderson Mine, but you share this trail with some off-road vehicles (all-terrain vehicles and motorcycles). Enjoy a hike of any length, and soak in the views.

DIRECTIONS Take U.S. Highway 70 west from Denver and exit at Empire for Berthoud Pass/Winter Park. Drive through Empire toward the pass. When you come to the first sharp turn to the right, exit to the left for Henderson Mine. Continue north on the mine road until you reach the designated parking area. The road is closed at the trailhead that serves both the Jones Pass Trail and the Butler Gulch Trail. Travel west through the trees on the joint trail until a junction at approximately 0.3 mile. Bear right for the Jones Pass Trail or left for the more difficult and advanced Butler Gulch Trail.

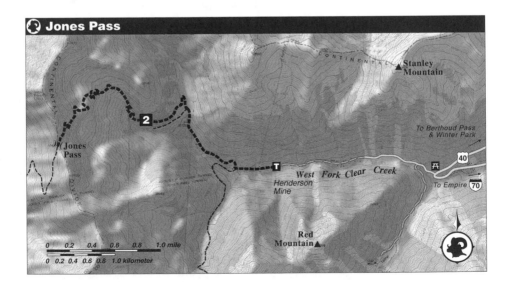

You have some glimpses of the ridge-line as you travel through the trees. At a little less than 0.5 mile you break out of the trees and enjoy the panorama of the valley and soaring ridgeline. Avalanche runout zones are observable on the steep slopes to the west. The trail steepens as it switchbacks. It then travels through a varied landscape of high mountain meadows and trees. You can go all the way to the summit of the pass or turn around whenever you wish.

TRIP 3 Silver Dollar Lake Trail

Distance	Up to 3.0 miles, Out-and-back
Difficulty	Easy
Elevation Gain	1000 feet (starting at 11,000 feet)
Trail Use	Mountain biking, leashed dogs OK
Agency	Clear Creek Ranger District, Arapaho National Forest
Map	Trails Illustrated *Idaho Springs, Georgetown, & Loveland Pass*

HIGHLIGHTS This short, fairly easy trail to a pristine lake surrounded by soaring mountains is one of the best trails on Guanella Pass and is easy driving distance from Denver.

DIRECTIONS Take Interstate 70 west from Denver. Take Exit 228 for Georgetown, and drive into town, following signs to Guanella Pass. On the first road past Guanella Pass Campground, turn right and park. The picnic ground turnoff is on the right side of the road.

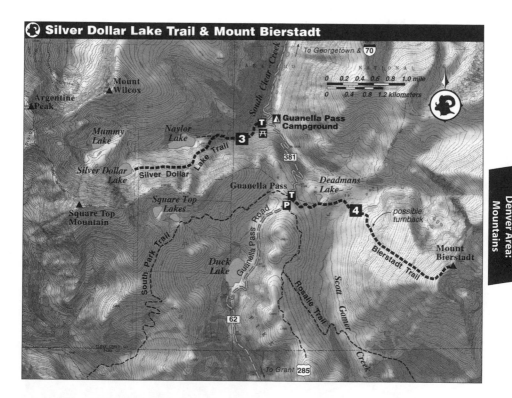

Silver Dollar Lake Trail & Mount Bierstadt

Denver Area: Mountains

Take the road approximately 0.4 mile to the trailhead, which is on the left and well marked. The road to the trailhead is steep. Once you reach the trailhead, the route levels somewhat, and you follow a small creek for a short distance. The trail then leaves the drainage, tracking to the right (west), and winds through the trees back toward the road. It then climbs out of a hollow and along a narrow section with a small drop-off until you emerge from the trees to a spectacular view of the lake and the surrounding rock wall cirque that towers above. From the lake you can climb one of the surrounding 12,000- to 13,000-foot peaks, with a good topographic map and compass and mountaineering preparation.

TRIP 4 Mount Bierstadt

see map on p. 269

Distance	6.0 miles to summit, Out-and-back
Difficulty	Varies, depending on distance hiked
Elevation Gain	2930 feet to Mount Bierstadt (starting at 11,130 feet)
Trail Use	Mountain biking, leashed dogs OK
Agency	Clear Creek Ranger District, Arapaho National Forest
Map	Trails Illustrated *Winter Park, Central City, & Rollins Pass*

HIGHLIGHTS One of Colorado's most accessible 14ers and much shorter and easier than Longs Peak, Mount Bierstadt can be climbed almost any time of the year and is a short drive from the Denver metro area. Safe, short excursions in the awe-inspiring terrain at the base of the Evans-Bierstadt massif can also be rewarding. The town of Georgetown is always a treat to visit and has a variety of food and beverage opportunities.

DIRECTIONS Take Interstate 70 west from Denver to Georgetown. Take Exit 228 for Georgetown and head toward town. Turn right toward Georgetown at the first four-way stop. Pass through Georgetown before climbing west and then south out of town toward the pass. Look for the Guanella Pass Trailhead for Bierstadt on the left (east) side of the road when you break out into the open and see the striking view of the Evans-Bierstadt massif to the east.

At 14,060 feet Mount Bierstadt is one of Colorado's highest mountains. As with any 14er, high altitude is challenging, but you can take a nice 2-mile hike (round-trip) before encountering lung burn. Plus the panoramic setting is superb.

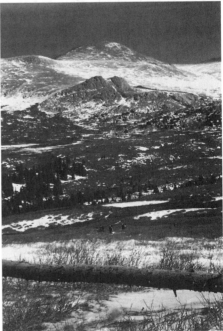

The route up Mount Bierstadt

Start at the Guanella Pass Trailhead and go as far as you like. Your starting time and company will determine the scope of your adventure. It is not advisable to climb high mountains alone or start late and expect to summit safely. The first part of the trail actually goes downhill for 1 mile. Just using the first mile as an out-and-back trek is worth the trip. At that point you are near Scott Gomer Creek at around 11,400 feet. You previously would have encountered challenging willows and marshes here, but now there is an easy-to-follow trail and footbridge through the willows.

The trail is well marked with cairns all the way to the summit, but you sometimes have to look for them with a keen eye to stay on course. I recommend using one of the many books providing detailed routes on the 14ers for a complete description of the route. From the parking lot the trail actually descends to Gomer Creek and a series of footbridges and boardwalks to help you avoid what was once a dreaded grove of willows and marsh. After you have made your way across the boardwalk, look for the cairns that mark the switchbacking trail to the top. You will come to a saddle about 200 feet below the summit, where you will want to take a breather before the final summit push.

South Park Trail on the other side of the road from the Bierstadt Trail can be used for another short out-and-back trek with great views. It starts out on a short hill, travels around 100 yards or so on a flat area, and then descends before climbing again. After another 100 yards it starts to meander and climb steeply.

TRIP 5 Baker Mountain

Distance	2.0 miles, Out-and-back
Difficulty	Moderate
Elevation Gain	448 feet (starting at 12,000 feet)
Trail Use	Option for kids, leashed dogs OK
Agency	White River National Forest
Map	Trails Illustrated *Vail, Frisco, & Dillon*

HIGHLIGHTS Baker Mountain with a steep but short hike straight uphill from the top of Loveland Pass is an easier summit to achieve than its neighbors Sniktau Mountain and Grizzly Peak. You start at 12,000 feet and only have to climb about 500 feet in the thin air. Although not as distinctive as its neighbors, it's much easier to summit.

DIRECTIONS From Denver take Interstate 70 west to the Loveland Pass exit just before the Eisenhower Tunnel. Drive to the parking areas on top of the pass; arrive early to beat the crowds and the thunderstorms. Carpool if possible. Baker Mountain and its loftier compadres, Sniktau and Grizzly, are all on the south side of the pass, left if you are traveling west. Park on either side of the road and climb south from it.

The start of the trek is the same for all three mountains (Baker, Grizzly, and Sniktau) for the first 0.3 mile. Go straight uphill on the broad trail wide enough to be a road. You are immediately treated to awesome 360-degree views. The first 0.3 mile gains more than 200 feet—you feel every step at this elevation.

If you are well prepared, take a right and go southwest at the first

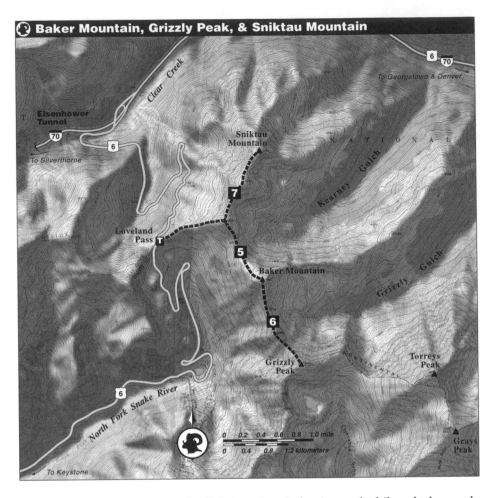

Baker Mountain, Grizzly Peak, & Sniktau Mountain

trail intersection. You travel slightly downhill at first as you traverse the steep slope on a trail that provides good footing and no exposure. You will feel like an eagle or hawk soaring through the air and looking down on the traffic and A-Basin ski area. There are some hearty Indian paintbrush flowers along the trail in season. After 0.25 mile the trail starts to climb, at first gradually and then more steeply. You lose a bit of elevation and then gain around 150 feet over the first 1.5 miles.

Then the real climbing begins as you clamber up a steep slope to the saddle gaining 100 feet in 0.25 mile. You have a great view from the saddle that makes the whole trip worthwhile—the huge valley between Loveland Pass and the Grays and Torrey massif makes you feel like you have already summited. This is a good turnaround point if members of your party aren't partying. Baker Mountain is to the right (west). There is an easy trail to follow, though the going is slow as you reach a couple of level spots on the way up and catch your breath. As you get near the top, you have a view of the Gore range to the northwest. The trail traverses around Baker and stays lower than the summit for a more direct route to Grizzly Peak.

If Baker is your goal, leave the trail and track left (south) toward Baker's unremarkable summit. The view is great, but the summit is not honored in any way since some argue it is just a high point in the 12,000- to 13,000-foot high ridge that it shares with Sniktau. The latter is very visible with its sinuous route and three false summits to the northeast.

Great for Kids

If you are a family hiking with small children or are unaccustomed to high altitudes, climb as high as you want to, take a few snapshots, enjoy the views, and reverse course. Altitude can cause dizziness and headaches, so ascend slowly.

TRIP 6 Grizzly Peak

Distance	5.0 miles, Out-and-back
Difficulty	Moderate
Elevation Gain	1637 feet (starting at 11,990 feet)
Trail Use	Leashed dogs OK
Agency	White River National Forest
Map	Trails Illustrated *Vail, Frisco, & Dillon*

HIGHLIGHTS This mountain looks like a grizzly bear in comparison to the soft, round, teddy bear shapes of Sniktau and Baker mountains. It is a spectacular ridge walk and steep scramble at the end that is clearly worth the effort for the views. It requires a bit of a roller-coaster climb since the ridge between Baker and Grizzly drops more than 150 feet and that altitude has to be regained going and coming. Although you can continue to Grays and Torrey Peaks from Grizzly, that would be a very long trek.

DIRECTIONS From Denver take Interstate 70 west to the Loveland Pass exit just before the Eisenhower Tunnel. Drive to the parking areas on top of the pass; arrive early to beat the crowds and the thunderstorms. Carpool if possible. Baker Mountain and its loftier compadres, Sniktau and Grizzly, are all on the south side of the pass, left if you are traveling west. Park on either side of the road and climb south from it.

The start of the trek is the same for all three mountains (Baker, Grizzly, and Sniktau) for the first 0.3 mile. Go straight uphill on the broad trail wide enough to be a road. You are immediately treated to awesome 360-degree views. The first 0.3 mile gains more than 100 feet—you feel every step at this elevation. Take a right and go southwest at the first trail intersection. You travel slightly downhill at first as you traverse the steep slope on a trail that provides good footing and no exposure. You will feel like an eagle or hawk soaring through the air and looking down on the traffic and A-Basin ski area. There are some hearty Indian paintbrush

flowers along the trail in season. After 0.25 mile the trail starts to climb, at first gradually and then more steeply. You lose a bit of elevation and then gain around 150 feet over the first 1.5 miles.

Then the real climbing begins as you clamber up a steep slope to the saddle gaining 100 feet in 0.25 mile. You have a great view from the saddle that makes the whole trip worthwhile—the huge valley between Loveland Pass and the Grays and Torrey massif makes you feel like you have already ummited. This is a good turnaround point if members of your party aren't partying. Baker Mountain is to the right (west). There is an easy trail to follow, though the going is slow as you reach a couple of level spots on the way up and catch your breath. As you get near the top, you have a view of the Gore range to the northwest. The trail traverses around Baker to the northwest and plunges down to the first saddle between the peaks. Edge your way as low as possible around the first hump and then drop down a bit lower before you have to climb up steep switchbacks to the summit of Grizzly.

see map on p. 272

TRIP 7 Sniktau Mountain

Distance	4.0 miles, Out-and-back
Difficulty	Moderate
Elevation Gain	1637 feet (starting at 11,990 feet)
Trail Use	Leashed dogs OK
Agency	White River National Forest
Map	Trails Illustrated *Vail, Frisco, & Dillon*

HIGHLIGHTS The most popular peak climb from Loveland Pass heads across the undulating southwest ridge of Sniktau and passes with at least three false summits on the way up. Each step provides its own rewards—you don't have to summit to take in the view. This hike has the most sustained view of Interstate 70 and the Eisenhower Tunnel of the three choices from this trailhead, but the highway noise fades and the views of Grays, Torrey, and Grizzly peaks make the trek worthwhile.

DIRECTIONS From Denver take Interstate 70 west to the Loveland Pass exit just before the Eisenhower Tunnel. Drive to the parking areas on top of the pass; arrive early to beat the crowds and the thunderstorms. Carpool if possible. Baker Mountain and its loftier compadres, Sniktau and Grizzly, are all on the south side of the pass, left if you are traveling west. Park on either side of the road and climb south from it.

From the parking area on the southwest side of State Highway 6, climb up either of the two paths. Go straight up the steep ridge, and ignore the side trail that departs to the right (west) for Baker and Grizzly about 0.3 mile uphill. Climb until you reach the ridgeline and the first "summit," where you even see a bit of a wind break. Many hikers enjoy the trail to that point and head back to their vehicles—an achievement since you will have climbed 1000 feet in short order just to reach that point.

If you want to continue to the peak, take a left and waltz up the wide ridge to the north side of the next "summit" at

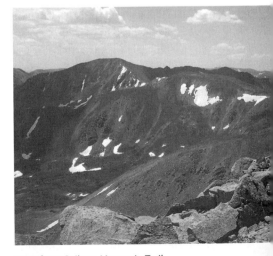

View from Sniktau Mountain Trail

13,152 feet. Although you will feel good about making the next "top," you will likely be unhappy to see the descending rocky path you have to follow down about 100 feet to a saddle before you start climbing again. You ascend 200 feet over the next 0.3 mile, bearing left to avoid unnecessary scrambling, and are rewarded with such great views of Grays, Torrey, and Grizzly that you will be tempted to make it a three-summit day.

> **Great for Kids**
>
> An easier trek than any of these three mountains that still has great views goes up from the other side of the road and follows the northwest side of the ridge to gain a view of the Loveland Pass Ski Area and Continental Divide. The trail immediately climbs 100 feet but then mellows as it more gradually climbs another 100 feet while offering a commanding view of the underrated Loveland Ski Area.

TRIP 8 Lily Pad Lake

Distance	3.0 miles, Out-and-back
Difficulty	Easy
Elevation Gain	200 feet (starting at 9700 feet)
Trail Use	Great for kids, leashed dogs OK
Agency	White River National Forest
Map	Trails Illustrated *Vail, Frisco, & Dillon*
Note	Bikes are prohibited, and dogs must be on leash because of the wilderness designation.

HIGHLIGHTS This hike takes you to a delightful series of small lakes and ponds in Eagle's Nest Wilderness on a path that is lavishly decorated with wildflowers in the early summer. Few hikes offer this much beauty with such easy access and minimal effort.

DIRECTIONS Even though the trail is in the wilderness, the trailhead is next to urban development and easy walking distance from many condominiums in Silverthorne. There is even a local bus service that you can take advantage of since the parking lot is small.

From Interstate 70, take the Silverthorne exit and go north on State Highway 9. Turn west on Ryan Gulch Road. Take the road until it ends in a loop, where there is a parking area for Buffalo Pass and Lily Pad Lake trailheads. Lily Pad Lake Trail is an unpaved road to the right of a paved road, with a cable hung from red posts across it.

Proceed west from the parking area toward the far trailhead and take the unpaved (right), closed road. The only steep section is at the very beginning of the hike and lasts less than 0.25 mile, so don't be dismayed if you have tykes in tow. Once you crest the top of hill, you see a large brown pipe sticking out of the top of a water storage tank on the left. Bear right/straight to reach the Eagle's Nest Wilderness boundary as the trail descends. The trail levels, enters a thick lodgepole pine forest, and then crosses a footbridge at 0.25 mile that takes you over wetlands in the early summer. The trail then climbs on a short, rocky section. It then roller coasters along and finishes downhill at the first pond that is surrounded by evergreens and offers a small peephole to the bright blue sky and wispy clouds floating by. The trail turns left (south) and goes downhill, and

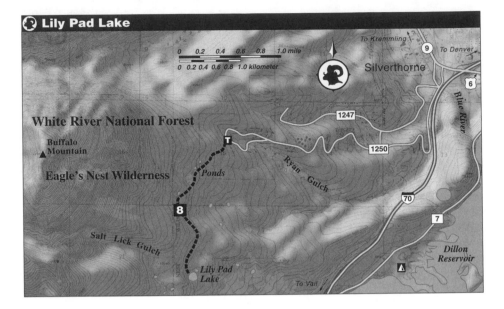

you see a variety of wildflowers in season including chiming bells.

The trail rolls gently as it turns southwest at 0.5 mile, where you can savor the vivid green of a pretty wetlands meadow accented by aspens. At around 0.75 mile you are encircled by wildflowers in season as the trail descends to 9600 feet and parallels the meadow before going southwest uphill. You cross the drainage again in very thick trees, good shelter on a hot day. The trail climbs up and tops out at around 9800 feet, and you see another trail entering as you begin to descend.

You roller coaster through a mixed forest, finishing downhill at Lily Pad Lake, which is covered by some of the thickest and hardiest lily pads in the state. If you are lucky, they will be blooming.

Climb over the next small hill for a spectacular view of an often snow-capped peak reflected in a clear, lily-pad-free and somewhat larger lake. Take your pick for superb settings for a snack, water, or lunch break before returning. When you do, be careful to bear right as you go uphill and don't take the closed trail on the left.

TRIP 9 Lake Constantine

Distance	10.0 miles, Out-and-back
Difficulty	Moderate
Elevation Gain	1400 feet (starting at 10,300 feet)
Trail Use	Backpacking, camping, fishing, leashed dogs OK
Agency	White River National Forest
Map	Trails Illustrated *Vail, Frisco, & Dillon*
Facilities	Restrooms at trailhead

HIGHLIGHTS This very popular trail features the constant distractions of wildflower riots and nonstop views, wildflower carpets in season, the soaring rocky ridge of Whitney Peak (13,271 feet), and pretty wetland meadows.

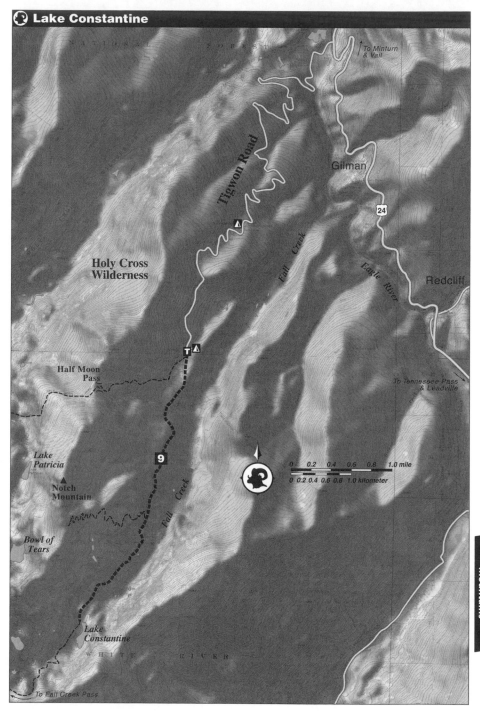

Lake Constantine

To Minturn & Vail

Gilman

Tigwon Road

Holy Cross Wilderness

Fall Creek

Eagle River

Redcliff

24

Half Moon Pass

T

To Tennessee Pass & Leadville

Lake Patricia

9

Notch Mountain

Fall Creek

Bowl of Tears

0   0.2   0.4   0.6   0.8   1.0 mile
0 0.2 0.4 0.6 0.8 1.0 kilometer

Lake Constantine

WHITE RIVER

To Fall Creek Pass

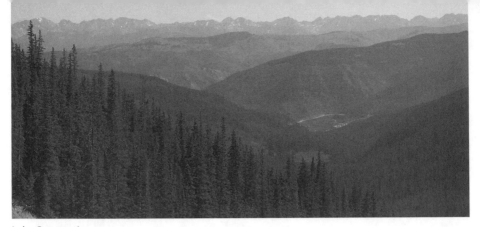

Lake Constantine

DIRECTIONS Take Interstate 70 west of Vail to Minturn and then turn south onto State Highway 24. From Interstate 70 drive approximately 5 miles south on Highway 24 to Tigwon Road and turn right (west). Take the very rough and rocky dirt road 8.5 miles to the trailhead and Half Moon Campground. You don't need a four-wheel-drive vehicle, just one that easily negotiates potholes and rocks. At the end of the road there are signs for Half Moon Pass, the route for 14,000-foot Holy Cross Mountain, Half Moon Campground, and Fall Creek. Take the Fall Creek Trail that is slightly downhill from the privy. Don't be dismayed by the crowds at the trailhead—most are going to conquer the Holy Cross Mountain.

The trail goes only a short distance before an intersection with trails that go to the Half Moon Campground and Trail. Go south on the Fall Creek Trail and in just 0.25 mile you enjoy a striking view of the ridgetop of Notch Mountain. If it is spring or early summer savor the off-white vetch flowers bordering the trail after 0.5 mile. The trail climbs 400 feet over the first mile or so, levels, and then descends. You will become very familiar with this pattern on this roller-coaster hike, as the trail climbs up to 10,900 feet and then descends.

As the trail descends, it breaks out of the thick tree cover and traverses an avalanche chute. You have a sweeping view of the Gore Range to the northwest and Fall Creek far below. You then enjoy the first of many stream crossings and are likely to encounter the mosquitoes that go with it. Brace yourself for the wildflowers: chiming bells, parry primrose, geraniums, columbines, and pink

Indian paintbrush, too. The trail is wide open to sun and views at the 2-mile mark and has climbed to 11,000 feet when it descends again. Then, just for variety, a steep uphill switchback heads through thick trees, including ponderosa pine and some aspen.

When you reach a trail intersection for Notch Mountain to the right, go straight as the trail levels at around 11,150 feet. The stately conifers fall off the hillside into the creek bottom with the soaring rocky ridge for a backdrop. The trail travels southwest and begins another slow descent from 11,160 feet. You can hear the cascading stream, which you soon cross on a broad fallen tree, dodging wildflowers and more mosquitoes. The trail then enters a rock garden, and you encounter an easy rock scramble up to around 11,200 feet. After more rocking and rolling, you reach the lakeshore meadows. Take your pick of routes to the water for a picnic.

TRIP 10 Wyoming Trail (#1101)

Distance	4.5 miles, Out-and-back
Difficulty	Moderate
Elevation Gain	1000 feet (starting at 10,038 feet)
Trail Use	Horseback riding, leashed dogs OK
Agency	Hahn's Peak Ranger District, Routt National Forest
Map	Trails Illustrated *Rabbit Ears Pass & Steamboat Springs*
Facilities	Restrooms
Note	Bikes are prohibited because the trail enters Mount Zirkel Wilderness in 0.25 mile.

HIGHLIGHTS This very enjoyable, rolling, easy trail from the top of Buffalo Pass at around 10,000 feet that rolls along next to the Continental Divide, offering beautiful high mountain vistas in all directions, particularly the Zirkel Range.

DIRECTIONS From Steamboat take Lincoln Avenue to 3rd Street and turn north. Turn right onto Fish Creek Falls and then left on Amethyst Drive. In 1.5 miles turn right on Strawberry Park Road (323). Drive 2.5 miles to Buffalo Pass Road (38) and turn right. Follow it 12.9 miles to the Summit Lake parking lot. The trail is across the road and is labeled "Trail 1101."

The trail heads downhill northwest from the parking lot and immediately traverses past a small creek. It is a gradual climb, a good thing at 10,000 feet. You see beautiful meadows and wetlands below and stroll next to stately fir trees, reaching the wilderness boundary in 0.25 mile, where you can see the Flattops in the distance to the west. The trail levels temporarily at 10,150 feet. Early in the season you are likely to encounter patches of snow and abundant mosquitoes. The trail then climbs steadily over the next 0.5 mile up to 10,500 feet, and the spectacular Zirkel Range comes into view.

Over the next 0.5 mile the trail descends 300 feet next to a wetland. It then roller coasters uphill, and in another

Author on the Wyoming Trail

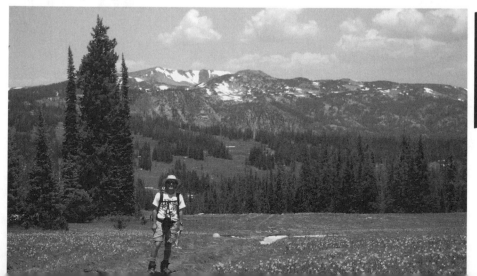

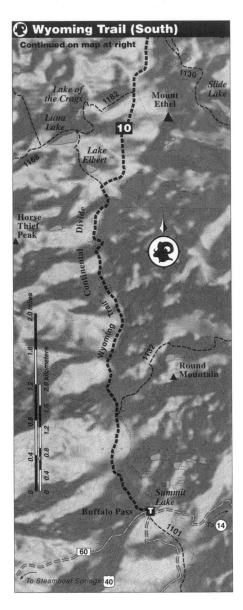

0.25 mile you cross the Newcomb Creek Trail and see a Continental Divide marker. The trail then switchbacks steeply uphill again for 0.5 mile, topping out at 10,500 feet. You can see the Rabbit Ears of pass fame if you look behind you. At the top of the hill, you get an even better view of the tundra- and snow-covered summits of the Zirkel Range, if you peek through the trees. The moisture gives the fir trees a healthy green glow and fragrant, soft needles. This is a good turnaround point since the trail plunges downhill in another 0.25 mile.

TRIP 11 Hinman Creek Trail (#1177)

Distance	6.0 miles, Out-and-back
Difficulty	Moderate
Elevation Gain	800 feet (starting at 7800 feet)
Trail Use	Mountain biking, horseback riding, leashed dogs OK
Agency	Hahn's Peak Ranger District, Routt National Forest
Map	Trails Illustrated *Rabbit Ears Pass & Steamboat Springs*

HIGHLIGHTS If you want to visit a wonderland of quaking aspens, rampant wildflowers, and giant fir trees, this is the trail for you. You can hike until you reach a spectacular canyon overview highlighted by Hahn's Peak. You can also visit lily-pad-decorated Hinman Lake along the way.

DIRECTIONS Take Highway 40 west of Steamboat Springs about 2 miles and turn right onto County Road 129. Travel north about 18 miles to the Seedhouse Road (FDR 400 or CR 64) and turn right. Continue for about 4.5 miles and turn left on to FDR 430 and park.

Start your hike on four-wheel-drive road FDR 430 and walk approximately 1.5 miles to the Hinman Creek (#1177) Trailhead. The road is impassable for anything other than a small four-wheel-drive so you might as well enjoy the walk. As you climb you emerge from the aspen groves and wind through aspen-bordered meadows, carpeted by dazzling wildflowers, including Queen Anne's lace. After about 1 mile you see informal campsites and it is worth a brief detour to enjoy the stream, as well as the wetlands and low foothills of the

Hinman Lake with lily pads on the Hinman Creek Trail

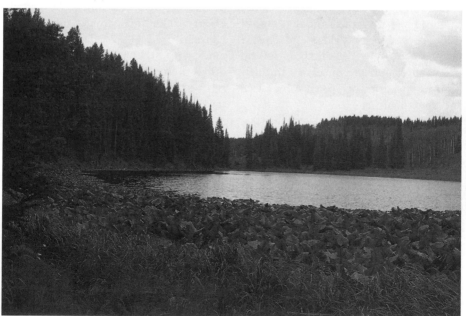

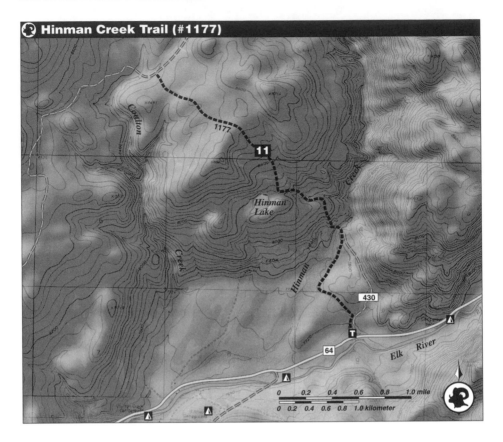

Park Range. You then reach the actual trailhead and cross the creek on a sturdy U.S. Forest Service bridge (no stream fording necessary). You climb out of the trees and, if they are in season, through head-high clumps of Queen Anne's lace and delphiniums.

The trail steepens and switchbacks, climbing up to an aspen grove at 7900 feet and leveling into a broad meadow that is often a wonderland of quaking aspen and brilliant wildflowers. You then climb up to 8000 feet and roller coaster down before going back up to 8100 feet where it levels. If you bear left at the next side trail (1183), you can enjoy a short detour to pretty Hinman Lake and its lily pads. Continue straight/right for the Hinman Trail (1177). The trail climbs quickly up to 8200 feet and levels again into a pretty meadow where you can see signs of the Hinman fire and some distant peaks in the Park Range. Stay right at the next trail junction (with #1188) as your trail continues, crosses Hinman Creek, and then follows Scott Run up into Diamond Park at 8400 feet. The north end of the trail is another 0.25 mile and 200 feet to where you enjoy the dramatic canyon overlook and Hahn's Peak, as well as views of the burnt forest.

TRIP *12* West Summit Loop 1A

Distance	3.5 miles, Loop
Difficulty	Moderate
Elevation Gain	500 feet (starting at 9320 feet)
Trail Use	Mountain biking
Agency	Hahn's Peak Ranger District, Routt National Forest
Map	Trails Illustrated *Rabbit Ears Pass & Steamboat Springs*
Note	Since the West Loop trails on Rabbit Ears are heavily used, the U.S. Forest Service requests that you leave your furry friends at home. The number of dogs on these trails usually outnumber humans, and the wilderness experience is in jeopardy unless people start to voluntarily comply with the request.

HIGHLIGHTS The west end of Rabbit Ears Pass is the best starting point for this loop and a real treat for beginners or novices, although there are also good intermediate-level trails too. They feature gradual climbs, beautiful vistas, views of the Yampa Valley, and generally well-marked but little-used trails. On a clear day you are treated to sweeping views of the Elk Valley to the north, the low hills of the Zirkel range to the east, and the Flattops to the south. The easier of the two loops offers beautiful views of the Yampa Valley and the Flattops and a variety of ascents and descents along the way that take you through groves of quaking aspens.

DIRECTIONS From Fort Collins, go west on State Highway 14 over Cameron Pass, crossing the Continental Divide, and drive down the other side 30 miles to Walden. Then drive south another 30 miles to State Highway 40. Take a right to and pass Muddy Pass Lake. Soon you will reach the east summit of Rabbit Ears Pass.

From Denver take Interstate 70 west to Dillon and then State Highway 9 to Kremmling where you can pick up Highway 40. It is 27 miles to Muddy Pass and the intersection with Highway 14. Stay on 40 and you will be on the pass.

These trailheads are 13 miles east of Steamboat. If you are driving west on the pass to Steamboat, watch for the last parking area on the right (with a large sign), approximately 12 miles from the intersection with State Highway 14. There are places to park on both sides of the road. Park on the north side for the Loop 1A, where you have the option of trying intermediate Loop 1B. The south side of the highway features trails not covered in this book that are less well marked but are also nice for out-and-back treks.

Go to the west end of the parking lot to a trail sign and a trail to the north (right) up a short hill. Though the hill is short, it immediately makes you aware that you are at 9400 feet and that pacing yourself is important. At the top of the short hill, go right (east) or left (west) onto the loop trail. The easiest out-and-back, the route to the left (clockwise), has some very pleasing scenery and a good view of the Flattops but doesn't offer the great views that climbing the ridge offers.

If you plan to complete the entire loop, I suggest traveling counterclockwise since the trail is easier to follow. Go right and slightly downhill (200 feet) on a former road, so it is a broad, easy start followed by a gradual 400-foot climb to the ridge-line at 9700 feet for great views.

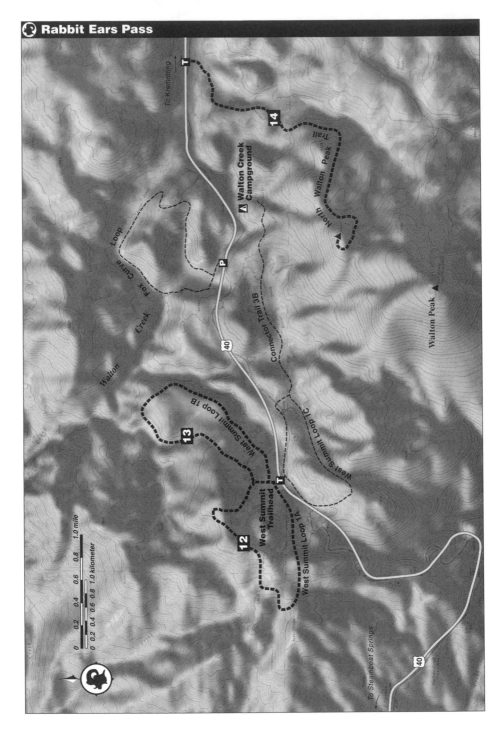

Rabbit Ears Pass

To Kremmling

14

Walton Peak Trail

North Walton Peak Trail

Walton Creek Campground

Loop

Fox Curve

Walton Creek

Walton

P

Connector Trail 3B

40

Walton Peak

West Summit Loop 1B

13

West Summit Loop 1C

West Summit Loop

West Summit Trailhead

12

West Summit Loop 1A

To Steamboat Springs

40

0   0.2 0.4 0.6 0.8 1.0 mile
0 0.2 0.4 0.6 0.8 1.0 kilometer

You parallel State Highway 40 for a very short stretch. The trail then takes a sharp left uphill through and across a beautiful meadow area rimmed by stately aspen and pine trees. It is very wet in late spring or early summer. Your goal is the beautiful grove of aspen trees at the top of the hill. Angle northeast and then northwest to avoid the willows and wetlands. As you climb the hill, you are in an area where Loops 1A and 1B overlap. At the intersection, bear left for 1A and continue your climb through the grove of aspen trees. Continue to climb northwest on the trail to reach the ridgeline at 9700 feet. On a clear day you are treated to spectacular views of Elk Valley to the north, the low hills of the Zirkel range to the east, and the Flattops to the south.

> **Great for Kids**
>
> If you are a beginner or there are young children in your party, the point where you reach the ridgeline might be a good place to return to the car, retracing your steps. When I had young children, this was usually as far as my family hiked, and everyone was happy.

To continue on Loop 1A, take the trail west and south to enjoy a short ridge walk followed by a significant downhill that descends to 9400 feet. The trail offers a nice variety of forested and open meadow trekking. When you reach the telephone line, the trail turns sharply left to return to the trailhead and take you back to your car.

TRIP 13 West Summit Loop 1B

Distance	4.0 miles, Loop
Difficulty	Moderate
Elevation Gain/Loss	500 feet (starting at 9320 feet)
Agency	Hahn's Peak Ranger District, Routt National Forest
Map	Trails Illustrated *Rabbit Ears Pass & Steamboat Springs*
Note	Since the West Loop trails on Rabbit Ears are heavily used, the U.S. Forest Service requests that you leave your furry friends at home. The number of dogs on these trails usually outnumber humans, and the wilderness experience is in jeopardy unless people start to voluntarily comply with the request.

HIGHLIGHTS This is the tougher of the two loops because of the number of ascents and descents. This trail starts easily going downhill and then into a meadow next to State Highway 40 (with the same trailhead as Loop 1A) and then climbs gradually and then somewhat steeply to a great view of the Hahn's Peak area west and north of Steamboat.

DIRECTIONS From Fort Collins, go west on State Highway 14 over Cameron Pass, crossing the Continental Divide, and drive down the other side 30 miles to Walden. Then drive south another 30 miles to State Highway 40. Take a right to and pass Muddy Pass Lake. Soon you will reach the east summit of Rabbit Ears Pass.

From Denver take Interstate 70 west to Dillon and then State Highway 9 to Kremmling where you can pick up Highway 40. It is 27 miles to Muddy Pass and the intersection with Highway 14. Stay on 40 to reach the pass.

These trailheads are 13 miles east of Steamboat. If you are driving west on the pass to Steamboat, watch for the last parking area on the right (with a large sign), approximately

12 miles from the intersection with State Highway 14. There are areas to park on both sides of the road. Park on the north side for the Loop 1B, where you have the option of trying the easier Loop 1A. The south side of the highway features trails that are less well marked but are also nice for out-and-back treks.

Though this trail doesn't climb as high as Loop 1A (though you can include a side trip to the top of the ridge if you'd like), it is more challenging because of its more varied terrain that steeply ascends and descends through thick trees and open meadows. When you reach the intersection near the aspen grove, turn right (northeast) rather than left (north-west). You continue to climb through the trees and then reach some meadow areas with nice views as you reach the high point. You then descend to 9200 feet and skirt a wetlands area. The trail turns sharply to the right and then goes south and west back to the start. The last 0.5 mile parallels State Highway 40, so an out-and-back route might be preferable.

TRIP 14 North Walton Peak

see map on p. 284

Distance	5.0 miles, Out-and-back
Difficulty	Moderate
Elevation Gain	650 feet (starting at 9500 feet)
Trail Use	Mountain biking, leashed dogs OK
Agency	Hahn's Peak Ranger District, Routt National Forest
Map	Trails Illustrated *Rabbit Ears Pass & Steamboat Springs*

HIGHLIGHTS This bumpy dirt road to the top of North Walton Peak can be hiked or mountain biked. It is more fun on a mountain bike since it is a good two-track road with a good gravel-and-dirt surface. It is a relatively easy, gradual climb through the rolling hills, aspen groves, and beautiful meadows of Rabbit Ears Pass. At the top you will be rewarded with a stunning view of the Continental Divide and the famous Rabbit Ears to the east. You might encounter a vehicle, so be watchful when rounding curves. The winter trails are overgrown, so bushwhacking is the only summertime alternative to the road.

DIRECTIONS The trailheads for North Walton Peak and Walton Creek are approximately 5 miles west of the intersection of State Highways 14 and 40 at Muddy Pass and approximately 18 miles east of Steamboat Springs. From the primary parking lot, drive approximately another mile east and look for the unsigned forest service road on the right/south side of the highway. Once you turn on to the gravel road you can park on a wide spot after the first 200 yards. The first section of the road was very rough at the time of this writing, so drive slowly because of challenging clearance over the rocks. A four-wheel-drive vehicle is not needed, but reasonable clearance is.

The dirt road climbs gradually for the first 0.25 mile through thick tree cover, and then begins to climb more steeply. Don't be discouraged since this doesn't last, as the road levels and climbs gradually over most of the first 1.5 miles. Over the next 0.25 mile, the views open up to the south, with beautiful meadows and abundant wildflowers. The next 0.5 mile is a gradual climb. You will see nice

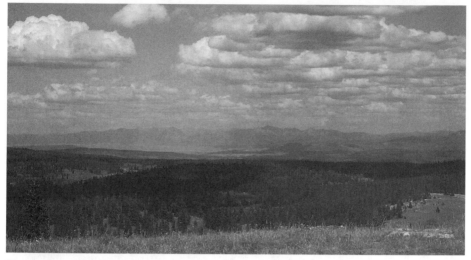

View from top of Walton Peak

groves of aspens and spruce trees around the 1-mile mark, ideal spots for shady picnic or rest spots.

The trail begins to climb in earnest again, for the next 0.5 mile, then leveling for 0.5 mile, before the steepest section begins. The last 0.5 mile is very steep, but the views to the east improve with every foot of elevation gained. The road winds sharply to the north/right, and then east as it climbs, finally leveling next to the tower. You will enjoy spectacular views that include the Rabbit Ears, the distant Front Range Mountains of Rocky Mountain National Park to the northeast, and the Gore Range to the southeast.

TRIP 15 Spronk's Creek Trail

Distance	2.1 miles, Out-and-back; 4.2 miles to Crosho Lake Trail, Out-and-back
Difficulty	Easy to moderate
Elevation Loss	600 feet (starting at 8000 feet)
Trail Use	Leashed dogs OK
Agency	Yampa Ranger District, Routt National Forest
Map	*Yampa Ranger District,* Trails Illustrated *Flat Tops NE & Trappers Lake*

HIGHLIGHTS This relatively short but beautiful trail through a pretty aspen forest has nice views of the southern part of the Yampa Valley. It is lightly used but offers a subtle beauty. You start on a rolling trail, go downhill to the creek bottom, and then finish by climbing the gradual hill back out.

DIRECTIONS Take State Highway 131 south from Route 40 to Phippsburg. You'll drive through Oak Creek, which has a grocery store, gas station, pharmacy, and good restaurants. When you are close to the south boundary of Phippsburg, slow down and take the first right, County Road 16, west to Dunckley Pass Road, which is closed several miles

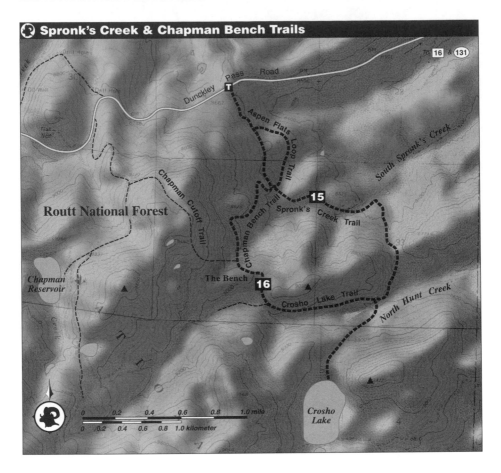

Spronk's Creek & Chapman Bench Trails

Routt National Forest

Chapman Reservoir

The Bench

Crosho Lake

ahead in the winter. Though this road is paved, you soon reach gravel Dunckley Pass Road (not the first intersection you reach), where you bear or turn right.

Alternatively, from Interstate 70 watch for State Highway 131 just west of Vail and Beaver Creek. Turn north on Highway 131 at the Wolcott exit. It is at least an hour's drive on dry roads to Phippsburg from I-70. You pass through Yampa, which has a grocery store, and a gas station. When you have almost reached the south boundary of Phippsburg, slow down and look for the first left; that is County Road 16 that takes you to the Dunckley Pass Road. Though this road is paved, you soon reach the gravel Dunckley Pass Road at the first intersection you come to. Bear or turn left (west) at the intersection.

The trails are on the left, if you are driving west, just beyond the cattle guard. There is a U.S. Forest Service stand with a large display map that usually contains individual trail maps.

This trail rolls fairly gently downhill for the first 0.5 mile or so and then goes down to the creek area more steeply. The Yampa Valley is visible to the east 0.25 mile from the start on the left (east) side of the trail. On the left a flat spot provides a nice overlook of the aspen forest rolling to the valley below and of Rattlesnake Butte, next to the Dunckley Pass Road. At around the 0.5-mile mark you encounter

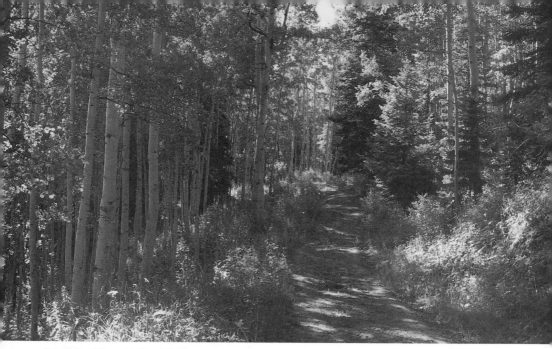

Aspen-lined Spronk's Creek Trail

the Aspen Flats Loop Trail. You can go either right or left around the Flats Trail to continue to Spronk's Creek; the left (east) side of the loop is the better one for the creek. The next trail you encounter is the Spronk's Creek Trail as it goes downhill to the usually dry drainage. Bear left at all intersections to be sure you end up on the correct trail; stay on the right edge of the meadow and drainage. The draw narrows as you close in on the bottom, and the drainage takes you to the bottom of the hill and the barbed wire fence that marks private property.

When you bottom out, either retrace your route back to the trailhead or bear right (west) uphill along the fence on the Crosho Lake Trail. You have the choice of adding 1 mile to the round-trip by continuing on to Crosho Lake or enjoying the magnificent wetlands valley that connects with the Chapman Bench Trail (Trip 16).

TRIP 16 Chapman Bench Trail

Distance	2.1 miles, Out-and-back, 4.2 miles if combined with the Spronk's Creek Trail, Semiloop
Difficulty	Moderate
Elevation Gain	800 feet (starting at 8600 feet)
Trail Use	Leashed dogs OK
Agency	Yampa Ranger District, Routt National Forest
Map	*Yampa Ranger District,* Trails Illustrated *Flat Tops NE & Trappers Lake*

HIGHLIGHTS Starting from the same trailhead as Spronk's Creek, this more challenging option charges uphill while Spronk's Creek Trail goes downhill. It offers nice views of the valley and, when you reach the heights of the Bench, superb views of the Dunckley

Flattops and a beautiful high mountain vale. The trail is a steady, fairly steep climb that switchbacks uphill on an old road. This trail is not recommended for small children or the marginally fit.

DIRECTIONS Take State Highway 131 south from Route 40 to Phippsburg. You'll drive through Oak Creek, which has a grocery store, gas station, pharmacy, and good restaurants. When you are close to the south boundary of Phippsburg, slow down and take the first right, County Road 16, west to Dunckley Pass Road, which is closed in the winter. Though this road is paved, you soon reach gravel Dunckley Pass Road (not the first intersection you reach), where you bear or turn right.

Alternatively, from Interstate 70 watch for State Highway 131 just west of Vail and Beaver Creek. Turn north on Highway 131 at the Wolcott exit. It is at least an hour's drive on clear roads to Phippsburg from I-70. You pass through Yampa, which has a grocery store and a gas station. When you have almost reached the south boundary of Phippsburg, slow down and look for the first left; that is County Road 16 that takes you to the Dunckley Pass Road. Though this road is paved, you soon reach the gravel Dunckley Pass Road at the first intersection you reach. Bear or turn left (west) at the intersection.

The trails are on the left, if you are driving west, just beyond the cattle guard. There is a U.S. Forest Service stand with a large display map that usually contains individual trail maps.

This trail is a very rewarding adventure if you take your time and bring lots of water since you will work up a good head of steam chugging uphill. The mountainside gets lots of late morning sun and can get quite toasty. After the trail stops switchbacking, it climbs steadily through the very tall pine, fir, and aspens, cresting temporarily in a small meadow. Your options are right (north) or left (south). Before choosing either option, go straight through the trees to the edge of the ridge and enjoy one of the better views in the Dunckley's. This is a good place to stop for photos and a rest break or snack. If you retrace you steps back to the trailhead at this point, you will have enjoyed a good two-plus-hour excursion out-and-back and largely up- and downhill.

If you continue on the trail to the right (north), you wind considerably through the thick tree cover and eventually top out on the Bench and not very far from Dunckley Pass Road were you a crow in flight. You will hear a bit of road noise.

If you bear south or left, it is a mellower downhill and excellent high mountain meadow scenery. The trail goes downhill through the trees close to the western edge of the ridgeline. You eventually bottom out near the Spronk's Creek Trail and can then make a climb back out to the trailhead. (See the Spronk's Creek description in Trip 15.) You are well rewarded for the effort by the colorful mixture of magnificent meadows, colorful wetlands, and stately aspen, pine, and fir trees. The climb back out is certainly easier than the climb up to the Bench area, but it might seem longer or more difficult than it is because it is at the end of your trip.

If you do want to complete the whole loop, allow at least 3 hours; it might take you most of the day if you want to stop for snacks or a picnic along the way. The trail bottoms out and then meanders to the Crosho Lake turnoff. Keep going straight to reach the fence that demarcates the Spronk's Creek turnaround, where you pick up with the description in Trip 15, or take a quick detour to see Crosho Lake, too.

TRIP 17 Mandall Lakes Trail (#1121)

Distance	8.4 miles, Out-and-back
Difficulty	Moderate
Elevation Gain	1840 feet (starting at 9760 feet)
Trail Use	Horseback riding, leashed dogs OK
Agency	Yampa Ranger District, Routt National Forest
Map	Trails Illustrated *Flattops*
Facilities	Campground 2 miles south of trailhead
Note	Bikes are prohibited because the trail enters Flattop Wilderness after 0.5 mile.

HIGHLIGHTS This spectacular trek through aspen glens and conifer forest heads through gorgeous wildflower meadows to pristine mountain lakes with an inspiring Flattop ridgeline backdrop.

DIRECTIONS From Yampa, travel south-southwest on Routt County Road 7 approximately 7 miles to FDR 900. Travel another 7 miles on FDR 900 to Bear Lake Campground. The trailhead is located across the road from the entrance to the campground.

The Mandall Lakes Trail is located in the Flattops, southwest of Yampa. The trail climbs through the Mandall Creek drainage, enters the Flattops Wilderness, and then passes Slide Mandall and Black Mandall lakes. The parking area is on the east side of the road, and the trail is hard to spot uphill in the trees. You immediately have a photo opportunity view of a Flattop Mountain created 40 million years ago by 12 million years of volcanic activity and then worn down. The road/trail starts steeply but mellows as it tracks south with spring wildflowers everywhere in steep meadows. Columbines and larkspur, as well as bright yellow daisies, usually border the gradual switchbacks. You climb 100 feet in the first 0.25 and then reach the Flattop Wilderness boundary in 0.5 mile.

The trail climbs more steeply with sweeping switchbacks to the north and

A hiker near Slide Mandall Lakes

Mandall Lakes Trail (#1121)

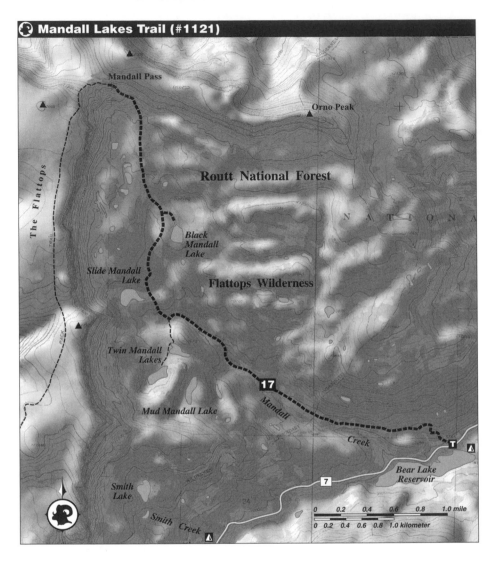

transforms from aspen grove to meadow at 9900 feet. Wild roses cheer you in season as you climb at the rate of 100 feet per 0.1 mile to a great lake view at 10,200 feet. You then descend 200 feet into a meadow and switchback gently 0.25 mile with great views of the Flattops' massif. Turn right (west) at the next trail intersection to travel along Mandall Creek, which you cross several times. Your climb alternates between gentle and steep and passes beaver dams, wildflowers, and a rushing mountain stream. In a couple miles, you come to the first of the lakes at around 10,400 feet. Declare victory and turn around whenever you wish.

TRIP 18 Twin Lakes Reservoir & Colorado Trail

Distance	5.0 miles, Out-and-back
Difficulty	Easy
Elevation Gain	Negligible (starting at 9400 feet)
Trail Use	Mountain biking, great for kids, leashed dogs OK
Agency	Leadville Ranger District, San Isabel National Forest
Map	Trails Illustrated *Aspen & Independence Pass*

see map on p. 294

HIGHLIGHTS Don't be fooled by the somewhat funky state of Leadville and the surrounding area where mine waste and tailings dominate the scenery. This trail is 17 miles southwest of Leadville near the road that leads to Independence Pass. It is surrounded by superb views of a towering ring of mountains: Mount Elbert (highest peak in the state), Parry Peak, 13,000-foot Rinker and Twin Peaks, and 13,461-foot Quail Mountain. It is an easy out-and-back trek in a great setting that is ideal for families or for a quick jaunt, with a beach and swimming.

DIRECTIONS Take Interstate 70 west from Denver and then either Highway 91 (from the Copper Mountain turnoff) or Highway 24 (from Minturn west of Vail) south to Leadville. From Leadville take Highway 24 south 14-plus miles to Highway 82, and turn right or west toward Aspen. After approximately 3 miles you reach the eastern edge of Twin Lakes Reservoir. After about 3 miles watch for a gravel road that goes left (south) below the dam. It is just before you cross a bridge. Continue on the gravel road around a wetlands area until you see the Colorado Trail. Bear right to the trailhead at the fork in the rough dirt road.

This rolling out-and-back trail allows you to walk around the southern edge of Twin Lakes Reservoir and also enjoy the ruins of the ghost town of Interlaken that is between the Twin Lakes. It is a spectacular setting with views of the southern flank of the Mount Elbert Massif and Mount Hope, both to the north, and west and south to Twin Peaks and Quail Mountain. There are even some beaches along the way if you want to take a dip in the chilly water. If you go to the ghost town, it is around 4 miles round-trip. If you decide to go farther, you will pass a wetlands area and then the second of the Twin Lakes. The Colorado Trail goes south at the western end of the second Twin Lake.

TRIP 19 Black Cloud Trail to Mount Elbert

Distance	Up to 10.0 miles, Out-and-back
Difficulty	Moderate to challenging, depending on distance and goal
Elevation Gain	1100 feet to treeline, 4740 feet to Mount Elbert (starting at 9700 feet)
Trail Use	Leashed dogs OK
Agency	Holy Cross Ranger District, White River National Forest
Map	Trails Illustrated *Breckenridge & Tennessee Pass*

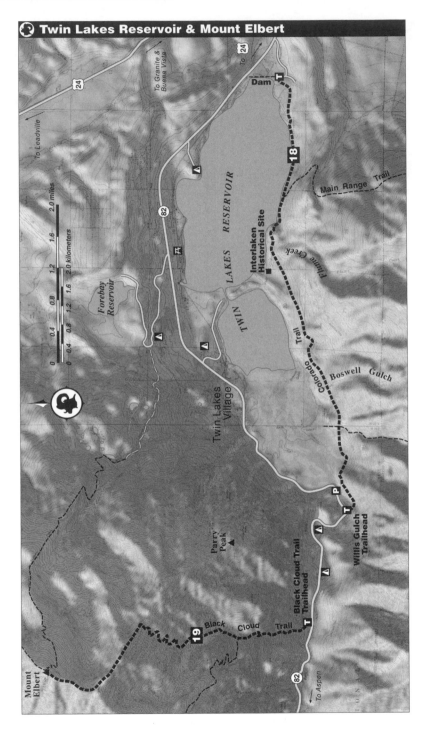

Twin Lakes Reservoir & Mount Elbert

HIGHLIGHTS Beat the crowds on an unusual, less-traveled, somewhat longer route up Mount Elbert on a spectacular, but steep trail and use your map, compass (or GPS), and mountaineering skills in the process. As you climb you will have superb views of 14,000-foot La Plata Peak to the south.

DIRECTIONS Take Interstate 70 west from Denver and then either Highway 91 (from the Copper Mountain turnoff) or Highway 24 (from Minturn west of Vail) south to Leadville. From Leadville take Highway 24 south 14-plus miles to Highway 82, and turn right or west toward Aspen. Follow Highway 82 for approximately 3.5 miles (0.5 mile past the Twin Peaks Campground). The trailhead is on the north (right) side of the highway approximately 4 miles west of Twin Lakes Village. It is very difficult to see, as only a small brown U.S. Forest Service sign marks it. If you reach the Mount Elbert Lodge without seeing it, then you missed it. You can use this route to climb Elbert if you are a good navigator.

D on't attempt to summit Mt. Elbert in this direction unless you are an experienced mountaineer because it involves some route-finding. Unless you have good route-finding skills, you will have to climb the south summit of Mt. Elbert (14,134 feet) and then descend into the saddle between the two summits, before climbing the main north summit (14,443 feet). You will then have to reclimb the south summit on the way back for extra fun. I recommend either a trip to treeline where you can enjoy spectacular views of Elbert's southern flank and the other majestic 14er in the neighborhood, La Plata Peak (14,361) that is across the valley and or that you climb the south summit of Mt. Elbert, an unofficial 14er. You will also see part of the impressive 13,000-foot duo, Twin Peaks, in the distance next to La Plata. Essentially you can enjoy a nice steep out-and-back trek to treeline with great scenery by taking on part of this route.

The first 0.75 mile is very steep, but the vertical climb eases a little after that. You will enjoy the sounds of the cascading stream of Black Cloud Creek and get

Hiker on the south summit of Mt. Elbert

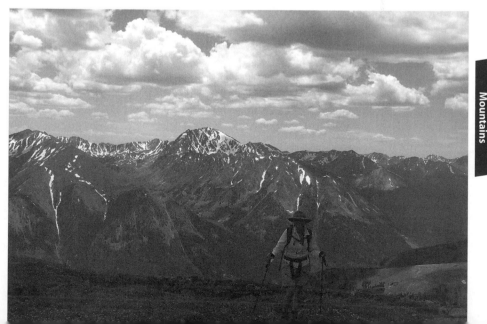

10th Mountain Huts & Trail Association

During World War II, Camp Hale near Tennessee Pass was the training center for the elite 10th Mountain Division troops who fought courageously in the Alps. After the war, many of the veterans returned to Colorado to found the Aspen, Breckenridge, Vail, Steamboat, Loveland, A-Basin, and Winter Park ski areas. They also converted the training huts they used during the war into European-style climbing huts for backcountry skiers and snowshoers. Now hikers and mountain bikers use them as well.

Staying in the 10th Mountain Division Huts is a terrific way to explore the high country any time of the year. There are dozens of huts, and they stretch from Vail Pass to Aspen. Reaching some of the huts is a challenging long-distance trek, while others are close to civilization and can be reached by the reasonably fit. For more information and reservations, visit the 10th Mountain Trail Association website (www.huts.org).

glimpses of small waterfalls. Approximately 1 mile from the trailhead at around 10,600 feet, you break out of the beautiful aspen and lodgepole pine forest and enjoy great views of the aforementioned peaks across the valley in the distance behind you. The trail then flattens for the next 0.25 mile or so. Shortly after that, around 10,800 feet, there is a footbridge across Black Cloud Creek to the west side of the creek, and you enjoy your first good look at Elbert's massif.

The trail then enters the lodegpole pine part of the forest and flattens again as it heads toward treeline from around 11,000 feet and then crosses back to the east side of the creek. The trail becomes difficult to follow, but bear somewhat to the right (east) until you burst out of the trees and get a truly stunning view of Elbert's southern ridge. You are standing at the edge of a massive avalanche runout zone—don't attempt this trail during snow seasons. The trail stays along the edge of the trees and continues to climb to the north and then west; follow the tree blazes that mark the trail and the ruins of an old miner's cabin around 11,500 feet that was obliterated by a fire. Ignore the faint trail you will see to the east. The trail climbs north and then crosses the creek to the west again on a log bridge and then ventures into the cleared out avalanche zone. It then starts to switchback much more steeply at the edge of the open area as it turns sharply right (east). Take the switchbacks until you have a satisfactory view of La Plata. At that point I suggest a lunch or snack and photography session before you turn around.

If you want to climb the south summit, continue as the switchback takes you east and then into a straight uphill surge that veers back to the west in the ever-thinning trees. Oddly enough, treeline is much higher on this slope than in most places, as you climb beyond 11,700 feet. The steep, loose switchbacks continue up the steep south slope of Mt. Elbert for another 2000 feet to a broad, flat ridge that is another possible lunch destination at 13,600 feet. The 360-degree views are superb—Leadville and the Gore Range to the north and the Collegiate Peaks to the south. From there it is another mile to the south summit and 1.5 miles one-way to the actual summit, a long day regardless of destination.

TRIP 20 Vance's Hut Trail

Distance	Up to 6.0 miles, Out-and-back
Difficulty	Moderate
Elevation Gain	1100 feet (starting at 10,400 feet)
Trail Use	Mountain biking, leashed dogs OK
Agency	Holy Cross Ranger District, White River National Forest
Map	Trails Illustrated *Breckenridge & Tennessee Pass*

HIGHLIGHTS This easy-to-follow trail features superb views of the Holy Cross Wilderness Area, Mount Elbert, the Mount Massive massif, and Ski Cooper. Vance's is one of the most accessible huts; it is only three miles from the trailhead at Ski Cooper/Tennessee Pass. Many fallen trees across the trail makes this more challenging for mountain bikers.

DIRECTIONS Drive north approximately 8 miles from Leadville to Tennessee Pass. Where you see Ski Cooper on the left (east) side of the road, pull into the parking lot and, as you near the main lodge, look for a small one-story building on the right (south) side of the road, west side of the parking lot. It is the Nordic ski and snowshoe rental hut in the winter. The trailhead is the road across from the Nordic building that descends into the drainage toward Chicago Ridge. It is 100 yards from the main lodge on the left (north) edge of the ski area. Drive down the dirt road, bear left at the fork, and drop your gear for overnight trips. You cannot park at the end of the road overnight. The ski area gate locks up at 4:30 PM during the summer months, so plan your day trips accordingly, and park in the parking lot above the trailhead. The hut is open from mid-August through April 30. It is closed in late spring and early summer.

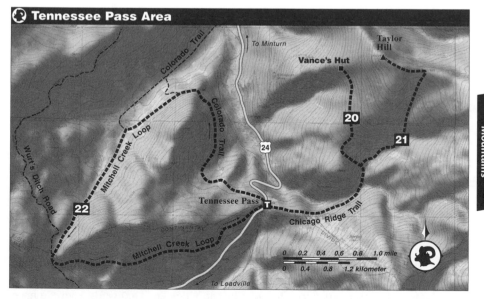

Follow the road or trail downhill about 0.6 mile until you reach a fork; bear left for Vance's Hut. (The 10th Mountain Trail was not marked at the time of this writing.) The road dead ends, and the trail goes left (north) and crosses the irrigation canal. You will have to cross the stream to the north on either the water diversion dam or through the stream itself.

Once you cross the stream, look for the double track, actually an old logging road, that climbs gradually uphill along the edge of the trees on the left. There is an open wetlands and meadow area on the right (east) where the trails separate. The Chicago Ridge Trail continues straight up the drainage to the right, while the hut trail climbs sharply uphill to the left (west) on the old road. After edging along the trees, the trail (road) turns west and then northwest and enters the trees. Watch for blue diamond trail markers in the trees; the road continues to the left (west), and the trail turns away to the right (north) marked only by the

blue diamonds, but the track is faint. The trail emerges from the trees across a nice steeply sloped meadow, and you reenter thick tree cover for a gradual slog up 700 feet to the top of the ridge as the trail switchbacks. Look sharply to see the trail markers. There are widely spaced blue diamonds but, because of the switchbacks, they are easy to miss. Once you reach the top of the ridge, the trail levels considerably and you see views of the mountains peeking through the trees. Be careful when detouring around or climbing over lots of fallen trees.

In another 0.5 mile from where the switchback ends, the trail rounds the ridge and opens up to a beautiful meadow with spectacular views of the Holy Cross Wilderness Area, Turquoise Lake, Mount Elbert, and the Massive massif down-valley. This is a good place to turn around since the trail goes steeply downhill to the left (west). You can't see the hut—it is hidden in the trees on the left side of the meadow around 200 yards downhill.

TRIP 21 Taylor Hill Trail

see map on p. 297

Distance	Up to 6.0 miles, Out-and-back
Difficulty	Moderate
Elevation Gain	1325 feet (starting at 10,400 feet)
Trail Use	Mountain biking, leashed dogs OK
Agency	Holy Cross Ranger District, White River National Forest
Map	Trails Illustrated *Breckenridge & Tennessee Pass*

HIGHLIGHTS Climbing Taylor Hill gives you an even better panorama of the area than the 10th Mountain Trail. You get a close-up look at Chicago Ridge and the spectacle of the Holy Cross Wilderness and the Sawatch Range to the south.

DIRECTIONS Drive north approximately 8 miles from Leadville to Tennessee Pass on U.S. Highway 24. Where you see Ski Cooper on the left (east) side of the road, pull into the parking lot and, as you near the main lodge, look for a small one-story building on the right (south) side of the road, west side of the parking lot. It is the Nordic ski and snowshoe rental hut in the winter. The trailhead is the road across from the Nordic building that descends into the drainage toward Chicago Ridge. It is 100 yards from the main lodge on the left (north) edge of the ski area.

ollow the road or trail downhill about
0.6 mile until an intersection with
the turnoff for Vance's Hut. (The 10th
Mountain Trail was not marked at the
time of this writing.) The road climbs
higher while the trail goes to the left or
north and crosses the irrigation canal.

The trail then climbs gradually uphill
along the edge of the trees into an open
wetlands and meadow area where the
trails separate. The Taylor Hill Trail continues straight up the drainage right
(northeast), and the Vance's Hut Trail
tracks to the left (northwest). Watch for
tree blazes. Stay on the left side of the
Piney Gulch stream as it follows the creek
and weaves through some open meadows
and trees. When you reach a secondary
drainage coming in from the left, turn
north and shoot for the saddle on the
east side of Taylor Hill. Make your own
switchbacks to the saddle; this steepest section of the trek requires patience,
given the altitude. From the top of the
saddle, follow the ridgeline west and
northwest to the summit of Taylor Hill
for a real treat. Enjoy the panorama and
have a nice break before retracing your
steps to the trailhead.

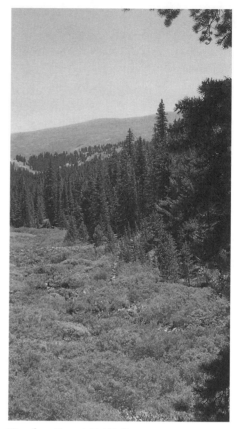

View from Vance's Hut Trail

TRIP 22 Mitchell Creek Loop

see
map on
p. 297

Distance	2.5 miles to kilns, 6.0 miles total, Loop
Difficulty	Easy
Elevation Gain/Loss	600 feet (starting at 10,400 feet)
Trail Use	Mountain biking, option for kids, leashed dogs OK
Agency	Holy Cross Ranger District, White River National Forest
Map	Trails Illustrated *Breckenridge & Tennessee Pass*

HIGHLIGHTS The top of this pass is an unexpected treasure trove of great trails for hiking
and biking. Its railroading history dates back to the narrow gauge lines of the 19th century, and modern freight service lasted until late in the 20th century. The Mitchell Creek
Loop uses the Tennessee Pass portion of the Colorado Trail. Part of this trail is a former
railroad bed and offers great views of the Holy Cross Wilderness and Homestake Peak. It
is a good trail for beginners but interesting enough in location and terrain to be fun for
all hikers at all levels.

DIRECTIONS Drive north approximately 8 miles from Leadville to Tennessee Pass on U.S. Highway 24. The trailhead is at the end of a large parking lot on the west side of Tennessee Pass across the road from Ski Cooper.

This part of the Colorado Trail is an old railroad grade that descends about 200 feet gradually while traveling first to the northwest. For the first 0.6 mile you enjoy great views of Homestake Peak. After approximately 0.25 mile you pass old charcoal kilns and continue on the old road as you pass the Powderhound Trail junction. The trail then levels out and turns right to the north. It begins to climb again and goes back up to 10,000 feet, flattens, and then rounds a bend, and the Colorado Trail turns off to the right and goes west and north.

The Mitchell Creek Loop Trail splits off to the left and then travels southwest into the Mitchell drainage, where it bottoms out and levels around 9850 feet. After about 1 mile the railroad grade ends, and the terrain becomes more difficult as it begins to climb again. The trail crosses the drainage and enters the trees around the 3-mile mark. The trail climbs steadily up to 10,600 feet and intersects Wurt's Ditch Road. The trail travels downhill on the road approximately 0.25 mile to the intersection with the Colorado Trail. When the trail rejoins the Colorado Trail, it turns sharply to the left and starts to go back to the east and north. You then have two stream crossings. The trail goes gradually up- and then downhill to the pass at 10,400 feet. Go straight at the junction with the Treeline Trail, and enjoy your trip back to the trailhead.

> **Great for Kids**
>
> An easy, short, and scenic option for families with kids and other people looking for short hikes is going round-trip to the ruins of the kilns. You will see some nice mountain views, have a wide easy two-track trail to ramble on, and have good photo opportunities when you reach the ruins. Be careful to keep the kids off of the kiln rocks for their own safety and the preservation of the site.

TRIP 23 Colorado Trail: West Branch

Distance	Up to 11.4 miles (round-trip) to Jefferson Creek Campground, Out-and-back
Difficulty	Easy to moderate, depending on distance traveled
Elevation Gain/Loss	800 feet (starting at 10,000 feet)
Trail Use	Mountain biking, option for kids, leashed dogs OK
Agency	South Park Ranger District, Pike National Forest
Map	Trails Illustrated *Tarryall Mountains & Kenosha Pass*
Facilities	Restrooms near trailhead and a campground

HIGHLIGHTS Kenosha Pass is a splendid location for gazing down upon the unique high country plains of South Park and the soaring mountains that surround and majestically frame it. The Colorado Trail is accessible from Kenosha Pass, and you get the benefits of starting off at 10,000 feet. Superb views of South Park and the 14,000-foot peaks of the Mosquito Range are just off-trail. It is very popular with both mountain bikers and hikers.

Colorado Trail

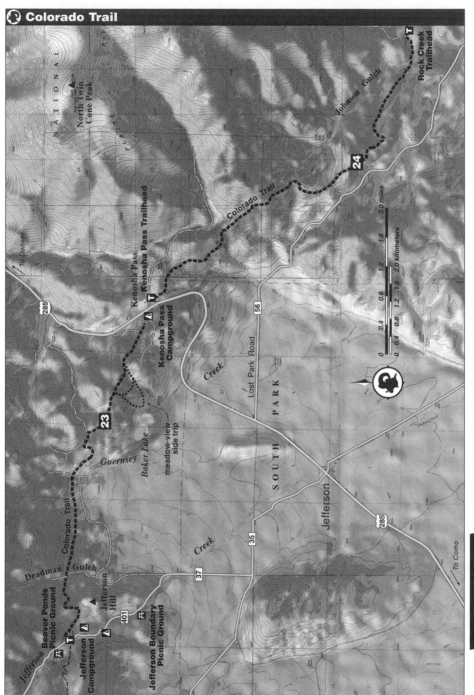

North Twin
Cone Peak

NATIONAL

To Denver

285

Kenosha Pass

Kenosha Pass Trailhead

Kenosha Pass
Campground

23

Guernsey

Baker Lake

meadow-view
side trip

Deadman Gulch

Colorado Trail

Jefferson Beaver Ponds
Picnic Ground

Jefferson Hill

Jefferson
Campground

401

Jefferson Boundary
Picnic Ground

Jefferson

37

35

Creek

Creek

Lost Park Road

SOUTH PARK

56

Colorado Trail

Johnson Gulch

24

Rock Creek
Trailhead

285

To Como

2.0 miles

0   0.4   0.8   1.2   1.6   2.0

0   0.4   0.8   1.2   1.6   2.0 kilometers

You can choose short, easy family hikes or more ambitious treks. It is often not clear of snow and dried out until mid- to late June in heavy snow years.

DIRECTIONS Kenosha Pass is approximately 65 miles southwest from Denver on Highway 285. Park on the east side of the highway outside of the Kenosha Pass Campground. Assume at least 1½ hours of drive time from Denver.

From the west side of the highway, you see a sign for the Colorado Trail. From the road, bear left around the restrooms and keep going; do not walk into the campground area on the right, and you eventually come to another sign for the Colorado Trail. Go to the right (north) on the trail. You are in a very thick tree tunnel at first as you climb steadily but gradually for 0.5 mile. You gain another 100 feet before it levels off and then starts to go downhill before emerging from the trees. You are treated to an eagle-high-overview of South Park. This is a great spot for a photo or snack break. The trail is on the part of the slope that slants to the south, so it features intense summer midday sun, with a pleasant breeze—don't forget your sunscreen.

After about 200 yards of downhill travel, it reenters trees. You lose around 250 feet if you walk all the way down near Baker Lake—the low point of this section of the trail. You regain all of the lost elevation, plus another 250 feet, gradually if you continue toward Jefferson Creek. Baker Lake is just short of 1.5 miles from the trailhead; if you turn around there,

> **Great for Kids**
>
> The first 2 to 3 miles of the trail climb very gradually, and the trail emerges out of the trees to a panoramic view of South Park and the massive backdrop of the 14,000-foot wall of 14ers in the Mosquito Range with some scenic glimpses of the Tarryall Range to the east, too. Since the trail travels at first gradually and then steeply downhill to the west from this point, you might want to have a snack or water break and then turn around. Going to Baker Lake will require a relatively long, moderate uphill climb on the return.

you will have about a 3-mile trek round-trip and about 350 feet in total elevation gain.

From Baker Lake you climb steadily but gradually as you cross Guernsey Creek and Deadman Gulch and meander into and out of the trees on your way to Jefferson Creek Campground at around 10,300 feet. As always, be cautious and turn around early if the weather changes and cumulus clouds start forming.

TRIP 24 Colorado Trail: East Branch

see map on p. 301

Distance	Up to 14.4 miles to Rock Creek Trailhead, Out-and-back
Difficulty	Easy to moderate, depending on distance traveled
Elevation Gain/Loss	800 feet (starting at 10,000 feet)
Trail Use	Mountain biking, leashed dogs OK
Agency	South Park Ranger District, Pike National Forest
Map	Trails Illustrated *Tarryall Mountains & Kenosha Pass*
Facilities	This fee area ($5 in 2007) has restrooms and a campground.

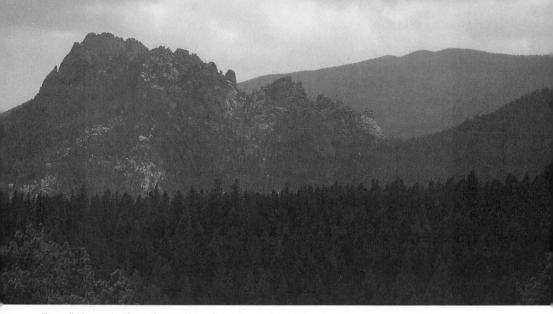

Tarryall Mountains from the Rock Creek segment of the Colorado Trail

HIGHLIGHTS This segment of the Colorado Trail is on the east side of Highway 285. The entire Colorado Trail can be used for an out-and-back outing of any length up to 30 miles or a one-way car shuttle of around 15 miles. The trail features sweeping views of South Park, and the Mosquito Range as it rolls gently through some thick aspen glens—great for viewing fall or summer colors.

DIRECTIONS Kenosha Pass is approximately 65 miles southwest from Denver on Highway 285. Park on the east side of the highway outside of the Kenosha Pass Campground. Assume at least 1½ hours of drive time from Denver.

The trail starts uphill and then levels near a log bench and railroad history marker. The area's railroad history is remarkable; four different railroads operated in the area: the Denver, South Park, and Pacific over the pass; the Denver-Rio Grande from Pueblo; the Colorado-Midland from Woodland Park; and the Colorado & Southern through Jefferson and Como.

After leveling, the trail rolls gently through a thick and beautiful stand of aspens, making this an ideal spot for fall or summer colors. The forest thins in about 0.5 mile, and you get great views of South Park and the Mosquito Range. An informal side trail on the right (south) of the main trail leads down to a small meadow that is good for picnics, as well as enjoying the view.

The trail gradually climbs 360 feet over the next mile, topping out at around 10,360 feet, leaving traffic noise behind. It levels at around the 1.5-mile mark, offering even better views of the east side of South Park. The forest transitions into conifers as the trail descends gradually and then more steeply into the valley—a good place to turn around. The views back to the trailhead are even better since you are directly facing the towering 13,000- and 14,000-foot mountains on the horizon. You can backpack to the Rock Creek Trailhead.

TRIP 25 Boreas Pass Road

Distance	Up to 10.0 miles, Out-and-back
Difficulty	Easy to challenging, depending on distance
Elevation Gain	1600 feet (starting at 9900 feet)
Trail Use	Mountain biking, leashed dogs OK
Agency	South Park Ranger District, Pike National Forest
Map	Trails Illustrated *Tarryall Mountains & Kenosha Pass*

HIGHLIGHTS This dirt-and-gravel road is passable for passenger cars that can handle rocks, bumps, and a steep climb. The pass offers superb views of part of South Park, the Tarryall Mountains, Breckenridge, and the Ten Mile range. I suggest you mountain bike it, but you will share the road with lots of vehicles unless you start at the crack of dawn. The pass is a treat that also gives you the easiest access to Bald Mountain and Boreas Peak, both 13ers.

DIRECTIONS Como is approximately 75 miles southwest of Denver on U.S. Highway 285. Take the Como exit from Highway 285 and drive west through Como. Approximately 5 miles from Highway 285, turn onto Boreas Pass Road on the right (north) side of the road. It isn't plowed in the winter but is usually usable by high-clearance vehicles in summer—be prepared for a rough, rocky road.

Drive if you must, but mountain biking the first few miles from Como is a real treat, if you get up early before the vehicle traffic begins. The first long hill is a lung and leg burner and then it mellows. The views of South Park are spectacular. Go as far as you wish and then enjoy the quick ride down. Test your brakes before descending, you'll need them!

TRIP 26 Gold Dust Trail: Southern Segment

Distance	4.0 miles, Point-to-point or out-and-back
Difficulty	Easy
Elevation Gain	100 feet (starting at 9900 feet)
Trail Use	Leashed dogs OK
Agency	South Park Ranger District, Pike National Forest
Map	Trails Illustrated *Tarryall Mountains & Kenosha Pass*

HIGHLIGHTS Would you like to roller coaster on a gentle trail with great views in every direction and streamside beauty? Then this trail segment is for you. Mountains of various sizes and shapes, as well as very pretty riparian areas, surround this lightly used trail with two segments. You can enjoy streams, trees, views, and wildlife without a great deal of exertion or difficult route-finding. The road to Boreas Pass is the route to the trails, so it is a well-maintained gravel road that won't have you bouncing off the ceiling of your vehicle.

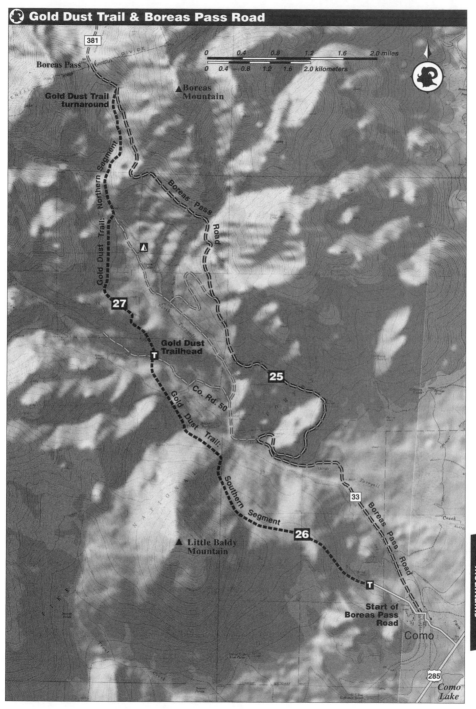

Gold Dust Trail & Boreas Pass Road

381

Boreas Pass

Gold Dust Trail turnaround

Boreas Mountain

Gold Dust Trail: Northern Segment

Boreas Pass Road

0   0.4   0.8   1.2   1.6   2.0 miles
0   0.4   0.8   1.2   1.6   2.0 kilometers

27

Gold Dust Trailhead

T

Co. Rd. 50

Gold Dust Trail

25

33

Boreas Pass Road

Southern Segment

Little Baldy Mountain

26

Creek

NATIONAL

T

Start of Boreas Pass Road

Como

285

Como Lake

DIRECTIONS Como is approximately 75 miles southwest of Denver on Highway 285. Go right (west) at the Como turnoff and then drive 5.5 miles west on the good gravel road to reach the trailheads.

The trail starts at Church Camp Road in the town of Como and travels northwest around the shoulder of Little Baldy Mountain, eventually intersecting with County Road 50 west of the Boreas Pass turnoff. The trail crosses scenic Tarryall and Silverheels Creeks before intersecting with the road. The hike can be done as an out-and-back or as an easy car shuttle for a one-way trip by dropping one car at the intersection with County Road 50 and then returning to the trailhead or vice versa.

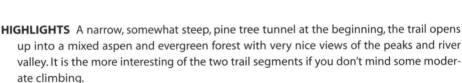

TRIP 27 Gold Dust Trail: Northern Segment

Distance	10.0 miles, Out-and-back
Difficulty	Moderate
Elevation Gain	550 feet (starting at 10,000 feet)
Trail Use	Leashed dogs OK
Agency	South Park Ranger District, Pike National Forest
Map	Trails Illustrated *Tarryall Mountains & Kenosha Pass*

see map on p. 305

HIGHLIGHTS A narrow, somewhat steep, pine tree tunnel at the beginning, the trail opens up into a mixed aspen and evergreen forest with very nice views of the peaks and river valley. It is the more interesting of the two trail segments if you don't mind some moderate climbing.

DIRECTIONS Como is approximately 75 miles southwest of Denver on Highway 285. The trail begins west of Como and the Boreas Pass turnoff approximately 5.5 miles from Hwy. 285. It is easy to miss the brown U.S. Forest Service sign on the north side of the road because it is back from the road and parking is a bit farther west (0.3 mile) past the trailhead, which is well marked. This more interesting and challenging option climbs all the way up to the Boreas Pass Road.

The first 0.5 mile is in thick tree cover as the trail switchbacks from lowland to highlands and then opens up, offering some peekaboo views of the surrounding foothills. The next climbs reaches a ridgetop with even better views of the hilly environment. This makes a good turnaround point for families. The trail descends into a beautiful forest glade. It then roller coasters and climbs steeply to the Boreas Pass Road. Allow at least half of a day for the round-trip. The view from near Boreas Pass Road is well worth the effort.

TRIP 28 French Pass Trail

Distance	Up to 6.0 miles, Out-and-back
Difficulty	Moderate
Elevation Gain	1400 feet (starting at 10,600 feet)
Trail Use	Leashed dogs OK, option for kids
Agency	South Park Ranger District, Pike National Forest
Map	Trails Illustrated *Breckenridge & Tennessee Pass*
Facilities	Campground on the way to the trailhead

HIGHLIGHTS One of the prettiest hikes in the state offers everything: a beautiful riparian area, a riot of nonstop wildflowers, and panoramic peak views. However, it also features a very healthy bug population because of the abundance of water and the lush vegetation that goes with it, so take precautions. The pass goes all the way to Breckenridge, but you'll need a car shuttle on the other side, unless you are prepared to add 10 miles to the end of the hike. You can also summit two 13ers: Bald Mountain or Guyot Peak. The former, which is described below, is a steep, beautiful climb, the latter an "exciting" knife-edge ridge walk.

DIRECTIONS Take Highway 285 south over Kenosha Pass toward Fairplay. After you descend approximately 3 miles from the pass, you reach Jefferson; turn right (west) onto County Road 35. In about 2.5 miles you come to County Road 54 (Michigan Creek Road), bear right (west) and continue past the Michigan Creek Campground in about 2 miles. Continue on County Road 54 toward Georgia Pass. Check your odometer and drive 2.25 miles past the campground to a curve and creek crossing, where there is an opening for informal camping. You can park in the flat spot before crossing the creek. The trailhead sign is in the trees, southwest of the parking area.

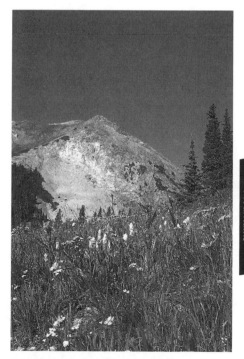

Bald Mountain from French Pass Trail

Most of the trail is a wide, two-track, old mining road. The beginning is easy mountain biking, but then the trail becomes very rocky and stays that way for most of the trek. Although for many stretches, it isn't rocky, the descent to Breckenridge is even rockier; don't bike it unless you are a rock hound. The rocks are very passable on foot and easily avoided. The trail begins across the road from the parking area to the west at a large sign that reads TRAIL 651. It zigzags through tall spruce and fir trees with lots of wildflowers from the outset.

French Pass & Bald Mountain

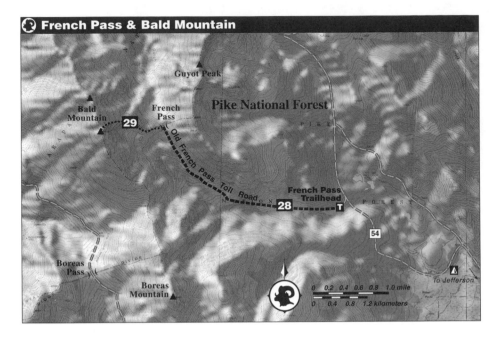

Guyot Peak

Bald Mountain

French Pass

Pike National Forest

29

P I K E

A R A P A

Old French Pass Toll Road

French Pass Trailhead

28 T

54

Boreas Pass

DIVIDE

Boreas Mountain

P O R E S T

To Jefferson

0 0.2 0.4 0.6 0.8 1.0 mile

0 0.4 0.8 1.2 kilometers

Great for Kids

The trail climbs very gradually and opens up to great mountain views in the first 0.5 mile, making it a good scenery stroll if you want a short out-and-back with young children or a relaxing hike.

You start off around 10,600 feet with soaring ridgelines around 12,000 to 13,000 feet above, bathed in reds, yellows, and greens of every shade, and of course the typical, dazzling, bright blue sky. As the trail swings from an S shape to a W shape, it flattens and becomes a gorgeous meadow stroll. The trail climbs around 400 feet in the first mile and then swings northwest, passing a huge pile of talus that was once a ridgeline. After 1.5 miles, around 11,000 feet, the trail acquires the rocks that make biking it bumpy. At this point you can see the pass dead ahead (west-northwest); to the southwest is Black Powder Pass, which is a tough bushwhack. The northwest ridge across the valley is a tall arm of Guyot, hidden

out of view high above. The peak just to the left (southwest) of French Pass is an impressive, cliff-slashed subpeak of Bald Mountain.

The trail takes a sharp right off the mining road into the drainage and across a magnificent meadow of wildflowers. Listen to the sparkling sounds of the water as you journey downhill, north-northeast and then northwest as you cross two streams. The flies and mosquitoes love the water (and you, too). The wildflowers are in full riot, requiring sunglasses, as you climb out of the drainage parallel to the creek. The trail bears left across another bright meadow and tracks, affording you a terrific sweeping view of the riparian valley, the ridgeline with multiple peaks across the way, and the impressive hulk of Bald Mountain.

Around 2 miles the trail takes another sharp right (northeast), but this time it climbs 130 feet in 0.25 mile, briefly testing your legs and lungs and giving you an even better view. It then tracks through low willows, climbing ever more steeply until it takes you to the bottom of a steep dirt-and-scree mound that is often covered by snow late into the summer.

You climb 600 feet over the last mile, but the view from the top of the pass is well worth it, with the tempting slopes of Bald Mountain on the left and the sharp slope of Guyot on the right. Also visible are the distant members of the Mosquito range and the route flying downhill into a verdant valley, which ends in trendy Breckenridge. Enjoy the cool breezes of 12,046 feet, have lunch or at least a snack, savor your accomplishment, and enjoy your reverse-course views of South Park and the Tarryall Mountains.

TRIP 29 Bald Mountain

Distance	8.0 miles, Out-and-back
Difficulty	Challenging
Elevation Gain	2079 feet (starting at 10,600 feet)
Trail Use	Leashed dogs OK
Agency	South Park Ranger District, Pike National Forest
Map	Trails Illustrated *Breckenridge & Tennessee Pass*

HIGHLIGHTS One of the (technically) easier 13ers to access and climb with commanding views of Breckenridge, the Ten Mile and Gore ranges, and the Tarryall Mountains, as well as the intimidating knife edge of Guyot Peak. It can be climbed from either Boreas Road, or the more pristine and less busy French Pass route. If you have made it to the top of French Pass with 3 to 4 hours (total) set aside for hiking and no thunderstorms in sight, you can make this summit.

DIRECTIONS Take Highway 285 south over Kenosha Pass toward Fairplay. After you descend approximately 3 miles from the pass, you reach Jefferson; turn right (west) onto County Road 35. In about 2.5 miles you come to County Road 54 (Michigan Creek Road), bear right (west) and continue past the Michigan Creek Campground in about 2 miles. Continue on County Road 54 toward Georgia Pass. Check your odometer and drive 2.25 miles past the campground to a curve and creek crossing, where there is an opening for informal camping. You can park in the flat spot before crossing the creek. The trailhead sign is in the trees, southwest of the parking area.

From the top of French Pass, contour southwest up the grassy tundra slope to 12,240 feet, and then make your own switchbacks up the very steep tundra slopes, speckled with wildflowers. Go west-northwest up the southeast ridge and enjoy the grand view of the cliff faces, as well as the exposure. You can see the summit of Guyot and its exceedingly narrow ridge. After 0.25 mile look to the right (west) for cairns that guide you away from the cliffs toward the summit that is out of view on the far right. The subpeak on the left is unfortunately a false summit—avoid climbing it. Traverse away from the southeast ridge and cliff faces and avoid climbing the humps on the ridge. Pick your way through the rocks and scree, and try to preserve your feet and ankles by staying on tundra when possible. If you aren't alone, spread out to lessen the impact on the tundra and flowers. You will encounter several bands of rock that require care and a bit of determination.

After picking your way through the series of rock bands, you are able to use welcome but very steep tundra again for your climb, as you reach 13,100 feet. Aiming for the saddle dead ahead, you have to dance with a steep scree slope for the last 150 feet of the 13,500-foot saddle. The view of Breckenridge and the Ten Mile Range from the saddle is great but does not include the actual summit out of view to the right (northwest), over the scree pile next to you. Contour around it, and follow the rolling, rocky ridge to the actual summit.

TRIP 30 Limber Grove Trail

Distance	3.0 miles, Out-and-back
Difficulty	Easy
Elevation Gain	600 feet (starting at 10,300 feet)
Trail Use	Leashed dogs OK
Agency	South Park Ranger District, Pike National Forest
Map	Trails Illustrated *Breckenridge & Tennessee Pass*

HIGHLIGHTS This rocky, but easy trail traverses talus slopes and reaches a grove of 1000-year-old limber pine trees that have been sculpted by wind, snow, and ice into gnarled works of natural art. The exposed wood grain and twisted shapes of these ancient trees are worth the talus scramble and rough road. The trail travels between the Four Mile and Horseshoe campgrounds.

DIRECTIONS Go 1.4 miles south of Fairplay on Highway 285 to County Road 18 (Four Mile Road) and turn right (west). Take the very rough, washboard road 9.4 miles to just past the access road for Four Mile Campground. Park on the south side of the road near the trailhead.

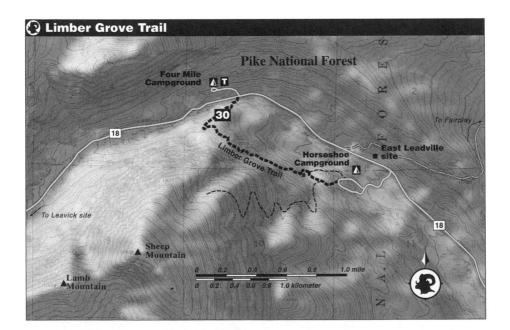

Don't take this trail unless you have good high-top hiking boots or don't mind cleaning rocks and dirt out of your shoes. You will be crossing steep talus slopes that require good footgear. The trail travels southwest from the trailhead, crosses Four Mile Creek, and then climbs fairly steeply about 100-plus feet onto a low ridge of Sheep Mountain, where you have nice views and continue to climb more gradually. It then travels slightly downhill, through the limber grove and then descends all the way to Horseshoe Campground. Refrain from cutting, breaking, and touching the tress to save them for future visitors. Since the limber grove is closer to Four Mile Campground than to Horseshoe, you don't have to take the entire 3-mile round-trip if you have problems with the scree and talus.

TRIP 31 Salt Creek Trail (#618)

Distance	Up to 18.0 miles north (Out-and-back), 6.0 miles south (Out-and-back)
Difficulty	Easy to moderate, depending on distance traveled
Elevation Gain	1000 feet (starting at 10,300 feet)
Trail Use	Mountain biking, horseback riding, backpacking, option for kids, leashed dogs OK
Agency	South Park Ranger District, Pike National Forest
Map	U.S. Forest Service *Salt Creek Trail (#618)*

HIGHLIGHTS This gorgeous, roller-coaster trail rolls around near the scenic Buffalo Peaks Wilderness with the high, rounded, impressive peaks looming in the distance. Expect a rich variety of flora with a forest of aspens and ponderosa and limber pine, bright lichen on scattered rocks, evergreen forests, riparian valleys, and foothills vistas. This trailhead can be used for enjoyable short out-and-back hikes in either direction; a long thru-hike to the north that would be an excellent, easy, point-to-point backpack with a car shuttle; or a very long, challenging dayhike. The description below covers two separate dayhikes.

DIRECTIONS Take Highway 285 about 18 miles south of Fairplay. Turn right (west) onto Salt Creek Road (Forest Road 435). The narrow, but well-maintained road does not require a high-clearance or four-wheel-drive vehicle unless it is very wet and muddy. It can become impassable in heavy, sustained rain. Take the road to an intersection 2.5 miles in and bear right for another mile where it dead-ends at the trailhead.

Buffalo Peak from the Salt Creek Trail

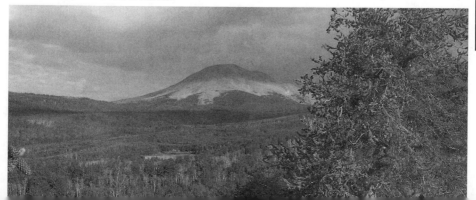

Y ou have a choice between hiking either northeast or southwest, both of which I describe. Think twice about driving the length of this road if it has been raining heavily; the mud can make the road passable only by four-wheel-drive vehicles. If it is dry, however, passenger cars can easily make the trip.

Southwest Route

This 1-hour round-trip takes you immediately uphill through a mixed aspen and conifer forest. You crest the small hill in about 0.25 mile and are treated, as

> **Great for Kids**
> The first mile of the Southwest Route is ideal for a short excursion. Bear southwest for the initial uphill stretch that is very short, and then enjoy immediate views to the north. Go downhill on a very gradual switchback. Cross a small stream as the trail continues its gradual downhill trend, with good tree cover for protection from the elements. Stop for a snack break, and then reverse course while the uphill return is easy.

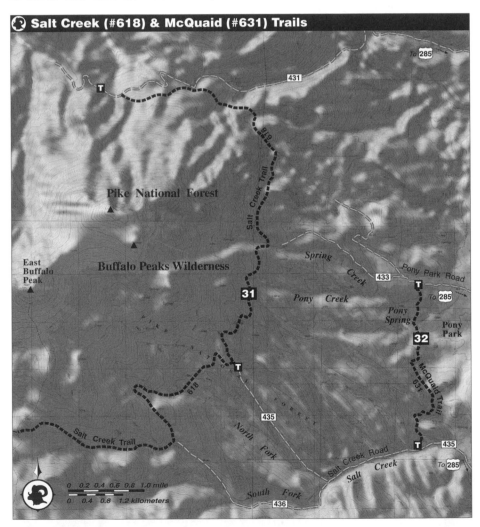

Salt Creek (#618) & McQuaid (#631) Trails

the trail turns north, to a spectacular view of Buffalo Peak, rolling waves of forested hillsides in every direction, and a rich green valley below. The trail travels downhill 100 feet and is edged by elegant ponderosa pines interspersed with aspens and limber pines. Large lichen-encrusted rocks and abundant wildflowers complete the landscape—one of the prettiest panoramas in the state.

The trail reaches the bottom of the hill and crosses a drainage. It then climbs west-northwest, crosses a meadow, and travels southwest with every shade of green displayed off to the horizon and distant peaks in sight. At a sign reading TRAIL 618, the trail turns right and joins Trail 435 1B, a four-wheel-drive road that is still in use. At this point you can either join the road and the vehicles on it as it climbs out of the valley to a pass or reverse course to the trailhead.

Northeast Route

This section of the trail travels downhill out of the parking area for a short stretch before beginning a gradual climb for 0.5 mile through a very thick stand of healthy quaking aspen. The slightest breeze sets them off to provide an optical delight. You cross some small wildflower-dominated meadows, before coming to a trail intersection at 0.75 mile that indicates that the Salt Creek Trail goes either straight north or east. Right (east) looks like a more developed trail, and, after climbing a short hill, you are rewarded with a great view of a reservoir and the Tarryall Mountains to the east.

From this point you could climb onto the ridge just above the trail and gaze upon Buffalo Peaks to the west and the reservoir and the Tarryall to the east. The trail then turns north and travels gradually downhill into the thick tree cover, losing the view but gaining lots of welcome shade on a hot summer day. The trail continues to roll and offer intermittent views. Watch the time and distances you travel, remember that you have to climb the hills again on the return, and turn around when the spirit moves you.

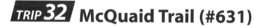 **McQuaid Trail (#631)**

Distance	Up to 6.0 miles, Out-and-back
Difficulty	Easy
Elevation Gain	500 feet (starting at 9480 feet)
Trail Use	Mountain biking, horsing around, leashed dogs OK
Agency	South Park Ranger District, Pike National Forest
Map	U.S. Forest Service *McQuaid Trail (#631)*

HIGHLIGHTS This trail isn't as comely as the Salt Creek or French Pass trails, but it's easier to access, has pleasing scenery, and is an easier hike. It roller coasters gently through the eastern foothills of the Buffalo Peaks with nice foothills views, crosses interesting streambeds, and winds through a fairly open and sunny mixed lodgepole, ponderosa pine, Douglas fir, and quaking aspen forest.

DIRECTIONS Take Highway 285 south from Fairplay 18 miles south to the Salt Creek Road (FDR 435). Check your odometer when you turn so you can look for the hard-to-see trailhead in 3 miles. It will be on the right/north side of the road hidden by trees. There is a small field for parking just short of the trailhead on the left (south) side of the road and a short road down to a pond also on the left (south) side for parking or informal camping. You can pull off on the side of the road if you'd prefer, but be careful not to block this narrow roadway. You can also access the trail from the four-wheel-drive Pony Park Road, 15.5 miles south of Fairplay.

The trailhead mentions two trail options that intersect in 3 miles: #434 for mountain bikes and #433 for hikers. The trail climbs gradually from the trailhead through hills covered largely by lodgepole pines. As it reaches the 0.5-mile mark, aspen join the pretty scene, and two large fallen trees block the trail, making mountain biking it more interesting.

The trail then descends into a dramatic drainage glade, and crosses a trickle before rolling uphill for a nice view, at approximately 1 mile; with foothills stretching to the east above a meadowed valley. You then descend to a gate and go north into a valley that opens up into meadows; roll along as far as you wish before turning around. The way back will surprise you with a great view of Buffalo Peak and the lichen-covered rocks you likely missed on the way out.

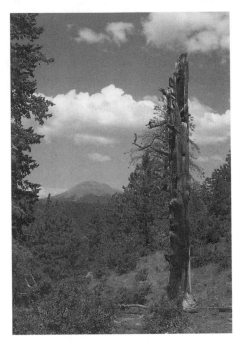

Buffalo Peak from the McQuaid Trail

Chapter 13

Colorado Springs Area

The Colorado Springs area offers many recreational options, from hiking and climbing on Pike's Peak to rambling through the easy, but busy trails at Garden of the Gods and many other parks and open spaces closer to and a bit farther from the city lights.

Fox Run Regional Park

Below 7000 feet in elevation, this park is just outside Monument and very close to Colorado Springs but offers shade and cooler temperatures on hot days. It features some of the thick tree cover of the Black Forest area. Fox Run is next to the infamous Monument Hill that closes Interstate 25 during many snowstorms, so keep your forecast up-to-date in the early spring and late fall.

Most of the park's almost 400 acres is part of the Fallen Timber Wilderness Area. The three trails are all short and easy. You can enjoy nice views of Pikes Peak from some areas, though most of the trails are thickly wooded. The tree cover blocks the wind but also limits the views.

Garden of the Gods

This soaring rock garden is not to be missed. Sculpted by the gods, the glowing sandstone and dizzying cliffs stand as monuments to humankind's relatively short stroll on the planet. A variety of short, easy trails wind among the striking red rocks often with snow-capped Pikes Peak looking over their shoulder. There is a small mountain biking area, and there are bike lanes on all paved roads.

Pikes Peak

No trip to the Colorado Springs area would be complete without exploring some of the trails on Pikes Peak, even if you don't want to summit. You can always drive to the top after your hike if you don't want to climb at least 3000 feet to make it an official summit. You can hike any round-trip distance on the Barr Trail or do the same thing from the top.

Mueller State Park & Wildlife Area

This state park is a treat with the western slopes of the Pikes Peak Massif on the east and the Sangre de Cristo Mountains, the distant and enticing backdrop for its west side. The park is on top of a plateau almost 10,000 feet high with trails going downhill from the top. You can savor a colorful tapestry of aspen, pine, fir, and spruce trees, and most of the trails feature good views.

The park is open year-round, as is one of the campgrounds, and it is a delightful place to spend a night or two, though facilities are limited to pit toilets in the winter. The park trail map can be a little confusing because it shows so many trail options, but the trails are well marked and are clearly designated for use by hikers, cyclists, or equestrians. The visitors center is closed during the week in the winter but is always open on weekends, and there is a self-service entry station near the campgrounds. I like using the campgrounds as a starting point because they are the highest point along the access road. A look at the map for this state park and wildlife area shows you that there is an infinite number of possibilities for combining trails for various activities. Route-finding can be tricky since so many trails intersect; and while most of the trails are well marked, some are not. It is difficult to get lost, however, since going up generally takes you to the main road.

TRIP 1 Devil's Head Lookout

Distance	1.5 miles, Out-and-back
Difficulty	Moderate
Elevation Gain	940 feet (starting at 8808 feet)
Trail Use	Leashed dogs OK
Agency	Pikes Peak Ranger District, Pike National Forest
Map	*Pikes Peak Ranger District, Pike National Forest*
Facilities	Restrooms at trailhead and near the top; picnic area, campground, and many benches along the trail.

HIGHLIGHTS This spectacular viewpoint provides a commanding panorama from Pikes Peak to Mount Evans from a historic fire lookout tower built in 1912. The first woman fire lookout ranger in the U.S. Forest Service, Helen Dowe worked there from 1919 to 1921, and reported 16 fires in her first year alone. The tower was in a state of disrepair, until it was reconstructed in 1951 with the help of 100 men and 72 mules. Devil's Head is the last remaining Front Range lookout tower and is on the National Register of Historic Places.

The challenge is getting to the trailhead over the very rough, gravel Rampart Range Road. It doesn't require four-wheel-drive, except during downpours, but you'll need good shock absorbers and sound teeth for the sections of deep washboard. There is a campground that makes the long round-trip drive unnecessary. Rampart Range Road is an off-road vehicle mecca with trails paralleling almost the entire length of the road; so keep that in mind when you consider visiting; love 'em or leave 'em, you cannot avoid them. The Devil's Head trail is nonmotorized.

DIRECTIONS There is no easy way, but from Woodland Park you can drive north approximately 23 miles on Rampart Range Road. Woodland Park is approximately 15 miles west of Colorado Springs on State Highway 24. It is 16 miles round-trip from Indian Creek Campground from the north. Avoiding the 7 miles of rough road is well worth the backtracking. Indian Creek is southwest of Sedalia on County Highway 67. Assume at least 1½ hours from Colorado Springs with dry roads.

From the parking area, the wide, well-maintained trail employs long, sweeping switchbacks to reach the meadow and picnic area that is just short of the top. There are frequent wooden benches for rest stops and some signs. The picnic area

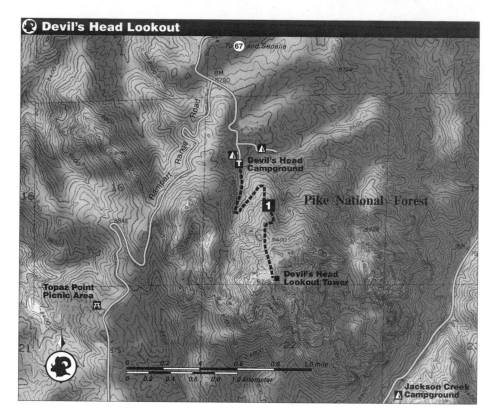

Devil's Head Lookout

To 67 and Sedalia

Devil's Head Campground

Pike National Forest

Topaz Point Picnic Area

Devil's Head Lookout Tower

Jackson Creek Campground

features restrooms, a pretty, well-shaded meadow, and a historic cabin still used by rangers. From there it is straight up on metal and wooden steps that surmount the impressive rock that is the base of the tower's lofty perch. You will enjoy great views of Pikes Peak from the top.

TRIP 2 Garden of the Gods

Distance	Up to 5.0 miles, Loop
Difficulty	Easy
Elevation Gain	300 feet (starting at 6200 feet)
Trail Use	Great for kids, wheelchair-accessible, mountain biking, leashed dogs OK
Agency	City of Colorado Springs
Map	*Garden of the Gods Park, City of Colorado Springs*
Facilities	Restrooms at trailhead

HIGHLIGHTS Circumnavigate one of Colorado's easily accessible scenic wonders—magical massive red rock sculpted by wind, water, and the sands of infinite geologic time. This short, easy route gives you a 360-degree view of this spectacular foothills rock garden. There are also wheelchair-accessible trails.

DIRECTIONS Take the Garden of the Gods exit west from Interstate 25 onto Garden of the Gods Road. Bear left on Mesa Road to 30th Street, and follow signs to the visitors center.

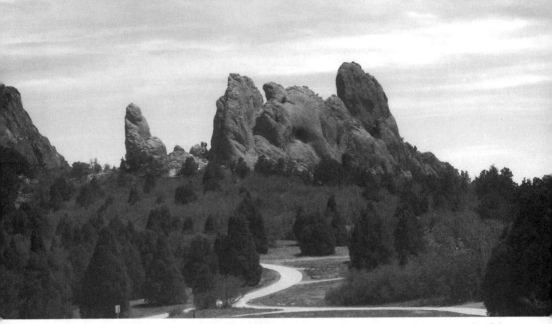

The magical rock formations in Garden of the Gods   *Joe Grim*

From the visitors center drive west on Gateway Road to Juniper Way Loop Road and turn right (north) to the main parking area on the north end of the park.

There are many short trail options within the park. This route links together the Palmer, Siamese Twins, Cabin Canyon, Scotsman, and Central Garden trails. From the main parking lot walk north, and cross Juniper Way Loop Road to intersect the Palmer Trail. Turn west and follow the trail as it rolls first northwest, then west, and finally south; paralleling Juniper Loop Road but far enough away to avoid the vehicles and noise. Walk slowly and enjoy the ever-changing views of the Tower of Babel rock face. The trail climbs very slowly for the first 0.5 mile before topping out on a narrow ridgeline with nonstop views of the rock formations. As you stroll south through fragrant pinyon pine trees, the Kissing Camels and Pulpit Rocks come into view to the east. The trail descends slowly to an intersection with a trail that goes east to the Central Garden Trails. If this is good enough for you, exit to the left and stroll around the paved garden trails.

Otherwise, continue south. The trail levels and travels next to the road for a short distance, before veering sharply to the west and climbing gradually uphill. At an intersection, go right (northwest) on the Siamese Twins Trail, a short tour around the toothsome twin rocks, to get farther from the road. Climb the gentle hill behind the rocks and feel like you have escaped to Utah's red rock canyons. After the short climb, you go gently downhill to intersect the Cabin Canyon Trail. Turn right (northwest) and descend into the shallow canyon that is more like a small arroyo, decorated with nice rock outcrops, through rolling terrain to where the trail turns left (south). After 0.3 mile the trail intersects with a trail that would cross the road to the Balanced Rock Trail. Turn left (northeast), for your return route, toward the Spring Canyon Trail-

Mountain Biking at the Garden

If you are a mountain biker, visit the Ute Trail bike loop, which is accessible from the South Garden parking lot. It is an easy approximately 4- to 5-mile loop, depending on how many side trails you include.

head. At the next intersection turn right, avoiding the Spring Canyon Trailhead and completing the rest of the Siamese

Twins Loop, unless you wish to lengthen your hike, and repeat the loop.

In 0.1 mile you reach a second intersection and turn left to cover the part of the Siamese Loop you haven't hiked, and return to the Palmer Trail in 0.2 mile. Turn right at the next trail intersection, and walk on a fairly level part of the trail toward the road and the Scotsman Picnic Area. In 0.2 mile you can cross the road, and enjoy a rest and snack at

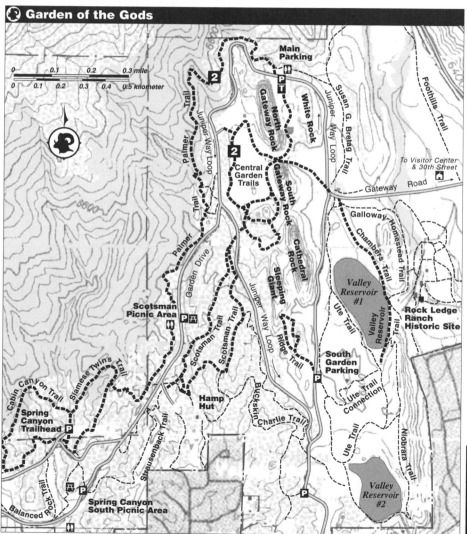

Garden of the Gods

the Scotsman. Take the Scotsman Trail north back to the Central Garden Area. It is a gradual uphill with great views of the Keyhole Window and Sleeping Giant formations. You also see Gray/Cathedral Rock peaking through—it is worth a short side trip to take it in. Once back in the Central Area you are up close and personal with the South Gateway Rock. Cut between the two major formations to make your way back to the Main Parking area, enjoying White Rock along the way.

TRIP 3 Pikes Peak

Distance	10.7 miles (Point-to-point) to 21.4 miles (Out-and-back) from summit, 12.0 miles for Barr Camp (Out-and-back)
Difficulty	Challenging
Elevation Gain	7500 feet to the summit, 3400 feet to Barr Camp (starting at 6600 feet)
Trail Use	Leashed dogs OK
Agency	Pikes Peak Ranger District, Pike National Forest
Map	*Pikes Peak Ranger District, Pike National Forest*
Facilities	Restrooms at the trailhead, Barr Camp at mid-point, and a restaurant and visitors center on top. Cog Railroad can be used in season for return trip.

HIGHLIGHTS No trip to the Colorado Springs area is complete without exploring some of the trails on Pikes Peak even if you don't want to summit. You can always drive to the top after your hike if you don't want to climb at least 3000 feet to make it an official summit (the minimum requirement of the Colorado Mountain Club). You can hike any round-trip distance on the Barr Trail or from the top. Barr Camp offers four different types of overnight accommodations.

DIRECTIONS From Colorado Springs drive west on Highway 24 to Manitou Springs. Take Ruxton to the Cog Railroad Depot and park. Follow signs to the Barr Trail.

Since there are several fine 14teener (local usage) books that describe, in glorious detail, the various routes up Pikes Peak, you can use this broad-brush overview for minor excursions or peak climbs. Buy a detailed book or check www.14ers.com for a detailed route description if you plan to climb to the summit. This description does not have a detailed ascent route. The primary route for the very hail and hearty is the Barr Trail. There is even a Pikes Peak Marathon and Half Marathon that wild-and-crazy fitness "fools" (OK, I'm jealous) use to run up and down the mountain. It is 13 miles one-way with a gain of 7500 feet. You can, however, take the Cog Railway back down if it's running, take the railway up and hike down, or have someone take the toll road ($10 per adult, $5 per child, or $35 per car in 2007) to pick you up from, or drop you off on, the top. Another option is to start at the top for an out-and-back, first down and then back up.

Your decision depends on the altitude you want to experience and enjoy on your hike. If you want to experience the slow-motion impact of immediate high altitude, from 14,000 to 13,000 feet, start on top and enjoy the spectacular panorama without the obstruction of trees, on the rocky, sometimes icy and snowy, switchback path at your feet. Keep in mind that you will be climbing back up what you go down, and it will be at least twice as

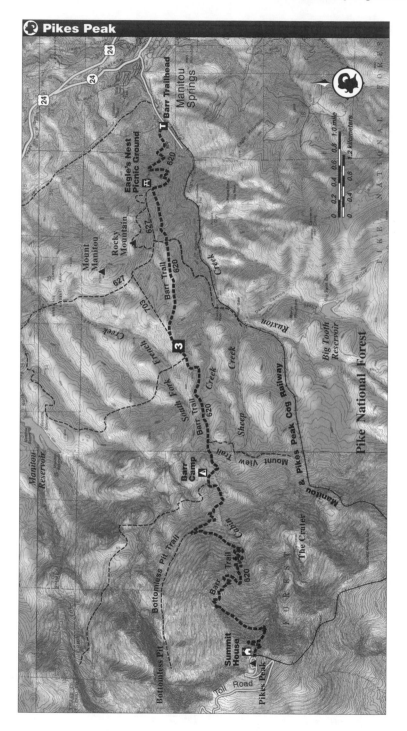

difficult. If you start at the bottom, you are encased in the beauty of the forest with peekaboo views all the way to Barr Camp, a challenging dayhike destination. I have enjoyed many briefer, satisfying jaunts up, and back, on the Barr Trail.

The first 3 miles of the Barr Trail is steep but has wide, sweeping switchbacks and a beautiful towering tree cover of ponderosa pine, white fir, and blue spruce, keeping it fairly cool on hot days. The elevation gain is around 2200 feet in that first section and might convince you that that is quite enough. You will have some intermittent views, back over your shoulder, of the city below.

When you reach the enormous rocks that frame the rock tunnel, you enjoy a much more gradual angle of ascent. The next 3 miles to Barr Camp climb a mere 1200 feet, making for a much more breathable climb. As you climb you get rewarding glimpses of the mountain's shoulder while savoring the ponderosa pine, aspens, and granite rock formations that frame the trail. Unless you can reach

> **Accommodations at Barr Camp**
>
> Barr Camp offers four overnight accommodations by reservation, with a limited amount of bottled spring water available each day:
>
> A bunkhouse-style main cabin sleeps 15 people. From Memorial Day Weekend to Labor Day, the main cabin is $25 per person per night; the rest of the year, it's $20 per person per night.
>
> Lean-to shelters, which each sleep 3 people, are $15 per person per night.
>
> Each of the upper private cabins, which have three double beds and sleep up to 12 people, can be rented as a whole unit and are $70 per night, plus $15 per person.
>
> Tent sites within the Barr Camp perimeter are $10 per person per night.

Barr Camp (10,200 feet) early in the morning, consider spending the night or turning around. You still have almost 4000 feet and around 5 miles and likely at least another 4 hours of high-altitude exertion to reach the summit, and you want to

View from the top of Pikes Peak   *Joe Grim*

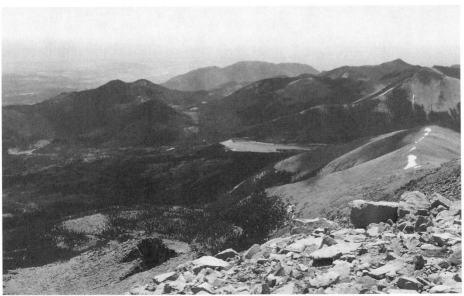

be there before noon to avoid thunderstorms. In another 900 feet, you reach the treeline and tundra, exposing you completely to the whims of the weather. The steep switchbacks begin, and you might encounter snow on the trail early or late in the season; so bring hiking sticks or an ice axe during the late spring or late fall. You will likely need extra layers of clothing since the temperature typically drops and the wind increases as you get closer to the clouds. As compensation, you will have the nonstop panorama of views only eagles enjoy, which seem to sweep across the mountains and plains all the way to Colorado's eastern border.

Mere mortals can summit an easier way (7 miles and 4100 feet) from the back (west) side of the mountain, near the Crags Area, though it involves crossing and paralleling the road for short stretches. If you have someone drop you off along the road, you can shave off part of that trail if you are less ambitious but still want to enjoy the vistas above treeline and retain some bragging rights for the coach potatoes back home.

With any mountain climb, a very early start is wise, since afternoon thunderstorms can start early in these cloud-top environments. Be prepared for very cold weather at any time of the year when you venture above 9000 feet; imagine a stiff breeze in a sleet storm if you will be far from shelter, and prepare accordingly.

TRIP 4 The Crags

Distance	1.0 to 3.5 miles, Out-and-back or Loop
Difficulty	Easy to moderate
Elevation Gain	800 feet (starting at 10,100 feet)
Trail Use	Option for kids, leashed dogs OK
Agency	Pikes Peak Ranger District, Pike National Forest
Map	Trails Illustrated *Pikes Peak & Canon City*
Facilities	This fee area ($5 in 2007) has restrooms.

HIGHLIGHTS The Crags are dramatic pinnacles, and the area is ideal for hiking or scrambling on the backside of Pikes Peak, and is across from Mueller State Park. Hiking through the valley is worth the price of admission, and the view from atop one of the pinnacles is breathtaking in more ways than one. You can see the Sangre de Cristo Mountains in the distance, as well as the backside of Pikes Peak and the interesting landscape of Mueller State Park and Wildlife Area. You can choose a short, easy jaunt up the valley to the base of the rocks or a steep scramble to the summit. The trail rolls and climbs gradually to the base of the Crags. It is straight uphill steeply from there to summit a crag. The area often stays snowy, wet, or marshy until mid- to late July because of the elevation in normal snow years.

DIRECTIONS To reach the Crags Trailhead, take Highway 24 from Colorado Springs to Divide. From Divide turn south on Highway 67 and drive 4 miles. Turn left on Forest Service Road 383, at a sign for the Crags Campground and Rocky Mountain Camp. The dirt road through the campground to the trailhead parking lot is narrow and deeply rutted.

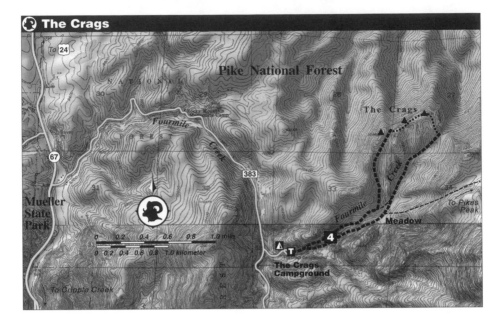

The well-marked trail goes up a few steps out of the parking lot. Follow it about 100 yards and you will come to a fork with two options. You can go straight up the valley, enjoying views and warm sun all the way, or cross the creek and stay in the cool tree cover until you reach the base of the Crags. The left (straight) branch is more open with excellent views after the first 0.25 mile. The right branch is a little more direct for climbing a pinnacle but has fewer views. You could go up on one branch and return on the other for variety.

If you want a tree-sheltered route, the latter choice is better if it is hot and sunny, but the views are obscured. It also has a short stretch of boulders that the trail circumvents. If you prefer the cool, deep forest green, look for a small footbridge and cross the creek on the right. Enjoy the streamside sounds and quaking aspens.

If you choose the left (straight) branch, you will have your first view of the Crags in just 0.25 mile. The trail then rolls and climbs and comes to a beautiful meadow area at approximately the 0.75-mile mark. From there the trail makes its way to the base of the Crags, an adequate destination for many. If you want to do a bit of climbing, reaching the top of the first ridgeline is rewarding since you get some views there. Use your judgment to determine whether to go all the way to a summit, based on how wet or dry the rock is and whether you feel like climbing straight uphill for a total of 3.5 miles.

Great for Kids

If you want a casual excursion, or have kids along, bear left up the valley on the main trail. You will have excellent views of the Crags rock outcrops in 0.25 mile and be at the foot of beautiful meadows in 0.75 mile or so. There are many options for picnics, as long as it isn't too early in the summer. The area often stays wet or marshy until mid- to late July because of the elevation, in normal snow years.

TRIP 5 What in a Name Trail

Distance	0.25 mile, Out-and-back
Difficulty	Easy
Elevation Gain	Negligible (starting at 9600 feet)
Trail Use	Great for kids
Agency	El Paso County
Map	*Fox Run Regional Park, El Paso County*
Facilities	The Rollercoaster Road Trailhead at the north end of the park and the Fallen Timbers Trailhead at the main entrance provide restrooms, parking, potable water, picnic units, and interpretive displays.
Note	Dogs, horses, and bikes are prohibited because the trail is too short and heavily used.

HIGHLIGHTS Fox Run Regional Park is an easy outing. This heavily used, family-excursion trail is perfect for photography because of its view of Pikes Peak. Circle petite Spruce and Aspen Lakes for waterfowl, and additional picnic options.

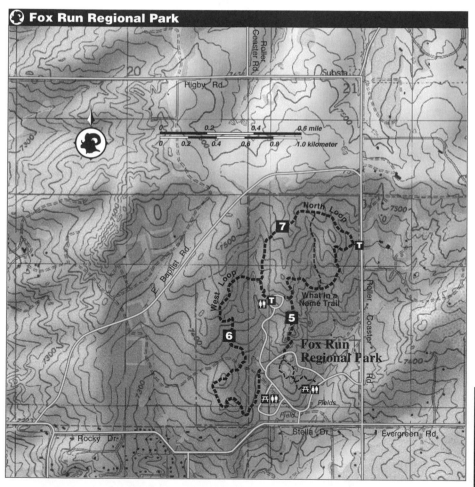

DIRECTIONS From Colorado Springs drive north on Interstate 25 and take the Monument exit. Take State Highway 105 east about 5 miles. Turn right onto Roller Coaster Road and take it south. You will pass signs for the park. Turn east (left) in Higby and then south back onto Roller Coaster Rd. You reach the north trailhead on the west side of the road after about 2 miles. Although there's no prominent sign for the park, it is an obvious parking area.

To reach the main entrance and the Fallen Timbers Trailhead, take Interstate 25 to exit 156A for Northgate Road. Turn east on Northgate Road and proceed for 3.5 miles. Turn north on Rollercoaster Road and continue for 1.5 miles to Stella Drive. From State Route 83, turn west on Northgate Road for 0.5 mile and then north on Rollercoaster Road for 1.5 miles to Stella Drive.

This trail is essentially an easy family outing, more of a stroll than a hike, and is probably the most heavily used trail in the park due to its easy access to parking. You can circle Spruce and Aspen lakes, which are small but pretty. The trail features lots of interpretative signs discussing flora, fauna, geology, and history. Definitely plan to find a shady spot for a picnic, or use the tables in the picnic areas. On a clear day, you even enjoy a distant view of Pikes Peak.

TRIP 6 West Loop

see map on p. 325

Distance	2.0 miles, Loop
Difficulty	Easy
Elevation Gain	100 to 200 feet (starting at 7000 feet)
Trail Use	Great for kids, leashed dogs OK
Agency	El Paso County
Map	*Fox Run Regional Park, El Paso County*
Facilities	The Rollercoaster Road Trailhead at the north end of peaceful Fox Run Park and the Fallen Timbers Trailhead at the main entrance provide restrooms, parking, potable water, picnic units, and interpretive displays.

HIGHLIGHTS If you want an easy mountain biking or walking option with lots of shade in the thick "black" forest, this is a good one. You will enjoy rolling hills, thick fragrant Ponderosa pines, and a view or two of Pikes Peak to the south. It is also possible, if you look carefully, to see red foxes, mule deer, Steller's jays, mountain chickadees, and nuthatches.

DIRECTIONS From Colorado Springs drive north on Interstate 25 and take the Monument exit. Take State Highway 105 east about 5 miles. Turn right onto Roller Coaster Road and take it south. You will pass signs for the park. Turn east (left) in Higby and then south back onto Roller Coaster Rd. You reach the north trailhead on the west side of the road after about 2 miles. Although there's no prominent sign for the park, it is an obvious parking area.

To reach the main entrance and the Fallen Timbers Trailhead, take Interstate 25 to exit 156A for Northgate Road. Turn east on Northgate Road and proceed for 3.5 miles. Turn north on Rollercoaster Road and continue for 1.5 miles to Stella Drive. From State Route

83, turn west on Northgate Road for 0.5 mile and then north on Rollercoaster Road for 1.5 miles to Stella Drive.

The West Loop trail rolls significantly, but not steeply, on its 2-mile circuit. It rolls in and out of the forested hills and provides a surface and terrain that is easy for beginner mountain bikers. You will enjoy a few glimpses of Pikes Peak along the way, and the forest is a real treat.

TRIP 7 North Loop

see map on p. 325

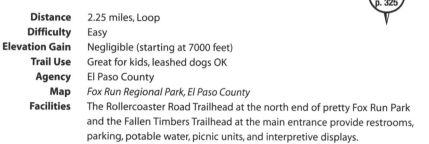

Distance	2.25 miles, Loop
Difficulty	Easy
Elevation Gain	Negligible (starting at 7000 feet)
Trail Use	Great for kids, leashed dogs OK
Agency	El Paso County
Map	*Fox Run Regional Park, El Paso County*
Facilities	The Rollercoaster Road Trailhead at the north end of pretty Fox Run Park and the Fallen Timbers Trailhead at the main entrance provide restrooms, parking, potable water, picnic units, and interpretive displays.

HIGHLIGHTS Enjoy the Ponderosa pines and tassel-eared squirrels, red foxes, mule deer, Steller's jays, mountain chickadees, and nuthatches that are residents of Fox Run Regional Park. This virtually flat trail is less intensely used than those on the south end of the park, so you are more likely to see wildlife and enjoy a bit of solitude.

DIRECTIONS From Colorado Springs drive north on Interstate 25 and take the Monument exit. Take State Highway 105 east about 5 miles. Turn right onto Roller Coaster Road and take it south. You will pass signs for the park. Turn east (left) in Higby and then south back onto Roller Coaster Rd. You reach the north trailhead on the west side of the road after about 2 miles. Although there's no prominent sign for the park, it is an obvious parking area.

To reach the main entrance and the Fallen Timbers Trailhead, take Interstate 25 to exit 156A for Northgate Road. Turn east on Northgate Road and proceed for 3.5 miles. Turn north on Roller Coaster Road and continue for 1.5 miles to Stella Drive. From State Route 83, turn west on Northgate Road for 0.5 mile and then north on Roller Coaster Road for 1.5 miles to Stella Drive.

This heavily forested trail offers stately ponderosa pines and is great for a family excursion with little kids or people not used to exertion and altitude. It features two adjoining, somewhat overlapping loops, each approximately 1 mile, that you can cover in either order. You can cut the distance in half by using only one of the two adjoining loops. There is excellent shade on this trail.

TRIP 8 Peak View, Elk Meadow, & Livery Loop

Distance	4.0 miles, Loop
Difficulty	Moderate
Elevation Gain/Loss	400 feet (starting at 9600 feet)
Trail Use	Option for kids, leashed dogs OK
Agency	Mueller State Park and Wildlife Area
Map	*Mueller State Park*
Facilities	Restrooms in campground

HIGHLIGHTS This trail (#19) is near a campground popular for its great views of the western slopes of Pikes Peak. The easy-to-locate, well-marked trailhead features a nice, open, out-and-back trail that heads downhill to the east outbound and uphill and west on the return as do most of the trails in Mueller State Park.

DIRECTIONS Take State Highway 24 from Colorado Springs to Divide (25 miles). From Divide turn south onto State Highway 67 and drive approximately 4 miles, the park will be on the right.

Peak View Pond is visible on the right as you descend through the colorful mixture of aspen and pine trees. It is worth a short detour to get some close-up shots of the pond. The easiest and shortest route is to take the ridge down the gentle slope about 0.25 mile to the intersection with the Elk Meadow Trail (#18).

If you are looking for a longer adventure, continue either north or south on the Elk Meadow Trail. If you take it south, it rolls gently and eventually climbs back

Pikes Peak from Mueller State Park

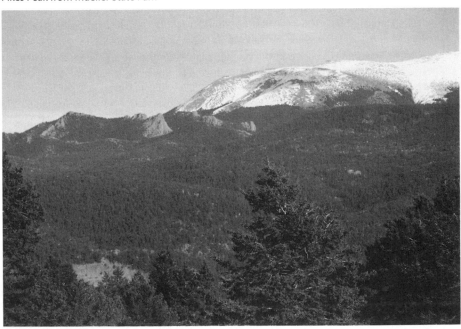

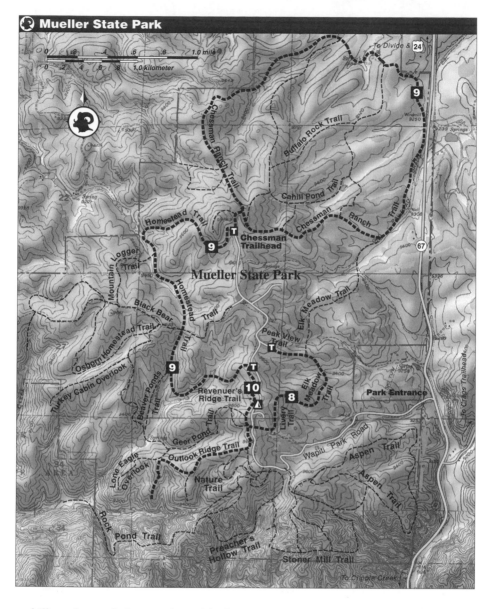

Mueller State Park

uphill to the road, intersecting with the Livery Trail (#20) and then meandering across the ridge to the Livery Trailhead. If you complete that loop, you go approximately 1.6 miles one-way. You are then about 0.5 mile from the Peak View Trailhead via the road.

Great for Kids

This trail is good for short outings with kids. Just turn around at the intersection with Elk Meadow Trail and then return to the trailhead. It's a pleasant 2-mile stroll.

TRIP 9 Homestead Trail

see map on p. 329

Distance	2.5 miles, Loop
Difficulty	Easy to moderate
Elevation Gain/Loss	300 feet (starting at 9600 feet)
Trail Use	Leashed dogs OK
Agency	Mueller State Park and Wildlife Area
Map	*Mueller State Park*
Facilities	Restrooms in campground

HIGHLIGHTS This aspen-lined trail can be covered as a loop or an out-and-back. Either way you enjoy a fairly hilly trail along the way that rolls, heading mostly downhill on the way out and uphill on the return, and have good views of the Sangre de Cristo Mountains.

DIRECTIONS Take State Highway 24 from Colorado Springs to Divide (25 miles). From Divide turn south onto State Highway 67 and drive approximately 4 miles, the park will be on the right. There are three trailheads from Wapiti Park Road for this trail—two in the campground area and a third downhill from the campground entry station. When I scouted it, I started at the one near the entry station.

At the trailhead you see several options with statistics listed for each. When you start from the campground entry area, you go gradually downhill and immediately see the Revenuer's Ridge Trail traversing the ridge off to the left. It looks like a hiking trail, while the Homestead Trail is so wide that it looks more like a service road. If it is a very clear day, the Sangre de Cristo Mountains are visible in the distance peaking through the trees. Descend fairly steeply to the wetland valley through a mixed aspen forest, cross the wetlands, and then climb up to the short ridge. The trail then rolls and intersects with Beaver Ponds Trail. When you top out, you are in a pretty grove of aspens—a good place for a snack or lunch. You then descend into another aspen-lined valley and intersect the Mount Logger Trail. The Grouse Mountain section is a great area to enjoy pine trees. An uphill climb brings you to the end of the campground road and the Chessman Trailhead.

TRIP 10 Revenuer's Ridge

see map on p. 329

Distance	2.25 miles, Semiloop
Difficulty	Easy
Elevation Gain/Loss	100 feet (starting at 9600 feet)
Trail Use	Leashed dogs OK, great for kids
Agency	Mueller State Park and Wildlife Area
Map	*Mueller State Park*
Facilities	Restrooms in campground

HIGHLIGHTS Although this trail stays high for the most part, it descends into some beautiful meadows along the way. You will enjoy nice views in all directions. This is one of few trails in Mueller State Park that isn't a significant uphill on the way back, so it is ideal for families with small children or group members who are less ambitious. The trail has multiple, easy access points, making it easy to hike as much, or as little, of the trail as you wish.

DIRECTIONS Take State Highway 24 from Colorado Springs to Divide (25 miles). From Divide turn south onto State Highway 67 and drive approximately 4 miles, the park will be on the right.

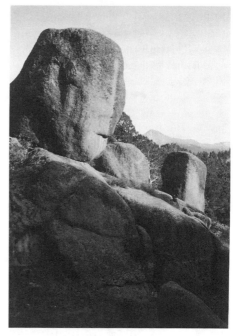

Revenuer's Ridge rock formation

Pick one of the trailheads along the road to access this trail: Black Bear is at Pisgah Point at the north end near the camper services building, the Homestead Trail can be accessed 0.5 mile south, and Geer Pond can be accessed 0.25 mile farther south, and the Outlook Ridge Trail, just south of the visitors center, is the southernmost access point of the trail.

If you start at the south end, near the visitors center, the trail stays high for 0.7 mile, paralleling the primary campground road, though the road is not visible. It then descends and crosses beautiful meadows and wetlands fringed by aspens. As it climbs gently out of the valley, it passes a striking rock formation and ends up near the camper services building.

TRIP 11 Rainbow Gulch Trail to Rampart Reservoir

Distance	3.0 miles to Rainbow Gulch, Out-and-back;
	11.0 miles to Rampart Reservoir, Loop
Difficulty	Easy
Elevation Gain	200 feet (starting at 9000 feet)
Trail Use	Fishing, camping, mountain biking, swimming,
	option for kids, leashed dogs OK
Agency	Pikes Peak Ranger District, Pike National Forest
Map	Trails Illustrated *Pikes Peak & Canon City*
Facilities	Restrooms and campgrounds

HIGHLIGHTS Easy access from Colorado Springs is the primary benefit of this recreational area. The reservoir is also in a beautiful foothills and mountain setting, with giant granite boulders; aspen, fir, and spruce trees; sun-drenched hillsides; and good views of Pikes Peak in the distance. The trail is great for children and novice mountain bikers since it rolls gently and has no challenging terrain. You will find that there are sections where you'll have to walk your bike to get around the picturesque boulders.

DIRECTIONS From Colorado Springs take State Highway 24 west 17 miles to Woodland Park. Stay on the highway for 3 miles, turn right at McDonald's onto Loy Creek Road (Forest Service Road 393) when you see the sign for Rampart Reservoir. Follow the reservoir signs to Rampart Range Road and turn right. Take it 2.5 miles south to Rainbow Gulch Road.

The Rainbow Gulch Trail is a gently sloping trail that takes you to the shoreline of the reservoir. The trail starts in a ponderosa pine forest and then opens up into a meadow before joining the trail around the lake. You can take the Rampart Reservoir Trail either due east on the south side of the reservoir or northeast to the north side of the reservoir. In either direction, the trail is essential the same—gently rolling with some rocky sections. You will come to trail intersections at times for side trails to picnic areas, campgrounds, or parking lots. When these

> **Great for Kids**
>
> The beauty of visiting this reservoir is the variety of short family hike options. Take a look at the map available at the reservoir, and pick a section that has a picnic area. Decide on a short out-and-back that includes a place to have a snack or lunch in a picnic area. Then bring along a snack, and use the picnic area as your turnaround point.

options arise, turn toward the reservoir to stay on the main trail.

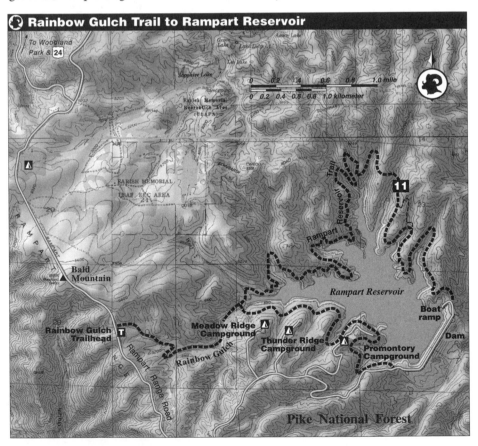

Rainbow Gulch Trail to Rampart Reservoir

Appendix 1
Best Hikes by Theme

Best Canyons
Big South, Poudre Canyon (Chapter 3: Trip 5)
Eldorado Canyon State Park (Chapter 10: Trips 21–23)

Best Fall Colors
Bear Lake, Rocky Mountain National Park (Chapter 6: Trip 8)
Wild Basin, Rocky Mountain National Park (Chapter 8: Trips 4–5)
Brainard Lake near Boulder (Chapter 9: Trip 2)
Rabbit Ears Pass (Chapter 12: Trips 10, 12, 13, & 14)

Best Lakes
Dream Lake, Rocky Mountain National Park (Chapter 6: Trip 9)
Monarch Lake near Grand Lake, Rocky Mountain National Park (Chapter 7: Trip 9)
Bluebird Lake, Rocky Mountain National Park (Chapter 8: Trip 5)
Brainard Lake, Indian Peaks (Chapter 9: Trips 5–9)
Lily Pad Lake near Silverthorne and Dillon (Chapter 12: Trip 8)

Best Peak Climbs
Mount Bierstadt (Chapter 12: Trip 4)
Grizzly Peak (Chapter 12: Trip 6)
Black Cloud Trail to Mount Elbert (Chapter 12: Trip 19)
Barr Trail up Pikes Peak (Chapter 13: Trip 3)

Best Rock Formations
Gem Lake and Lumpy Ridge, Rocky Mountain National Park (Chapter 6: Trip 1)
Chasm Lake near Diamond, Rocky Mountain National Park (Chapter 8: Trip 2)
Roxborough State Park (Chapter 11: Trips 5–7)
Garden of the Gods, Colorado Springs (Chapter 13: Trip 2)

Best Suburban
Poudre River and Spring Creek Trails, Fort Collins (Chapter 5: Trips 1–2)
Mount Sanitas, Boulder (Chapter 10: Trip 13)
Mesa Trail, Boulder (Chapter 10: Trips 15–16)
South Boulder Creek Trail, Boulder (Chapter 10: Trip 19)
Eldorado Canyon State Park, Boulder (Chapter 10: Trips 21–23)
White Ranch near Golden (Chapter 11: Trips 1–2)
Roxborough State Park, Denver (Chapter 11: Trips 5–7)
Garden of the Gods, Colorado Springs (Chapter 13: Trip 2)
South Valley Trail near Denver (Chapter 11: Trip 4)

Best Waterfalls

Alberta Falls, Rocky Mountain National Park (Chapter 6: Trip 13)

Adams Falls, Rocky Mountain National Park (Chapter 7: Trip 8)

Calypso Cascades and Ouzel Falls and Lake, Wild Basin, Rocky Mountain National Park (Chapter 8: Trips 4–5)

Best Wildflowers

Brown's Lake, Poudre Canyon (Chapter 3: Trip 15)

Pella Crossing near Boulder (Chapter 10: Trip 3)

Golden Gate Canyon State Park (Chapter 11: Trip 3)

Lake Constantine near Vail (Chapter 12: Trip 9)

Mandall Lakes Trail near Steamboat (Chapter 12: Trip 17)

French Pass near Fairplay (Chapter 12: Trip 28)

Best Wildlife

Ranger Lakes, Colorado State Forest (Chapter 4: Trip 5)

Cub and Fern Lakes, Rocky Mountain National Park (Chapter 6: Trips 4 & 5)

Appendix 2
Recommended Reading

Abbey, Edward. *Desert Solitaire: A Season in the Wilderness.* New York City: Simon and Schuster, 1968. Reprint, New York City: Ballantine Books, 1990.

Apt, Alan R. *Snowshoe Routes: Colorado's Front Range.* Seattle, WA: Mountaineers Books, 2001.

Borneman, Walter, and Lyndon Lampert. *A Climbing Guide to Colorado's Fourteeners, Third Edition.* Boulder, CO: Pruett Press, 1994.

Brower, David. *Let the Mountain Talk: Let the Rivers Run.* Gabriola Island, B.C.: New Society Publishers, 2000 (reprint).

Cox, Steven M., and C. Fulsass. *Mountaineering: The Freedom of the Hills, 7th Edition.* Seattle, WA: Mountaineers Books, 2003.

Dannen, Kent. *Hiking Rocky Mountain National Park.* Guilford, CT: Globe Pequot Press, 2002.

Dawson, Louis W. *Dawson's Guide to Colorado's Fourteeners: Northern Peaks.* Colorado Springs, CO: Blue Clover Press, 1999.

Dziezynski, James. *Best Summit Hikes in Colorado: An Opinionated Guide to 50+ Ascents of Classic and Little-Known Peaks from 8,144 to 14,433 Feet.* Berkeley: Wilderness Press, 2007.

Ells, James. *Rocky Mountain Flora.* Golden, CO: Colorado Mountain Club Press, 2006.

Fletcher, Colin, and Chip Rawlins. *The Complete Walker IV.* New York City: Alfred A. Knopf, 2002.

Foster, Lisa. *The Complete Guide to Hiking Rocky Mountain National Park.* Englewood, CO: Westcliffe Press, 2005.

Gascoyne, John. *The Best Fort Collins Hikes.* Golden, CO: Colorado Mountain Club Press, 2008.

Hagan, Mary. *Hiking Trails of Northern Colorado.* Fort Collins: Azure Publishing, 1994.

Jacobs, Randy, and Robert M. Ormes. *Guide to the Colorado Mountains, 10th Edition.* Golden, CO: Colorado Mountain Club Press, 2000.

Malocsay, Zoltan. *Trails Guide to Front Range Colorado.* Colorado Springs, CO: Squeezy Press, 1999.

Roach, Gerry. *Colorado's Fourteeners: From Hikes to Climbs, 2nd Edition.* Golden, CO: Fulcrum Press, 1999.

———. *Rocky Mountain National Park: Classic Hikes and Climbs.* Golden, CO: Fulcrum Press, 1988.

——— and Jennifer Roach. *Colorado's Thirteeners: From Hikes to Climbs.* Golden, CO: Fulcrum Press, 2000.

The Colorado Trail Foundation. *The Colorado Trail: The Official Guidebook, 7th Edition.* Golden, CO: Colorado Mountain Club Press, 2006.

Twight, Mark. *Extreme Alpinism.* Seattle, WA: Mountaineers Books, 1999.

Work, James C. *Windmills, the River, & Dust: One Man's West.* Boulder, CO: Johnson Books, 2006.

Appendix 3
Agencies & Information Sources

Colorado State Parks

Individual park websites can be accessed at http://parks.state.co.us/.

Colorado State Forest State Park
Phone: (970) 723-8366
56750 Highway 14
Walden, CO 80480

Eldorado Canyon State Park
Phone: (303) 494-3943
9 Kneale Road, Box B
Eldorado Springs, CO 80025

Golden Gate Canyon State Park
Phone: (303) 582-3707
92 Crawford Gulch Road
Golden, CO 80403

Lory State Park
Phone: (970) 493-1623
708 Lodgepole Drive
Bellvue, CO 80512

Mueller State Park
Phone: (719) 687-2366
P.O. Box 39
Divide, CO 80814-0039

Roxborough State Park
Phone: (303) 973-3959
4751 North Roxborough Drive
Littleton, CO 80125

National Forests & Parks

For general information about the Rocky Mountain Region of the U.S. Forest Service, visit www.fs.fed.us/r2/. A detailed map of the areas they manage can be found at www.fs.fed.us/r2/recreation/map/colorado/index.shtml.

Arapaho & Roosevelt National Forests
www.fs.fed.us/r2/arnf/
Phone: (970) 295-6600
2150 Centre Avenue, Building E
Fort Collins, CO 80526

Boulder Ranger District
Phone: (303) 541-2500
2140 Yarmouth Avenue
Boulder, CO 80301

Clear Creek Ranger District
Phone: (303) 567-3000
101 Chicago Creek Road
Idaho Springs, CO 80452

Sulphur Ranger District
Phone: (970) 887-4100
9 Ten Mile Drive
Granby, CO 80446

Medicine Bow-Routt National Forests
www.fs.fed.us/r2/mbr/
Phone: (307) 745-2300
2468 Jackson Street
Laramie, WY 82070-6535

Hahns Peak/Bears Ears Ranger Distrist
Phone: (970) 879-1870
Fax: (970) 870-2284
925 Weiss Drive
Steamboat Springs, CO 80487-9315

Laramie Ranger District
Phone: (307) 745-2300
Fax: (307) 745-2398
2468 Jackson Street
Laramie, WY 82070-6535

Parks Ranger Distrist
Phone: (970) 723-8204
Fax: (970) 723-4610
P.O. Box 158 or 100 Main Street
Walden, CO 80480

Parks Ranger District
Phone: (970) 724-3000
Fax: (970) 724-3068
P.O. Box 1210 or 2103 East Park
Avenue
Kremmling, CO 80459

Yampa Ranger District
Phone: (970) 638-4516
Fax: (970) 638-4635
300 Roselawn Avenue or P.O. Box 7
Yampa, CO 80483

Pike and San Isabel National Forests
www.fs.fed.us/r2/psicc/index.shtml
Phone: (719) 553-1400
2840 Kachina Drive
Pueblo, CO 81008

Leadville Ranger District
www.fs.fed.us/r2/psicc/leadville/
Phone: (719) 486-0749
Fax: (719) 486-0928
810 Front Street
Leadville, CO 80461

Pikes Peak Ranger District
www.fs.fed.us/r2/psicc/pp/
Phone: (719) 636-1602
Fax: (719) 477-4233
601 South Weber
Colorado Springs, CO 80903

South Park Ranger District
www.fs.fed.us/r2/psicc/sopa/
Phone: (719) 836-2031
Fax: (719) 836-3875
P.O. Box 219, 320 Hwy 285
Fairplay, CO 80440

White River National Forest
www.fs.fed.us/r2/whiteriver
Phone: (970) 945-2521
900 Grand Avenue or P.O. Box 948
Glenwood Springs, CO 81602

Holy Cross District
Phone: (970) 827-5715
24747 U.S. Highway 24
Minturn, CO 81645

Rocky Mountain National Park
www.nps.gov/romo/
1000 Highway 36
Estes Park, CO 80517
Phone Numbers
Visitor Information: (970) 586-1206
(8 AM–4:30 PM MST daily)
Visitor Information Recorded Message:
(970) 586-1333 (24 hours, updated
daily)
Visitor Information for the Hearing
Impaired (TTY): (970) 586-1319
(8 AM–5 PM MST daily)
Backcountry Office: (970) 586-1242
Campground Reservations:
(877) 444-677

Weather Forecasts

As mentioned elsewhere, mountain
weather is volatile and highly variable.
These sites will give you up-to-date forecasts and warnings: www.nws.noaa.gov
and http://radar.weather.gov/radar.

Huts & Yurts

10th Mountain Division Huts
www.huts.org
Email: huts@huts.org
Phone: (970) 925-5775
1280 Ute Avenue, Suite 21
Aspen, CO 81611

Never Summer Nordic, Inc.
www.neversummernordic.com/
Email: info@neversummernordic.com
Phone: (970) 723-4070
247 County Road 41
Walden, CO 80480

Appendix 4
Conservation & Hiking Groups

The Backcountry Snowsports Alliance
The Backcountry Snowsports Alliance represents winter backcountry users and advocates the preservation of nonmotorized areas on public lands. For more information, visit them online at http://backcountryalliance.org/.

The Colorado Fourteeners Initiative
The 54 mountains that comprise the 14,000-foot summits in Colorado have been impacted by the millions of people who climb them. The Colorado Fourteeners Initiative helps protect and preserve the trails and natural beauty of Colorado's 14ers. You can volunteer by visiting www.14ers.org/page.php.

Colorado Mountain Club
The club sponsors outings, conservation, and education year-round throughout the state, all of which are open to members and nonmembers. For local chapter and statewide activities, visit www.cmc.org/groups/groups.aspx.

Colorado Special Olympics
Special Olympics volunteers in Colorado assist with hiking, camping, cycling, skiing, and snowshoeing. For more information, visit the group online at www.specialolympicsco.org or at 410 17th Street, Suite 200, Denver, CO 80202. You can also call them at (303) 592-1361.

Colorado Trail Foundation
The Colorado Trail stretches almost 500 miles from Denver to Durango. The Colorado Trail Foundation (CTF) organized the volunteers who built the Colorado Trail, and continues to improve and maintain it. Enjoy the trail through the Adopt-A-Trail program, and help with maintenance. To enjoy volunteering visit: www.coloradotrail.org.

Diamond Peaks Ski Patrol
The patrol is affiliated with the National Ski Patrol, and volunteers patrol trails in the upper Poudre Canyon. For more information, visit them online at www.diamondpeaks.org/.

EDUCO
EDUCO offers outdoor experiences for children of all ages. For more information about them, visit www.educocolorado.org.

Friends of the Poudre
This organization has been fighting to protect and preserve the Poudre River for decades. They are currently opposing the destructive Glade Reservoir project. Visit them online at www.friendsofthepoudre.org.

The Nature Conservancy

The Nature Conservancy has preserved 600,000 acres in Colorado. Guided tours of some of the areas are offered. To find out more about their work in Colorado, visit www.nature. org/wherewework/northamerica/states/colorado/.

Poudre Wilderness Volunteers

Trail volunteers with this group patrol the upper Poudre Canyon for the U.S. Forest Service. For more information, visit them online at http://poudrewildernessvolunteers.com/.

Rocky Mountain Nature Association

The Rocky Mountain Nature Association (RMNA) supports the wilderness character of Rocky Mountain National Park (RMNP). RMNA sponsors a variety of nature seminars and field trips, which are listed at www.rmna.org/seminars_calendar.html. Donations to RMNA help RMNP with resource protection, capital construction, historical preservation, and education. Gifts are 100% tax deductible. Call them at (970) 586-0108, write them at P.O. Box 3100, Estes Park, CO 80517, or visit them at 48 Alpine Circle in Estes Park.

Rocky Mountain Sierra Club

The Sierra Club sponsors a wide variety of outings and presentations year-round, open to members and nonmembers. There are local chapters throughout Colorado. Visit the Rocky Mountain Chapter online at www.rmc.sierraclub.org/index.shtml or contact them at 1536 Wynkoop Street, 4th floor, Denver, CO 80202 or at (303) 861-8819.

Women's Wilderness Institute

The Women's Wilderness Institute offers wilderness courses, ranging from backpacking to rock climbing for girls ages 12 and up and for women. For more information about the courses and the institute, visit www.womenswilderness.org/womens_programs.html.

Index

Note: Italicized page references indicate photographs.

A

A-Basin Ski Area, 264, *265*
Alberta Falls, 128, *152*, 152–154, 154
Allenspark Trail, 183–185
Alpine Brook, 182
altitude sickness, 8–9
American Lakes, *76*, 77
American Lakes Trail, 76
Anne U. White Trail, 230
Antelope Trail, 222
Apache Peak, 189
Arapaho (tribe), 212, 225
Arapaho Glacier Overlook Trail, 205–208
Arapaho Peak, 256
Arrowhead Peak, 156, 158
Arthur's Rock, 98, *104, 105*
Arthur's Rock Trail, 101–106
Aspen Flats Loop Trail, 289
Aspen Lake, 325
Aspen Trail, 19–20
Audra Culver Trail, 110, 112
Audubon Peak, 189, 205, 256

B

backpacking, trails suitable for, 42, 47, 65, 69, 74, 159, 311
Baker Gulch, 169–170
Baker Lake, 302
Baker Mountain, 172, 264, 271–273, 274
Balanced Rock Trail, 318
Bald Mountain, 205, 307, *307*, 308, 309–310
Baldy Mountains, 28
Bancroft Peak, 267
Baptiste Trail, 193
Barber Lake Trail, 18, 22
Barr Camp, 322
Barr Trail, 315, 320–323
Bass Pond, 218
Bastille rock wall, 243
Bear Canyon, 235
Bear Lake, *1*, 128, 132, 135, 142, 143, *143, 148*
Bear Lake Trail, 152
Bear Peak, 235
Beaver Creek Trail, 64
Beaver Falls, 72
Beaver Meadows Resort, 23, *29*
Beaver Meadows visitors center, 127
Beaver Mountain, 164

Beaver Reservoir, *189,* 190, 192–193, *194,* 194–195
Beaver Road, 64
Beech Open Space area, 227
Belcher Hill Trail, 251–253
Bennett Creek, 72
Bierstadt, Albert, 128
Bierstadt Lake, 135, 138, 147, *151*, 151–152
Bierstadt Lake Trail, 149
Bierstadt Lake Trailhead, 152
Bierstadt Moraine, 154
Big South Trail, the, 41–42
Big Thompson Canyon, 121, 123, 150
bighorn sheep, 150
Bingham Hill, 88
Bingham Hill Road, 101
Bitterbrush Trail, 222
Black Bear Trailhead, 331
Black Canyon, 131
Black Cloud Creek, 295–296
Black Cloud Trail, 293–296
Black Lake, 128, 155–158, *158*
Black Mandall Lake, 291
Black Powder Pass, 308
Blackjack Trail Loops, 19
blisters, 5
Blue Grouse Trail, 256
Blue Lake, 48, *48,* 200
Blue Lake Trail, 47–48
Blue Sky Trail, 85, 86, 116–117
Bluebell Shelter, 239
Bluebird Lake, 186, 187
Bobcat Fire, 120, 121, 122, 123
Bobcat Ridge Natural Area, 118–119, 119–121
boots, 4–5
Boreas Pass Road, 304
Borneman, Walter, 179
Boulder, city of, 84, 189, 211
Boulder Brook, 156, 159
Boulder Brook Trail, 141, 142, 159
Boulder Creek, 247
Boulder Watershed, 208
Box Canyon, 76
Brainard Lake, *175,* 175–177, 196
Brainard Lake Road, 189–190, 193, 204
Braly Trails, 216
Breckenridge, 304, 307, 309
Brook Trail, 140
Brown's Lake, 60–61

Buchanan Creek, 177
Buchanan Pass, 192
Buckskin Trail, 31
Buffalo Pass area, 265
Buffalo Peak, *311, 314*
Buffalo Peaks Wilderness, 311
Burlington Northern-Sante-Fe/Amtrak rail line, 243
Button Rock Trail, 222

C

Cabin Canyon Trail, 318
Cache la Poudre River, *41,* 88
Cache la Poudre Wilderness, 32
Calypso Cascades, *178,* 186–187
Cameron Connection, 59–60
Cameron Pass, 32, *59,* 59–60
Cameron Peak, 47
Camp Dick, 192, 193
Camp Hale, 296
camping, 26, 37, 41, 69, 73, 123, 175, 181, 188, 190, 205, 331
Carpenter Peak, 251, 260–261
Cascade Creek, 177
Cathy Fromme Prairie Natural Area, 90, 91–93, *92*
Centennial Drive (Reservoir Road), 84, 96, 97–98, *100,* 100–101
Central Garden Trail, 318
Chambers Lake, 47
Chapin, Chiquita, and Ypsilon mountains, 134, *134,* 148, 165
Chapman Bench Trail, 289–290
Chasm Lake, 181–182, *182*
Chasm Lake Overlook, 182
Chatauqua Park, 237
Cheyenne (tribe), 212
Chicago Ridge Trail, 298
Chief's Head Peak, 156, 158
children, 7. *See also specific trails for options*
Chivington, John, 225
Cirque Meadows, 70
Cirque Meadows Road, 72
Clark Peak, 32, 45–46, 47, 48, 56, *82*
Clearwater Pond, 215, 216
Climax, town and mine pits of, 266
Climbing Guide to Colorado's Fourteeners, A (Borneman and Lampert), 179
clothing, 3–4
Cobalt Trail, 225–227
Collegiate Peaks, 296
Colorado Mountain Club, 12, *256*
Colorado River Trail, 167–169
Colorado Springs, city of, 84
Colorado State Park cabins, 73–74

Colorado State University (CSU), 67, 100
Colorado Trail, 261, 266, 293, 299, 300–302, 302–303, *303*
columbine, Colorado blue, *77*
Columbine Gulch, 249
Comanche Peak, 45, 64, 67, 69, 70, 72
Comanche Peak Wilderness, 32, 41, 62, 64, 124
Community Ditch Trail, 237
Como, town of, 266, 304, 306
Coney Creek, 187
Coney Flats Trail, 192–193
Coney Flats Trailhead, 193
Continental Divide, 133, *175,* 179, 187, 202, 215, 243, 244
Copeland Falls, 183
Copeland Mountain, 179
Cottonwood Glen Park, 90, 93
Cottonwood Marsh Trail, 218
Cow Creek Trail, 130, 131
Coyote Ridge, 86
Coyote Ridge Trail, 113–116, *115,* 116–117
Coyote Song Trail, 257–258
Coyote Trail, 254–256
Coyote Valley Trail, *171,* 172
coyotes, *135*
Crags, the, 323–324
Crags Campground Trail, 77
Crags Hotel, 243, 244
Crater Creek, 168
Crescent Meadows Trailhead, 248, 249
Crosho Lake, 290
Crosho Lake Trail, 289
Crosier Mountain Trail, *121,* 121–123
Cross Fall Creek, 70, 72
cross-country skiing, 106
Crown Point, 60
Crown Point Road, 39, 40
Cub Lake, 135–136, 138
Cub Lake Trail, 127, 137
Cub Lake Trailhead, 138

D

Dadd Gulch, 39–40
Dakota hogback sandstone, 251
Dancing Moose (cabin), 74
Deadman Gulch, 302
Deer Mountain, 132, 133–134, *134*
Deer Ridge, 128
dehydration, 9
Denver, city of, 84, 250
Devil's Backbone, 85, 86
Devil's Backbone Trail, 115, 116–117, *117*
Devil's Head Lookout, 316–317
Devil's Thumb Lake, 210
Diamond Park, 282
Diamond Peaks, *57,* 57–58, *58, 59,* 73, 74, 77, 80

Diamond Peaks Mountain Bike and Ski Patrols, 12
Dixon Dam, 101
Dixon Dam parking lot, 93, 95, 98
Dixon Reservoir, 93
dogs, 7, 126, 211, 283. *See also specific hikes and areas*
Doudy Draw Trail, 237–239
Dowdy Lake Connector Trail, 26
Dowdy Lake Trail, 26–27
Dowdy Lake Trailhead, 27
Dowe, Helen, 316
Dragonfly Pond, 215, 216
Drake, town of, 86
Dream Lake, 128, 143, 144–145, 148
Dream Lake Overlook, 147
Duck Pond, 218
Dunckley Flattops, 289–290
Dunckley Pass, 265
Dunraven and Lost Lake Trail, 86, 123–125
Dunraven Canyon, 124
Dunraven Creek, 65

E
Eagle Trail, 225–227
Eagle Wind Trail, 212, 213–215, *214*
Eagle/Cobalt Trailhead, 227–228
Eagle's Nest Natural Area, 85, 107–109
Eagle's Nest Rock, 107
Eagle's Nest Wilderness, 275
East Inlet Trail, 173–175
East Ridge Trail, 232
East Valley Trail, 106–107
Edora Park, 89
Edora Pool and Ice Center (EPIC), 84, 95
Eldorado Canyon State Park, 211, *243*
Eldorado Canyon Trail, 245–247, *247*
Eldorado Springs, 245
elk, 127, 128
Elk Meadow Trail, 328–329
Elk Trail, 254–256
Elk Valley Trail, 263
Emerald Lake, 128, 143, *144,* 144–145
Emmaline Lake and Trail, 67, 69–71
Environmental Learning Center, 84, 89
equipment, 3–4, 8
Estes Cone, 179–181
Estes Cone Trailhead, 142
Estes Park, 86, *121,* 131
etiquette, trail, 11–12
Eugenia Mine, 180

F
Fall Creek, 47
Fall Creek Trail, 278
Fall Mountain, 64, 67, 70, 72

Fall River Road, 128
Fallen Timber Wilderness Area, 315
Fallen Timbers Trailhead, 325
Fern Lake, 136–137
Fern Lake Trail, 127
Finch Lake, 183–185
Fish Creek, *64*
Fish Creek Trail, 62–65
fishing, 26, 42, 50, 65, 77, 123, 175, 190, 205, 215, 217, 254, 331
Flatirons, 217, 234, 235, 242
Flattop Mountain, 128, 145–148, *146,* 147, 265, 283, 291
Flattop Mountain Trail, *146 151,* 149
Flattop Peak, 142, 144
floods, flash, 123
Flowers Road, 64
food, 5–6
Foothills Trail (Boulder County), 228–229, 229–230
Foothills Trail (Fort Collins), 93–95, 96–97, 97–98, 99–100
Fort Collins, city of, 84
Fort Collins Trail System, overview, 84–85
Fountain Formation, 250
Fountain Valley Trail, 258–260, *260*
Four Mile Campground, 311
Four Mile Creek, 311
Fourth Lake, 173
Fowler Trail, 242–243, *243*
Fox Run Regional Park, 315, 325, 326–327, 327
French Pass Trail, 307, *307,* 307–309
Front Range, 1–2

G
Garden of the Gods, 315, 317–320, *318*
Gateway Park, 33
Geer Pond, 331
Gem Lake, 130, 131–132
Georgetown, town of, 264, 270
giardia, 6
Ginny Trail, 119–121
glaciation, 142
Glacier Basin, 140–142
Glacier Basin Campground, 128, 140, 141
Glacier Creek, 156
Glacier Gorge, 142, 149
Glacier Gorge Canyon, 156
Glacier Gorge Trail, 141
Glacier Gorge Trailhead, 128, 156, 159
Glacier Knob, 154
Glen Haven, town of, 86
Glen Haven Trails, 86
Goblin's Forest, 182
Gold Dust Trail, 304–306, 306
Golden Gate Canyon State Park, 250

Gomer Creek, 271
Gore Range, 264–265, 296, 309
Grand Ditch, 168
Grand Lake, 76, 148
Granite Pass, 156, 159, 160
Grass Creek Yurt Trail, *82*, 82–83
Grassy Hut (cabin), 74
Gray/Cathedral Rock, 320
Green Mountain, 234
Green Ridge Trail, 42–44
Green Rock Picnic Ground, 22
Greenfield Meadow Campsite, 256
Grey Peak, 256, 264
Grey Rock, 33, 34–36
Grey Rock Meadow, 34
Grizzly Peak, 264, 271–273, *273*–274, *274*
Gross Mountain Reservoir Road, 248
Guanella Pass, 264
Guanella Pass Trailhead, 271
Guernsey Creek, 302
Guyot Peak, 307, 308, 309

H

Half Moon Campground, 266, 278
Hall Ranch, 219–222, *221*
Hallet Peak, 142, *143*, 144, 145–148, *148*
Happy Jack, 17, 18, 19–20, *20*
Hawk Eagle Ridge, 243
Heil Valley Ranch, 222–225
Heil Valley Ranch Trailhead, *224*
Heron Lake, 215, 216, *216*
Herrington Trail, 113
Hewlett Gulch, *11*, 33, 36–37, *37*
Hidden Valley Trail, 227
high-altitude pulmonary edema (HAPE), 9
Hinman Creek Trail, *281*, 281–282
Hinman Lake, 281, *281*
Hogback Ridge Loop Trail, 228–229
Hollowell Park Trail, *138*
Holy Cross Wilderness Area, 264, 297, 298
Holzwarth Trout Lodge, 171
Homestead Peak, 299, 300
Homestead Trail, 237, 330, 331
horseback riding, trails suitable for, 24, 29, 31,
    36, 39, 62, 86, 99, 113, 118, 188, 215, 225,
    227, 251, 253, 263, 279, 281, 291, 311
Horseshoe Campground, 311
Horseshoe Park, 132–133, 150
Horsetooth Falls, 112–113
Horsetooth Falls Trail, 110, 112
Horsetooth Mountain Park, 86, 102
Horsetooth Reservoir, 93, 97, 99, *104*
Horsetooth Rock, 86
Horsetooth Rock/Soderberg Trail, 109–111
Hourglass Reservoir, 64
Howard Mountain, 168

hypothermia, 10

I

Illinois Pass, 82
Inca Trail, 30
Indian Creek Trailhead and Campground, 251,
    261, 263
Indian Mesa Trail, 213
Indian Peaks Wilderness, 188, 189–190
Inlet Bay, 86
insects and insect repellents, 6–7
Iron Mountain, 48–50, 52

J

James Peak, 256, 266–268
Jefferson Creek, 302
Jefferson Creek Campground, 302
Jewell Lake, 128, 155–158
Joe Wright Reservoir, 56
Jones Pass, 268–269

K

Kawuneeche Valley, 169
Kenosha Pass, 266, 300
Keyboard of the Wind, 155, 156
Keyhole Window, 320
Keystone Ski Area, 264
King's Lake, 210
Kiowa Peak, 208
Kissing Camels, 318
Knobtop Mountain, 150
Kriley Pond, 256

L

La Plata Peak, 295
Lagerman Reservoir, 217
Lake Agnes Nokhu Hut, 74
Lake Agnes Trail, 77
Lake Constantine, 264, 276–278
Lake Helene, 150
Lake Isabelle, 201–202, 203
Lampert, Lyndon, 179
Laramie Lake, 44
Larimer County, 84, 85–86
Lead Mountain, 168
Leadville, 265–266, 296
Lee Martinez Park, 84, 88
Left Hand Park Reservoir, 197
Left Hand Park Reservoir Road, 204
Left Hand Reservoir, 225, 226, 227–228
Libby Creek, 18
Libby Creek Campground Loops, 18
Libby Creek Canyon, 22
Libby Creek Trail, 21–22
Lichen Loop Trail, 224
lightning, 10

Lily Lake, 142
Lily Pad Lake, 275–276, *278*
Limber Grove Trail, 310–311
Lion's Park, 84, 88
Little Baldy Mountain, 306
Little Beaver Trail, 62–65
Little Matterhorn Mountain, 150
Little Raven Trail, 197, 204–205
Little Thompson Overlook Trail, 212–213
Little Yellowstone Canyon, 167–169, *168*
Livery Trail, 328–329
the Loch, 128, 154–155, *155*
Loch Vale Valley, 155, 156
Loggers Trail, 113
Lone Pine Creek, 25
Lone Pine Lake, 173
Lone Pine Trail, *27*, 27–28
Long, Stephen, 179
Long Draw Campground, 33
Long Draw Reservoir, 33
Long Draw Road, 33, 48
Long Lake Trail, 201
Longhorn Trail, 252, 254
Longs Peak, 86, 128, 133, 142, 145, 147, 149, 152, 155, 159, 179, 187, 205
Longs Peak Ranger Station, 181
Longs Peak Trail, 180
Lory State Park, 85, *85*, 101, 112–113
Lost Lake, 44, *44*, 86
Lost Lake and Dunraven Trail, 86, 123–125
Loveland Pass, 264, *265*, 271, 274
Loveland Pass Ski Area, 275
Lower Dadd Gulch, *39*, 39–40
Lulu Peaks, 76
Lumpy Ridge, 130, *131*, 132, 147
Lykin/Morrison Formation, 261
Lyon Overlook, 258
Lyons Formation, 242, 251

M
Mahler Mountain, 73, 79, 80, 81
Mahler Mountain Trail, 79–80
Mahler Peak, 56, 76, 79
Mandall Lakes Trail (#1121), *291*, 291–292
Maverick Trail, 252–253, 254
Maxwell Natural Area, 96–97, *97*
Maxwell Open Space, 96
McGraw Ranch, 130, 131
McGregor Ranch, *127*, 129–132, *131*, 147
McHenry's Peak, *157*, 158
McQuaid Trail, 313–314, *314*
Meadow Mountain, 187
Meadows Trail, 50, 52, 53–54
Medicine Bow Mountains, 17–18, 73, 82
Mesa Reservoir Trail, 227
Mesa Trail, 234–236, 236–237

Michigan Ditch, 79, 80
Michigan Ditch Trail, 60, 74–76
Middle Aspen Trail, 19–20
Middle St. Vrain, 190–192
Mill Creek Basin, 137–139, 147, 150
Mill Creek Link Trail, 102, 104, 113
Mills Lake, 128, 156
Mills Moraine, 182
Mineral Springs Gulch, 62
Minturn, town of, 265–266
Mitchell Creek, 199
Mitchell Creek Loop Trail, 299–300
Mitchell Lake, 199–200, *200*
Monarch Lake, 175–177, 202, 203
Montgomery Pass, 56–57
Montgomery Pass Trailhead, 57
Monument Hill, 315
Moore Park, 181
moose, *7*, 127
Moraine Park, 127–128, 137, 138, 142
Morrison Formation, 251, 261
Mosquito Range, 266, 300, 303
mosquitoes, 6
motorized recreation, trails with an option for, 21, 42, 81, 233
Mount Alto Picnic Area, 233
Mount Baldy Overlook, 27–28
Mount Bierstadt, *270*, 270–271
Mount Cirrus, 168
Mount Elbert, 266, 293–296, *295*, 297
Mount Ida, 165–167
Mount Ida trailhead, *165*
Mount Lady Washington, 128, 152, 156, 160
Mount Margaret Trail, *23*, 24–26, *25*
Mount Massive, 266, 297
Mount McConnel, 37–38
Mount Meeker, 179, 181, 187
Mount Nimbus, 169–170
Mount Richthofen, 60, 73, 76, 77, 78, 80
Mount Sanitas, *211*, 230–231, 232
Mount Stratus, 169–170
Mount Toll, 189, 199
Mount Wuh, 149
mountain biking. *See specific trails*
mountain lions, 7
Mueller State Park and Wildlife Area, 315–316, 323, *328*
Mule Deer Trail, 254–256, *256*
Mummy Pass, 69
Mummy Pass Trail, 70, 71–72
Mummy Range, 62, 64, 72, 128, 133–134, *134*, 140, 148, 159, 165
Mustang Trail, 252

N

National Center for Atmospheric Research (NCAR), 235, 237
Navajo Peak, 189
Nelson Loop Trail, 222
Nelson Ranch Open Space, 263
Neota Wilderness, 53
Nest Ridge, 243
Never Summer Range, 32, 33, 50, 73, 74, 77, 80, 81
Never Summer Yurts, 74
Newcomb Creek Trail, 280
Nighthawk Trail, 219
Niwot, Chief, 225
Niwot Mountain, 197, 204–205
Niwot Ridge, 204, 208
Nokhu Crags, 32, 56, 57, 60, 77
North Fork Trail, 65, 86, 123–125, *124*
North Lone Pine Trail, 27–28
North Longs Peak Trail, 128, 142, 154, 156, 159–160
North Loop (Fox Run Regional Park), 327
North Michigan Reservoir cabins, 74
North Park, 56, 74, 80
North Rim Loop Trail, 226, 227–228
North St. Vrain Creek, 187
North Twin Lake, 44
North Walton Peak, 286–287, *287*
Northside Atzlan Center, 88–89
Notch Mountain, 278
Notchtop Mountain, 150
Nymph Lake, 128, 143, 144–145

O

Odessa Lake, 149–150
Odessa Lake Gorge, 142, 150
Odessa Lake Trail, 147, 149
Ohlson, Kelly, 84
Outlook Ridge Trail, 331
Ouzel Falls, 186–187
Ouzel Lake, 186–187
Ouzel Lake Trail, *186*
Overland Trail Road, 88, 95, 101

P

paddling, trails with an option for, 26, 33
Palmer Trail, 318
Panorama Point, 254
Pauite Peak, 189, 193
Pawnee Pass, 177, 202–203
Pawnee Pass Trail, 202, 203
Pawnee Peak, 189, 202–203, *203,* 205
Peak View Pond, 328
Peak View Trail, 328–329
Pear Lake Trail, 185

Pella Crossing, 215–216
Pennock Creek, 65
Peterson Lake, 48
Peterson Lake Trail, 50
Pike National Forest, 251
Pikes Peak, 315, 320–323, *322, 328*
Pikes Peak Marathon and Half Marathon, 320
Pine Ridge Trail, 93
Pineridge Natural Area, 90, *93,* 93–95
Pingree Park, 32–33, *33,* 67, *71,* 72
Pingree Park County Road, 33
Pole Creek Trail, 19–20
poles, trekking, 5
Ponderosa Loop Trail, 224
Poplar Pond, 215, 216
Poudre Canyon, 32
Poudre Canyon Road (Highway 14), 33
Poudre Falls, 42
Poudre River, *165*
Poudre River Trail, 84, 86–89, *89*
Poudre Wilderness Rangers, 12
Powderhound Trail, 300
Powell Mountain, *155*
Powerline Road, 121
Profile Rock, *23*
Promontory Ridge, 256
Prospect Canyon, 154
Prospect Mountain, 62
Pulpit Rocks, 318

Q

Quartzite Ridge, 243

R

Rabbit Ears Pass, 265, 283, 286
Rabbit Mountain, 212, 214, *214,* 215
Rainbow Gulch Trail, 331–332
Rainbow Lakes, 190, 196–197
Rainbow Lakes Trail, 205–207
Rampart Reservoir and Trail, 331–332
Ramsey Peak, 69
Ranger Lakes Campground, 81
Ranger Lakes Trail, 81–82
Ranger Lakes Trailhead, 81, *81*
Rattlesnake Butte, 288
Rattlesnake Gulch Trail, 243–244
rattlesnakes, 7
Rawah Range, 23, 27, 32, 38, 47, 62, 82, *82*
Rawhide Trail, 254
Red Mountain, 109
Red Mountain Natural Area, 84, 85
Red Rock Lake, 197–198
Red Rock Picnic Area, 194–195, 196–197
Red Rock Trailhead, 197, 204
Red Rocks Lake, 190
Red Rocks Lake Trailhead, 193

Index

Red Rocks Trail, 230–232, *232*
Redgarden Wall, 243
Renegade Ridge Campground, 254
Renegade Trail, 29–31
Reservoir Ridge Natural Area, 98, *99*, 99–100
Reservoir Road (Centennial Drive), 84, 96, *97*, 97–98, *100*, 100–101
Revenuer's Ridge, 330–331, *331*
Ribbon Falls, *157*
Ricky Weiser Wetlands, 218
Ridge Loop, 19
Rim Campsite, 256
Ringtail Trail, 263
River Bend Ponds Open Space, 89
road biking, 86, 90, 91, 100, 143, 149, 154, 162, 164, 165, 167, 169, 171, 172, 175, 181, 183, 186, 188
road conditions, 9–10
rock climbing, trails with an option for, 34, 129, 159
Rocky Mountain National Park (RMNP), 1, 32, 76, 121, *121*, 126–128, 161–162, 178–179
Rocky Mountain Nature Association, 12
Rolland Moore Park, 84, 90
Rollercoaster Road Trailhead, 325
Roosevelt, Theodore, 17
Roosevelt National Forest, 32
Rotary Park, 96
Rotary Park Picnic Area, 98
Rotwand Wall, 243
Round Up Loop Trail, 252
Roxborough State Park, 250–251, *260, 262*
Royal Arch Trail, 239–240
running, trails suitable for, 86, 90, 91, 93, 96, 97, 99, 106, 107, 109, 113, 116, 118, 129, 215, 219, 225, 229, 234, 240

S
safety measures, 7–8
Sage Trail, 225–227
Salt Creek Trail (#618), *311*, 311–313
Sangre de Cristo Mountains, 315
Sanitas Valley Trail, 232
Saw Mill Pile Hill, 83
Sawatch Range, 298
Sawhill Pond, 218–219
Sawmill Creek Trail, 45–46
Sawmill Hikers Camp, 250, 253
Sawmill Trail, 253, 254
Sawmill/Specimen Creek, 168
Sawtooth Mountain, 193
Scotsman Picnic Area, 319
Scotsman Trail, 318, 320
Scott Gomer Creek, 271
Scott Run, 282
Settler's Quarry, 231

Seven Utes Lodge site, 78, 80
Seven Utes Mountain, 73, 80, 81, *81*
Seven Utes Trail, 78–79
Sharptail Trail, 263
Sheep Lake, 150
Shelter Rock, 177
Shipler Cabin, 168
Shirt Tail Peak, 243
Shoshone (tribe), 17
Shoshone Peak, 189
Siamese Twins Trail, 318–319
Sierra Club, 12
Signal Mountain Trail, 65–66, 124
Silver Creek, 81, 82
Silver Creek Meadows, 82
Silver Dollar Lake Trail, 269–270
Silverheels Creek, 306
Ski Copper, 297
Skyline Picnic Area, 97, *100*
Skyscraper Reservoir, 210
Sleeping Giant, 320
Slide Mandall Lakes, *291*
snakes, 7
Sniktau Mountain, 264, *265*, 271–273, *274*, 274–275
snowshoeing, *55*, 106
Snowy Lake, *3*
Snowy Range, *17*, 18
Soapstone Natural Area, 84
soapweed yucca, *85*
Soderberg Trail, 109–111
Sourdough Springs Equestrian Camp, 250
Sourdough Trail, *189*, 190, 193, *193, 196*, 196–197, 204
South Arapaho Peaks, 208
South Boulder Creek Trail, *240*, 240–241
South Boulder Creek Trailhead, 248–249
South Gateway Rock, 320
South Park, 300, 303, 304, 309
South Park Trail, 271
South Rim Trail, 262
South St. Vrain Trail, 193
South Twin Lake, 44
South Valley Park, 257–258
Spanish moss, 168
Sparkling Gem Lake, *127*
Spirit Lake, 173
Sprague Lake, 140–142, *141*, 160
Sprague Lake Picnic Area, 140
Spring Canyon Community Park, 92
Spring Canyon Trailhead, 318–319
Spring Creek, 84, 90
Spring Creek Trail, 89, 90–91, 93, 95
Spronk's Creek Trail, 287–289, *289*
Spruce Lake, 325
St. Mary's Glacier, 266–268

St. Vrain Creek Trail, 197
St. Vrain Mountain, 188
Stage Road campsites, 169
State Forest Moose Visitors Center, 78, 79–80
Static Peak, 78, 80
Steamboat Springs, 265
Stone Man Pass, 158
Storm Pass, 181
Storm Pass Trail, 140, 141, 142, 181
Storm Peak, 152, 160
Stormy Peaks, 72
Stormy Peaks Trail, *67*, 67–69
Streamside Trail, 241
Sugarloaf Mountain, 69
sun exposure and sunscreen, 6
Sunrise Picnic Area, 97, 98
Sunset Pond, 215, 216
Surprise Pond, 72
Swallow Trail, 258
Swallowtail Trail, 263
swimming, 331
Switzerland Trail, 233–234, *234*

T
Taft Hill Road, 92
Tarryall Creek, 306
Tarryall Mountains, 266, 302, *303,* 304, 309
Taylor Hill Trail, 298
Taylor Mountain, *155*
Teepee Mountain, 78
Tenmile Range, 264, 266, 304, 309
Tennessee Pass, 299
10th Mountain Huts & Trail Association, 296
Thatchtop Peak, 144
Thomas Hill, 263
Three-Bar Trail, 107, 109
Thunder Lake Trail, 173–175
Thunder Pass, 33, 56, 74, *76*
Thunder Pass Trail, 74–76, 168

ticks, 6–7
Timber Group Picnic Area and Park, 105, 106
Timber Trail, 104–106
Timberline Lake, 60, 61
Timberline Pass, 164
Toll Memorial Trail, 164–165
Tombstone Ridge, 164
Torrey Peak, 256, 264
Towhee Trail, 237
trail conditions, 10
Trail Ridge Road, 33, 76, 126, 128, 161–162
Trap Creek, 48, 50
Trap Lake, *7*
Trap Park Trail, 48–50
Trappers' Loop Trail, 29–31
Trappers' Pass, 31
Trappers' Trail, 29–31
Treeline Trail, 300
Turquoise Lake, 298
Twin Lakes Reservoir, 293
Twin Owls Trail, 130, 131
Twin Peaks, 295
Two Rivers Lake, 150
Tyndall Glacier, 145, 148

U
University of Wyoming Trail, 19
Upper Beaver Meadows, 162
Ute (tribe), 26
Ute Peak, 56
Ute Trail, *161,* 162–164

V
Vail, town of, 264
Valley Loop Trail, 118–119, 121
Vance's Hut Trail, 297–298, *299*
Vedauwoo, *14,* 18
Verna Lake, 173

About the Author

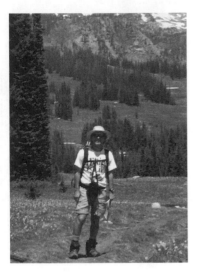

Alan Apt has been roaming Colorado's hills and dales for more than 30 years. He is the author of the bestselling guidebook *Snowshoe Routes: Colorado's Front Range*. He is a somewhat reformed peak bagger, who has climbed many of the state's highest summits but also thoroughly enjoys the lakes, vales, and rivers. He is an avid hiker, biker, snowshoer, backcountry skier, kayaker, and backpacker, and has trekked and climbed in the Andes, Alps, Himalayas, and Sierra Nevada.

Alan is a member of the Colorado Mountain Club and a Sierra Club trip leader, as well as a member of Friends of the Poudre. He is a former Ft. Collins city councilmember, who worked to create the city's Wind Power Program for the Natural Areas and Trails programs and to protect the Poudre River, and is currently on the city's Natural Resources Advisory Board. He is a Colorado Special Olympics and Eldora Ski Area Special Recreation Program volunteer. He is also a National Ski Patrol member, volunteering with the Diamond Peaks Ski Patrol and Snowy Range Ski Area. Alan is a former local columnist for the *Ft. Collins Coloradoan*. He is a technical book publisher by profession, and resides in Ft. Collins.